MedStudy

2nd Edition Pediatrics Board Review Core Curriculum

CME Application

P.O. Box 38148
Colorado Springs Colorado, 80937-8148
Phone: 719-686-7816
Fax: 719-520-5973

IMPORTANT NOTE: You must complete both sides of this form and submit it to MedStudy to receive CME credit. CME credit is available only to the original purchaser of this product. Issuance of a CME Certificate is subject to verification of product ownership.

AF697780

Verification of Credit

Pediatrics Board Review Core Curriculu

Release Date: January 15, 2006 **Expiration Date: January 15, 2009**

MedStudy is accredited by the Accreditation Council for Continuing Medical Education (ACCME) to provide continuing medical education for physicians.

MedStudy designates this activity for a maximum of 120 Category 1 CME credits towards the AMA Physician's Recognition Award. Each physician should claim only those hours of credit that he/she actually spent in the educational activity (one hour = one credit).

My signature on this document certifies my participation in the CME activity **MedStudy 2nd Edition Pediatrics Board Review Core Curriculum**. I have logged ____ credits and claim the same for AMA/PRA Category 1 CME (one hour = one credit; maximum credits: 120).

Signature ______________________ Date ______________

Printed Name: ______________________

Street Address: ______________________

City/State/Zip Code: ______________________

Telephone: ______________________

Fax: ______________________

Email: ______________________

Specialty: ______________________

CME processing fee: $40

Payment method: __ Check or money order (payable to MedStudy)
__ Visa __ MasterCard
Mail to: MedStudy
P.O. Box 38148
Colorado Springs, CO 80937-8148

Card # ______________________ Expiration Date ______________

Authorized Signature ______________________

Continued on other side

IMPORTANT: ALL questions on this Evaluation MUST be answered before CME credit can be awarded.

CME Learning Activity Evaluation

MedStudy 2nd Edition Pediatrics Board Review Core Curriculum

On a scale of 1 to 5, with 1 being POOR and 5 being EXCELLENT, please rate the following regarding your use of the product:

	POOR				EXCELLENT
I have a better grasp of subjects related to the ABP Certifying/Recertifying exam	1	2	3	4	5
I can better discuss accepted approaches to the diagnosis and therapy of conditions commonly seen by Pediatricians	1	2	3	4	5
I am better equipped to generate a comprehensive differential diagnosis based on a set of presenting signs and symptoms	1	2	3	4	5
I've been able to remedy weaknesses in Pediatrics and update and strengthen my overall knowledge in this area of medicine	1	2	3	4	5
I feel more confident in being prepared for a competency exam	1	2	3	4	5
The topic-by-topic format, Quick Quizzes, and other features made the books a viable mode of instructional delivery	1	2	3	4	5
The content was balanced and free of commercial bias	1	2	3	4	5

Please rate the quality of coverage for the following specialty/subspecialty areas:

	POOR				EXCELLENT
The Newborn	1	2	3	4	5
Childhood Development and Common Pediatric Disorders	1	2	3	4	5
Health Supervision	1	2	3	4	5
Adolescent Health	1	2	3	4	5
Genetics	1	2	3	4	5
Metabolic Disorders	1	2	3	4	5
Gastroenterology	1	2	3	4	5
Pulmonology	1	2	3	4	5
Cardiology	1	2	3	4	5
Infectious Disease	1	2	3	4	5
Nephrology	1	2	3	4	5
Endocrinology	1	2	3	4	5
Hematology	1	2	3	4	5
Oncology	1	2	3	4	5
Neurology	1	2	3	4	5
Rheumatology	1	2	3	4	5
Allergy & Immunology	1	2	3	4	5
Dermatology	1	2	3	4	5

The level of the content was __ Satisfactory __ Too advanced __ Too basic

The most valuable benefit of this product is: ______________________________

____

Main product improvement needed is (optional): ______________________________

____

____

Earn CME while you learn!

Up to 120 Category 1 CME credits available with the MedStudy 2nd Edition Pediatrics Board Review Core Curriculum

Release Date: January 15, 2006 **Expiration Date: January 15, 2009**

The MedStudy 2nd Edition Pediatrics Board Review Core Curriculum offers you the opportunity to earn up to 120 Category 1 CME credits towards the AMA Physician's Recognition Award.

This CME credit is provided by MedStudy. To apply for your CME credit, you must complete the **Verification of Credit** form found immediately following the next page. Then submit that completed form along with the $40 CME fee to MedStudy. All the necessary contact information is included on the Verification of Credit form. Please note that CME credit is available only to the original purchaser of this product, and issuance of CME credit is subject to verification of product ownership.

The Release Date for the MedStudy 2nd Edition Pediatrics Board Review Core Curriculum is January 15, 2006. To be eligible for CME credit, you must study the content in the books and submit your Verification of Credit form no later than January 15, 2009.

Accreditation

MedStudy is accredited by the Accreditation Council for Continuing Medical Education (ACCME) to provide continuing medical education for physicians. MedStudy designates this educational activity for a maximum of 120 Category 1 credits towards the AMA Physician's Recognition Award. Each physician should claim only those credits that he/she actually spent studying the MedStudy Pediatrics Board Review Core Curriculum (one hour = one credit).

MedStudy presents this activity for educational purposes only and does not endorse any product or content of presentation. Participants are expected to utilize their own expertise and judgment while engaged in the practice of medicine. The content of this educational activity is provided solely by contributors who have been selected because of their recognized expertise.

Learning Objectives

Effectively focus your studies on subjects relevant to the depth and scope of the ABP (American Board of Pediatrics) certifying or recertifying exam, and integrate this information for a successful exam outcome

- Identify and remedy weaknesses you might have in Pediatrics and strengthen your overall knowledge set
- Describe the clinical manifestations and treatment of diseases encountered by the Pediatrician
- Generate a comprehensive differential diagnosis based on a set of presenting signs and symptoms
- Effectively narrow the differential diagnosis list by utilizing the most appropriate laboratory studies, scans, etc.
- Completely discuss the accepted approaches to the diagnosis and therapy of conditions commonly seen by Pediatric practitioners

Method of Participation

Thoroughly read each section of the Core Curriculum, two to three times for maximum learning. Pay special attention to yellow-highlighted text, considered to be must-know facts for board examination. Use Quick Quiz questions to self-assess your learning (answers to Quick Quizzes found in yellow-highlighted text). Review figures and tables to reinforce the text reading and to see concise summaries of interrelated facts in key topic areas.

DISCLOSURE SUMMARY

MedStudy 2nd Edition Pediatrics Board Review Core Curriculum

It is the policy of MedStudy to ensure balance, independence, objectivity and scientific rigor in all its educational programs. All contributors/reviewers participating in this program are expected to disclose to the program users any real or apparent conflict of interest related to the content they have provided. This pertains to relationships with pharmaceutical companies, biomedical device manufacturers or other corporations whose products or services are related to the subject matter of the content topic, including off-label, experimental or investigational use of drugs or services.

MedStudy adheres to the ACCME's Essential Areas and Their Elements and Criteria regarding industry support of continuing medical education. Disclosures of contributors/reviewers and relevant commercial relationships have been documented below.

I. The following contributors/reviewers have openly disclosed inclusion of discussion of any off-label, experimental, or investigational use of drugs or devices in their provided content and/or have indicated any affiliations with organizations that have interests related to such content:

CONTRIBUTOR	AFFILIATION/DISCLOSURE(S)
Mark Corkins, MD	Serves on Speaker's Bureau for Dannemiller Memorial Education Foundation, TAP Pharmaceuticals Prevacid Pediatric Advisory Board, and Nestle Corporation Serves as Consultant for Pedia Med Pharmaceuticals Advisory Board Discusses off-label use of proton-pump inhibitors for children under 1 year of age
Stephen Kemp, MD	Receives Grant/Research support from Genentech, Inc., Pfizer, Novo Nordisk, and Tercica Serves as Consultant for Genentech, Inc., Eli Lilly, and Pfizer Serves on Speaker's Bureau for Eli Lilly, Pfizer, and Helix
Sriram S. Narsipur, MD	Serves on Speaker's Bureau for Ortho Biotech Discusses investigational use of immunosuppressants on the treatment of kidney disease and transplant (off-label for pediatric patients)
Larry Williams, MD	Receives Grant/Research support from Novartis and Genentech, Inc. Serves on Speaker's Bureau for Astra-Zeneca
Kimberly Jones, MD	Receives Grant/Research support from Corus Pharma, Genentech, Cystic Fibrosis Foundation, and Hill-Rom
Barbara Ostrov, MD	Receives Grant/Research support from Pfizer Serves on Speaker's Bureau for Merck, Pfizer, and Amgen Mentions newer medications likely to be approved in near future (as for RA, SLE, gout) and also meds used in rheumatic diseases, not specifically FDA approved, such as anti-inflammatory agents for Bechet's

II. The following contributors/reviewers have documented they have nothing to disclose:

Keith Boyd, MD
J. Thomas Cross, Jr., MD, MPH
Robert A. Hannaman, MD
Paul R. Haut, MD
Kim Keppler-Noreuil, MD
Ernest A. Kiel, MD
Amy Jo Nopper, MD
Arthur S. Pickoff, MD
Daniel Polk, MD
Thomas Krzmarzick, MD
Patricia Duffner, MD
Suzanne Whitworth, MD
Sara Copeland, MD

III. The following contributors/reviewers had not provided disclosures as of printing time:
NONE

Provider Disclosure Statement

As the provider of this continuing medical education activity, MedStudy Corporation documents that it does not have a financial interest, arrangement, or affiliation with any commercial organization that may have a direct or indirect interest in the subject matter of presentations given in this activity. This pertains to relationships with pharmaceutical companies, biomedical device and other commercial products manufacturers, and providers of commercial services.

MedStudy

2nd Edition

Pediatrics Board Review Core Curriculum

Book 1 of 4

Topics in this volume:

Health Supervision

Childhood Development and Common Pediatric Disorders

Adolescent Health

Infectious Disease

Authored by J. Thomas Cross, Jr., MD, MPH, FAAP and Robert A. Hannaman, MD

NOTICE: Medicine and accepted standards of care are constantly changing. We at MedStudy do our best to review and include in this publication accurate discussions of the standards of care and methods of diagnosis. However, the author, the advisors, the editors, the publisher, and all other parties involved with the preparation and publication of this work do not guarantee that the information contained herein is in every respect accurate or complete. We recommend that you confirm the material with current sources of medical knowledge whenever considering presentations or treating patients.

MEDSTUDY
1761 South 8th Street, Building H1
Colorado Springs, Colorado 80906
(800) 841-0547

Health Supervision

MedStudy

2nd Edition
Pediatrics Board Review
Core Curriculum

Health Supervision

Authored by J. Thomas Cross, Jr., MD, MPH, FAAP

Many thanks to

Keith Boyd, MD
Associate Chair of Education
Department of Pediatrics
Rush University Medical Center
Chicago, IL

Table of Contents

Health Supervision

OVERVIEW OF GROWTH

Pediatric Health Supervision is a cornerstone of pediatric health care and thus has a significant place on the Boards. Continuity of care is based on a developmental framework that recognizes the consistency of growth changes that occur throughout childhood. For the exam, you must know both normal patterns and common variations.

Two periods of rapid growth are observed: infancy and adolescence. The growth of most body tissues and organs parallels this pattern, with these notable exceptions:

- Brain growth is rapid during the first 6 years of life, with minimal change in head size after age 10.
- Lymphoid tissue volume increases rapidly before puberty and then declines steadily until one achieves adult levels.
- Growth of the reproductive organs is slow until puberty.

What determines growth? It involves genetic, environmental, and hormonal factors. Parental size and patterns of growth correspond well to both absolute size and timing of growth spurts. See Table 1-1 [Know] on predicting mid-parental height; for most children, adult height should be within 5 cm above or below the calculated midparental height. Maximal growth occurs in the spring and summer. We discuss endocrine control of growth in Endocrinology.

Table 1-1

PREDICTING MID-PARENTAL HEIGHT IN CHILDREN
Mid-parental height for Girls
$\frac{\text{(Father's height - 13 cm) + (Mother's height)}}{2}$
Mid-parental height for Boys
$\frac{\text{(Mother's height + 13cm) + (Father's height)}}{2}$

At each visit, weigh infants and younger children without their clothes using the same scale at each visit. (OK, this is what the books say; I know the real world is very different!) Measure length in the recumbent position until the age of 2. After 2 years of age, measure standing height. Measure head size using a tape measure around the greatest circumference of the occipitofrontal area.

Do not judge a single measurement of growing points (i.e., weight, height, and head circumference) as the only indicator of a growth problem. Remember that 5% of the population normally will be outside 2 standard deviations (2.5% will be > 95 percentile and 2.5% will be < 5 percentile)! The key is to evaluate the curves over time! Examples:

- If a child is genetically small (i.e., both parents are short or small), he will grow parallel to standard curves at or just below the statistically "normal" range of heights and weights. He will have a normal weight for height, a normal skin-fold thickness, and a bone age consistent with chronologic age.
- On the other hand, the child who suffered an event, such as a prolonged intrauterine hypoxic period leading to intrauterine growth failure, will typically be small for gestational age at birth and, over time, continue to fall further away from population means on all parameters.
- Postnatal onset of a growth problem will present as "falling off" the previously stable growth curves.

Crossing of percentiles during the first 2 years of life should always raise concern, but this pattern can also be consistent with normal growth variants, and thus, may be difficult to differentiate from growth failure. For example, a baby's size at birth is greatly influenced by maternal factors (maternal diabetes, etc.). Influence of these factors changes after birth.

Constitutional Growth Delay: When a child's birth weight and height are initially normal, but drop off proportionately during the first 2 years of life, this indicates constitutional growth delay. Height and weight eventually become parallel to growth curves at or just below the 3rd percentile for most of middle childhood. Eventually, the older child/adolescent grows rapidly and crosses percentiles to achieve normal adult height. The bone age is delayed for the child's chronological age but consistent with what is known as "height age" (the age at which the child's height is at the 50th percentile). These growth delays initially may cause concern, but they usually don't manifest as problems until adolescence, and then only if secondary sexual characteristics fail to appear. Also, head circumference is usually relatively spared compared to height and weight. Most of the time, constitutional growth delay is hereditary. "Longitudinal growth charts," which provide normative data for early, average, and late developing children, are helpful in differentiating these kids from those with other growth problems.

Other quick clues to consider in kids with growth problems:

- Intrauterine insult/genetic abnormality: Weight, height, and head circumference are all significantly below the curves.
- Structural dystrophies/endocrine etiologies: Head circumference frequently will be spared while height and weight are severely affected. (You can also see this, though, in genetic short stature and constitutional growth delay!)
- Caloric insufficiency: Head circumference and height are spared, but significant weight loss is occurring. Eventually, though, if caloric insufficiency is persistent and significant, height and head circumference will also suffer.

See Table 1-2—Quick Pearls to Remember about Growth for the Board exam! Especially know that height doubles by 3–4 years of age; full-term infants regain their birth weight within 2 weeks, double their birth weight by 4–6 months, and triple birth weight by 12 months of age.

Be sure to know that the standard head circumference of a full-term infant at birth is about 35 cm for girls and 36 cm for boys.

notes

Table 1-2
QUICK PEARLS TO REMEMBER ABOUT GROWTH
Weight
Birth weight is regained by day 10-14 of life
Birth weight doubles at 4 months
Birth weight triples at 12 months
Birth weight quadruples at 24 months
After age 2, normal weight gain is 5 lbs/year until adolescence
Length/Height
Birth length increases by 50% at 1 year
Birth length doubles by 4 years
Birth length triples by 13 years
After age 2, average height increase is 2"/year until adolescence
Head Growth
Largest rate of growth is between 0 and 2 months (0.5 cm/week)

FAILURE TO THRIVE

The term Failure to Thrive, or FTT, is a descriptive term with multiple definitions. It generally applies to weight or changes in weight, but FTT can also include failure to gain length/height and head circumference, depending on the severity and duration of the disorder causing the disruption in growth. See Table 1-3 for common definitions, but note that there is wide variation!

Table 1-3
DEFINITIONS OF FAILURE TO THRIVE (FTT)
One Point on the Growth Curve:
Weight < 3rd percentile
Weight for height < 5th percentile
Weight 20% or more below ideal weight for height
A Series of Points on the Growth Curve:
Weight gain < 20 grams/day from 0 to 3 months of age
Weight gain < 15 grams/day from 3 to 6 months of age
Downward crossing of ≥ 2 major percentiles

Note: For most cases of FTT, you will not find an identifiable organic etiology. Another clue for organic etiologies—they rarely present as just FTT! However, psychosocial and behavioral feeding problems are very common, and many texts recommend that they no longer be diagnoses of exclusion! Also, because many organic etiologies are reversible, although rare, it is very important to evaluate non-organic assessments for FTT at the initial evaluation.

What are the key components of evaluation?

- Review of past/present growth data (emphasis especially on pattern of growth)
- History and physical
- Developmental/behavioral assessment
- Feeding observation
- Assessment of child-parent interaction
- Selected laboratory studies based on findings above.

These can include CBC, Lytes, Cr, U/A +/- CX, total protein/albumin, and bone age (if height is also a problem).

The key question the Boards are likely to ask you: Should you hospitalize the child?

Here are clues to YES:

- Evidence of physical abuse/neglect
- High risk for abuse/neglect:
  - very disturbed parent
  - abnormal child interaction
  - poor parental functioning and/or
  - extremely stressful home environment
- Severe malnutrition
- Medically unstable
- Outpatient management failure
- Need for close observation

All of that said, most cases of FTT are caused by inadequate consumption of appropriate amounts and/or kinds of food, and you can manage most on an outpatient basis. These cases are frequently due to psychosocial and/or behavioral problems. If caloric intake appears to be adequate, search for a condition associated with caloric wasting or increased caloric requirements. Don't forget to have the parent explain formula preparation—a common cause of infant undernutrition.

Causes of excessive caloric losses:

- Gastrointestinal disorders (e.g. malabsorption)
- Renal disorders (e.g. renal tubular acidosis)

Causes of increased caloric requirements:

- Cardiopulmonary disorders (e.g. CHF)
- Malignancies
- Hyperthyroidism
- Chronic or recurrent infections (e.g. HIV)

If, on the Boards, you are asked to describe one of the best ways to identify specific behavioral or interactional problems, the answer is to watch a feeding session. Also ensure adequate calorie intake in the hospital if outpatient manage-

notes

Quick Quiz

1) What is the expected height of a girl, if the father is 182 cm and the mother is 152 cm?
2) In constitutional growth delay, is normal adult height achieved?
3) How soon does a child regain birth weight?
4) When does birth weight double? quadruple?
5) When does birth length double? triple?
6) When is the period of fastest head circumference growth?
7) At what percentile is FTT defined?
8) True or False: Downward crossing of 3 major percentiles would be considered "FTT."
9) Describe the reasons to hospitalize a child with FTT.
10) What causes most cases of FTT?
11) Name two benign causes of macrocephaly that occur in normal infants.

ment fails. If the child is not gaining weight with appropriate observed nutrition, you must suspect an organic etiology.

If severe psychosocial FTT is present, children may have gaze disturbances—"wary watchfulness" to total avoidance of eye contact and apathetic withdrawal. Infants may resist being held and prefer interactions with inanimate objects. Most will also exhibit developmental delays in the area of language and social behavior.

HEAD MALFORMATIONS

Micro and Macrocephaly are easily defined: head circumference (HC) 2 standard deviations below or above the mean, respectively. But don't forget that under this definition approximately 5% of children (2.5% on each end of the spectrum) will fall into this category. (Remember that bully in high school? He probably really did have a fat head!) For pre-term infants, plot gestational age rather than chronological age for HC. Also be aware that the catch-up growth of those with microcephaly will exceed their length/weight growth, and they may appear to have macrocephaly or hydrocephalus. The problem is that these premature kids are at increased risk for hydrocephalus. So be careful if the Boards present a premature kid with an enlarged head compared to the rest of his/her body! It could be normal or abnormal. Again, look at the growth pattern. If you're concerned, ultrasound is the diagnostic test of choice for macrocephaly.

So what do you do if you suspect abnormal head growth? The usual: Hx, PE, review of previous growth curves. Also review parental and sibling history, and check their head circumferences. Look for confounding factors in the history and exam—like developmental delay, focal findings, skin disorders, etc. If you confirm macrocephaly, the best initial diagnostic study is a head ultrasound, because hydrocephalus is the most likely diagnosis. For microcephaly, CT or MRI is the best test to help determine an underlying disease process. CT or MRI is better for microcephaly than ultrasound, because bone abnormality or lack of brain development is the most likely causes.

Microcephaly: This is usually a result of a primary or secondary defect in brain development. Remember that underlying brain growth is what leads to head growth. Normal intelligence can occur, but mental retardation is the norm. Primary microcephaly refers to the presence of a genetic or chromosomal condition in which mass and/or structural brain growth is abnormal. In secondary microcephaly, infections (pre/postnatal), toxins, and CNS injury arrest previously normal brain development. Remember that brain growth determines skull growth, so poor brain growth may result in premature fusion of the cranial fissures. You can differentiate this from primary craniosynostosis, which presents with both an abnormally shaped skull and palpably thickened suture lines; neither of these is present in conditions where lack of brain growth causes premature fusion of the cranial bones.

The finding of microcephaly at birth does not differentiate primary from secondary causes. However, an infant with a normal-size head at birth with subsequent development of microcephaly strongly suggests a secondary etiology. Perinatal injury to the CNS rarely causes head growth abnormalities before the age of 4–6 months. Usually these growth abnormalities are associated with multiple neurologic abnormalities. Head CT of infants with primary microcephaly is usually normal or shows brain abnormalities consistent with the specific etiology. Secondary microcephaly etiologies will frequently show up with abnormal CT scans.

Macrocephaly: This is usually due to excess CSF (hydrocephalus), excess brain tissue (macrencephaly or megalencephaly), thickening of the skull, or subdural or epidural bleed. Also, macrocephaly can be a normal variant (see below). Note that macrocephaly rarely presents alone in the face of inborn or acquired disorders! Megalencephaly means having excess brain tissue due to an increased size or number of brain cells. This could be just a normal anatomical variant without problems, but frequently it also occurs with syndromes or metabolic disorders. An infant with anatomic megalencephaly is generally born with a large head, whereas a baby with a metabolic etiology for megalencephaly will have a normal head size at birth that enlarges to macrocephaly during infancy. Usually, the metabolic form is associated with seizures, numerous developmental problems, and signs of increased intracranial pressure.

A benign cause of macrocephaly is enlargement of the subarachnoid space. This is fairly common in otherwise normal infants. The infant will have a large head (but within normal range) at birth, but the head circumference will subsequently exceed/parallel the 98th percentile. Head CT shows the enlarged subarachnoid space. You also may see normal or minimally increased ventricular size and a widened sulci and sylvian fissure. This is predominantly a male phenomenon, and also is frequently seen in the father.

notes

Genetic megalencephaly is another common variant similar to the previous findings, except that the head CT report is normal. Neither condition requires further workup unless neurologic / developmental problems develop.

Plagiocephaly: This is asymmetric head growth. It can be caused by alterations of internal and external forces that impact skull growth, or be due to abnormalities in bone formation. Note that most vaginally delivered infants have head molding that usually resolves during the first few weeks of life. Deformational flattening from lack of changes in head positions is the most common cause of an asymmetric head shape. This resolves without intervention as the head grows.

Note: There has been a large increase in the number of cases of posterior plagiocephaly due to the recommendation that sleeping infants be placed on their backs to reduce SIDS. It is important to differentiate this from asymmetric growth due to premature closure of one or more of the cranial sutures (e.g. craniosynostosis)! Remember that most sutures are closed by 12–24 months of age. Most are ossified by 8 years of age, and fusion is complete by early adulthood. With craniosynostosis, you get premature closure (or absence) of one or more cranial sutures. This causes a compensatory growth along the remaining open sutures in a direction parallel to the closed suture.

You can predict the head shape based on the sutures involved. It is mainly a cosmetic problem; however, associated ocular, neurologic, and intracranial pressure problems can occur.

If it involves only 1 suture, it is usually isolated and often occurs with a prevalence of .1%. 85% are in Caucasian kids with M:F ratio of 3:2. Sagittal suture involvement is most common (50%), followed by coronal and metopic. Closure of the lambdoidal suture is very rare. This would result in posterior plagiocephaly; thus, posterior plagiocephaly is almost always due to supine sleeping, not craniosynostosis!

Note again: If > 1 suture is involved, assume an association with a genetic disorder and the occurrence of resulting neurologic abnormalities.

Physical examination is very helpful in differentiating positional posterior plagiocephaly from craniosynostosis. In craniosynostosis, occipital flattening may accompany a flat ridge overlaying the fused lambdoid suture or the absence of a palpable suture. Compensatory growth causes frontal and parietal prominence on the side opposite the occipital flattening, and the child develops a trapezoid-shaped head. The ear on the same side as the fused suture will be displaced downward and backward. In contrast with positional posterior plagiocephaly, the head will be in the shape of a parallelogram, and occipital flattening will result prominently on the same side of the temporal and frontal areas. Also, the ear will be pushed forward and down away from the flattening. If you suspect a synostosis, order plain films. If these are inconclusive, a CT scan is the next step.

Positional posterior plagiocephaly is usually benign and resolves with time as the child spends less time on his/her back. Encourage the parents to keep the wakeful child in the prone position. Usually the condition will resolve in 2–4 months. For infants with severe or unremitting disease, a helmet may be beneficial. However, it requires using the helmet 22 hours a day! Helmet molding is most useful when initiated before 6 months of age. Treat synostosis with surgery between 6 and 12 months of age.

DEVELOPMENTAL MILESTONES

OVERVIEW

Tip on remembering "Developmental Milestones:" Think of your own children and hope they are "normal." (Personally, that's how I got through these questions on the examination). For these types of questions, I also recommend that, for the next several weeks when you see patients, perform developmental examinations (such as Denver II tool) to reinforce these milestones in your mind. See Table 1-4 through Table 1-10 (Developmental milestones). Know all of these and try to categorize them in your mind by action/response. Another strategy is to remember a handful of key milestones (two in each category, for example) and extrapolate from there. To reinforce these in your memory, incorporate questions to parents regarding their child's milestones as part of health maintenance visits, or develop an age-appropriate questionnaire for your parents.

If a parent asks about developmental delay, it is important to take the concerns seriously. Most parents overestimate rather than underestimate their child's skills.

Common things to remember for the Boards: if a child is ill or uncooperative, consider a "low score" invalid. Chronic disease or recurrent hospitalizations can cause developmental delay as well. For premature infants, continue age corrections until 18–24 months of age. Physical abnormalities (hearing, vision, etc.) or environmental factors (abuse/neglect) may present as a developmental delay. For speech delay, always check hearing first.

DEVELOPMENTAL DELAY

If you suspect developmental delay, conduct a full history and physical examination. This includes a complete review of systems, prenatal and perinatal history, and psychosocial/behavioral assessment. Guide laboratory testing with history/physical findings.

Generally, the following are recommended:

- For a newborn/infant: Always check any previous metabolic screening done by the State.
- For older children: Serum-lead level: Because even low levels can cause problems, also consider thyroid studies.

MRI of the Head may detect cerebral dysgenesis at any age in a child. Consider it if any of the following are present:

- Cerebral palsy
- Abnormal head shape or size
- Craniofacial malformation
- Loss or stagnation of developmental skills
- Neurocutaneous abnormalities
- Seizures
- IQ < 50

notes

Quick Quiz

1) What is the most common cause of plagiocephaly?
2) True or False: If more than 1 suture is closed prematurely, this is usually associated with other neurologic findings.
3) What is the recommended therapy for craniosynostosis?
4) Know Table 1-4 through Table 1-10—Developmental Milestones (Sorry, I know it is a lot).
5) You use the Denver II tool to evaluate a child while he is ill. If he does poorly, should you refer him for further intensive evaluation or repeat the test when he is well?
6) Describe when you should do metabolic screening.
7) True or False: Metabolic screening is required for every child with mental retardation.

Table 1-4

DEVELOPMENTAL MILESTONES: REFLEXES	
Moro	Absent by 3-4 months
Palmar Grasp	Absent by 2-3 months
Parachute	Present by 6-9 months

Table 1-5

DEVELOPMENTAL MILESTONES: HEAD CONTROL	
When lying down:	
Lifts head momentarily	1 month
Head up to 45 degrees	2 months
Head up to 90 degrees	3-4 months
When Pull to Sitting:	
Complete head lag	Newborn
No head lag	5 months
Lifts head off table in anticipation of being lifted	6 months

Table 1-6

DEVELOPMENTAL MILESTONES: ROLLING AND SITTING	
Rolling:	
Rolls front to back	4-5 months
Rolls back to front	5-6 months
Sitting:	
Sits with no support	7 months

Table 1-7

DEVELOPMENTAL MILESTONES: HAND/FINGERS	
Voluntary grasp (no release)	5 months
Transfers objects between hands	6 months
Uses thumb to grasp cube	6-8 months
"Mature" Cube grasp (Fingertip and distal thumb)	10-12 months
Plays pat-a-cake	9-10 months
Tower of 2 cubes	13-15 months
Tower of 4 cubes	18 months
Uses cup and spoon well	15-18 months

Table 1-8

DEVELOPMENTAL MILESTONES: SOCIAL	
Social smile	1-2 months
Smiles at mirror	5 months
Separation anxiety	6-12 months
Waves "bye-bye"	10 months
Dresses self (except buttons in back)	3 years
Ties shoe laces	5 years
Parallel play	1-2 years
Cooperative play	3-4 years
Can tell fantasy from reality	5 years

Metabolic screening: not recommended for asymptomatic children with idiopathic mental retardation.

Consider metabolic screening if the following symptoms are present with mental retardation:

- Episodic vomiting or lethargy
- Poor growth
- Seizures
- Unusual odors
- Loss of developmental skills
- Sensory abnormality (especially retina!)
- Acquired skin disorders

Tests for metabolic screening include: fasting plasma amino acids, blood lactate, ammonia, very long-chain fatty acids, and urinary oligosaccharides/mucopolysaccharides.

Table 1-9

DEVELOPMENTAL MILESTONES: AMBULATING	
Walking:	
Pulls to stand	9 months
Walks holding onto furniture	11 months
Walks without help	13 months
Walks well	15 months
Runs well	2 years
Stairs:	
Up and down stairs, 2 feet each step	2 years
Up and down stairs, 1 foot per step each way	4 years
Jumps:	
Jumps off ground with 2 feet up	2.5 years
Hops on 1 foot	4 years
Skips	5-6 years
Balances on one foot 2-3 secs	3 years
Balances on one foot 6-10 secs	4 years

Table 1-10

DEVELOPMENTAL MILESTONES: SPEECH AND LANGUAGE	
Coos	2-4 months
First words	9-12 months
Understands 1 step commands	15 months
Vocabulary of 10-50 words	13-18 months
2 word sentences	18-24 months
3 word sentences	2-3 years
4 word sentences	3-4 years

MENTAL RETARDATION

Statistically, mental retardation is represented by an IQ of 2 standard deviations below the population mean and is associated with delays in skills, including self-care, social interactions, and communication. This generally corresponds to an IQ of 70–75. "Mild" mental retardation is defined as an IQ of 50–75, and "moderate-to-severe" is an IQ of < 50. More recently, experts recommend basing classifying mental retardation on the child's ability to perform skills of daily living and function, and not on a "number."

"Mild" mental retardation occurs at a rate of 20–30/1000. It is often hereditary ("you should see his cousin Jesse"), occurs more commonly in low socio-economic groups, and is more common in boys. Of note, only 4–8% of those with mild mental retardation have associated identifiable chromosomal abnormalities.

Severe mental retardation occurs with a rate of 1–4/1000, is sporadic, more common in boys, and not associated with socioeconomic factors. 30% of these cases are due to chromosomal abnormalities. Trisomy 21 (Down syndrome) is the most common. History of CNS injury, such as from teratogens, infection and pre-, peri-, or postnatal insults, account for 15–20%. Another 10–15% will have cerebral dysgenesis on MRI. You will see multiple congenital anomalies with an identifiable syndrome in only about 4–5% of cases of severe mental retardation. Endocrine/metabolic etiologies account for 3–5%.

If mental retardation is present, do Cytogenetic Chromosome testing if any of the following are also found:

- Microcephaly
- Family history of mental retardation
- Family history of fetal loss
- IQ < 50
- Skin pigmentary abnormalities
- Suspected genetic syndrome

SPEECH/LANGUAGE DELAY

50% of children with delayed language development will have delays in other areas.

Common causes of Language Development problems:

- Hearing deficiency (always order the hearing test first!)
- Mental retardation
- Dysphasia
- Dysarthria
- Structural problems of the mouth/respiratory tract
- Child abuse/neglect

Stages:

0–10 months: Early Sounds

0–6 months: Localizes sounds, cooing—first at random and then interactively with adults. (Note: Acquisition of simple names such as "mama" and "dada" may occur this early.)

6–10 months: Consonants added to vowels to induce "babbling." (Note: deaf infants can coo, but don't "interactively" coo or progress to babbling.)

notes

Quick Quiz

1) True or False: Mental retardation is usually associated with chromosomal abnormalities.
2) Describe the clinical clues that a child is experiencing language development problems.
3) At what age should you be concerned when a child speaks NO words?

10–18 months: "Point and Name" Period

Rapid acquisition of names, especially those beyond "mama" and "dada."

12–18 months:Word-Comprehension Period

Child understands 75–100 words, follows simple commands and vocalizes "first words." "Pointing" with words is very important at this stage (e.g., pointing and saying, "car").

> 18 months: Word-Combination Period

The ability to combine words usually occurs after being able to speak > 50 words. First sentences are simple constructions, usually without prepositions, pronouns, and articles.

Language development is the most widely variable of all of the developmental areas! Children may be labeled as language-delayed when they actually are within acceptable limits. However, it is important to identify a child with genuine language development issues as early as possible!

Clinical evaluation of language skills is quite complicated and usually requires the assistance of an expert. However, look for these clues to possible language delay problems on the Board exam and in real life:

- Absence of babbling by 9–12 months
- Absence of any words by 18 months
- Absence of meaningful phrases by 24 months
- Speech that is unintelligible (to strangers) by 3 years
- Inability to use language to communicate after 3 years
- Difficulty with language comprehension after 3 years

If you suspect a language disorder, perform a hearing screen (behavioral or brainstem-evoked response audiometry). Again, review the history and exam (including prenatal history and labs), as well as psychosocial factors (abuse/neglect). Once you confirm a language disorder, begin specific treatments.

STATISTICS

OVERVIEW

Know statistics perfectly!

Screening is one of the most important aspects of a visit to a pediatrician. The value of screening is determined by many factors. You determine a good screening test by its sensitivity and specificity. Because these are so important, we will review these topics now.

THE BAYESIAN FOURSQUARE

Key: T = true, F = false, P = positive, N = negative

To make sense of the Foursquare used in answering sensitivity and specificity questions, let's go over the diagram in Figure

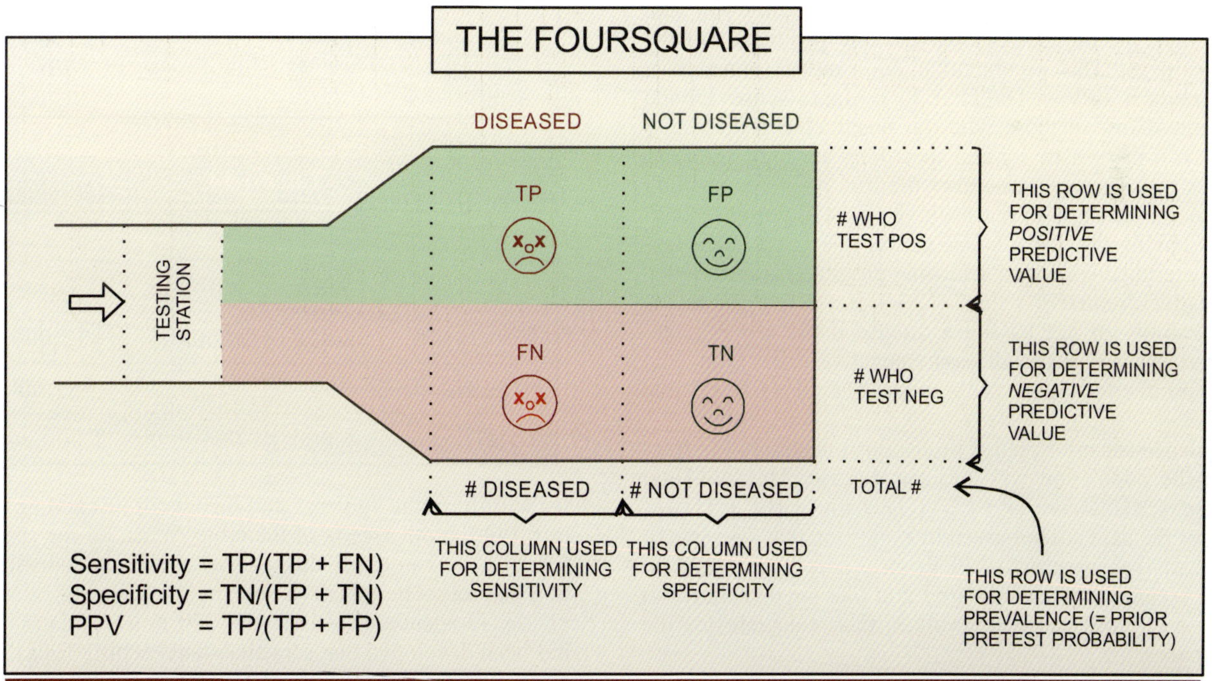

Figure 1-1: The Foursquare

notes

1-1. Assume we are testing a group of cattle for a deadly disease. They go through the testing station on the left, and you direct them either to the upper corral if their test is positive or to the lower corral if their test is negative. You then drive them all the way across the corral to the right, but this disease is so deadly, all the diseased cattle die before they get to the far right of the corral. So we are left with the four sets of cattle. The upper corral contains those who have the disease and tested positive (true positives = TP) and those who don't have the disease but tested positive (false positives = FP). The lower corral contains those who have the disease and tested negative (false negative = FN) and those who don't have the disease and tested negative (true negatives = TN). The Foursquare is very useful in determining sensitivity, specificity, and positive and negative predictive values.

Sensitivity takes into account only those who have the disease. Sensitivity = true positives (# of patients with disease who test positive) divided by the total # of patients with disease (those who test positive **plus** the false negatives); thus, sensitivity = TP/(TP+FN). Specificity takes into account only those who do not have the disease. Specificity = true negatives (# of patients without disease who test negative) divided by the total # of patients without the disease (those who test negative plus the false positives); thus, specificity = TN/(TN + FP).

To help remember: Sensitivity takes into account only those who have the disease, and specificity takes into account only those who do not have the disease. This means that each one is independent of the prevalence of the disease in the selected population! Disease prevalence is just the percentage of the population with the disease.

The "Positive-Predictive Value" (PPV) of a diagnostic test is the probability of disease in a patient with a positive test—i.e., PPV = P (disease | positive test). To figure this, you take into account the number of both the true positives and the false positives. This combination does reflect prevalence. The formula is PPV = TP/(TP + FP). Makes sense: Divide true positives by all those who test positive! If a disease is rare, even if the sensitivity and specificity are high, the false positives may greatly outnumber the true positives, making the chance much less that a positive test will correlate with actually having the disease. Use this as one of the main factors to determine whether a screening program is practicable.

The "Negative-Predictive Value" (NPV) of a diagnostic test is the probability of not having a disease if the test is negative—i.e., NPV = P (no disease | negative test). Using the foursquare, the formula is NPV = TN/(TN + FN). See Table 1-11.

The prevalence (or prior/pretest probability) is simply the fraction of the population who has the disease. This is (Total with disease)/Total, or (TP + FN)/((TP + FN) + (FP + TN)).

When all of the data are not given in a question that asks you to find sensitivity, specificity, PPV, etc., it is very useful to quickly sketch a foursquare-based grid like the one shown in Table 1-12. Insert the given values, then calculate for the blank spaces.

In Table 1-13 and Table 1-14 we solve the foursquare for the scenario in the next paragraph. First, after a bit of calculation, we will fill in the "givens" and then we'll just add or subtract to fill in the other cells of the table. When all the spaces are filled in, we can easily answer just about any statistics question that might be asked. [Know this stuff!]

Scenario: Incidence of asthma is 1/200 in a population. A test has been developed that screens infants at birth for asthma. In a test under consideration, if sensitivity = 99% and the frequency of abnormal tests in the population is 1.3%, what is

Table 1-11

	Disease	No Disease	Total
Abn tests	TP	FP	TP+FP
Nl tests	FN	TN	FN+TN
Total	TP+FN	FP+TN	

Table 1-12

I. Sketch this FIRST:

	with	without	Total
Abn tests			
Nl tests			
Total			

Table 1-13

II. Based on the GIVEN:

	with	without	Total
Abn tests	(1)	(3)	13,000
Nl tests	(2)	(4)	987,000
Total	5,000	995,000	1,000,000

Note that the 5,000 and 999,000 are the DENOMINATORS in the sensitivity and specificity equations!

Table 1-14

III.

	with	without	Total
Abn tests	4,950	8,050	13,000
Nl tests	50	986,950	987,000
Total	5,000	995,000	1,000,000

notes

Quick Quiz

1) A study shows a new treatment for acute lymphocytic leukemia improves survival by 60% and the study has a P-value of 0.2. Based on this "evidence," would you recommend this new treatment?
2) You have invented a test that is 90% sensitive and 95% specific for cystic fibrosis screening. If you tested 100 children with known cystic fibrosis, how many children would the test show as having this disease?
3) A new treatment for Wilms' Tumor improves survival by 30% compared to standard therapy, and the 95% confidence interval for the study is -5.9 to 10.0. Assuming treatments have the same side effects, would it be worthwhile to consider the new treatment?

the ratio of false positives to true positives, and is this a good screening test? To solve, first fill in the 4-square grid with all the known information.

If the population is not given, assume 1 million. 1/200 incidence = 5000 total persons with asthma. 0.013 x 1 million = 13,000 total abnormal tests. Just subtract to find the number without asthma (995,000) and the number of normal tests (987,000)—Table 1-13. Then figure out the other blanks in the order shown: 1, 2, 3, and 4. Blank (1) is the only one requiring thought:

Sensitivity = TP/(TP+FN) or .99 = TP/5000

So: TP = 4950. (Note that the 5000 and 995,000 are the denominators in the sensitivity and specificity equations!) The others are found by subtraction (Table 1-14).

Once you fill in the entire matrix, you can solve any problem, provided there is enough information. In this example, PPV = TP/(TP + FP) = 38%—NOT a good percentage for a screening test! If insufficient data are given to solve the problem, it will become apparent when you are unable to fill in all the blanks.

What happens if you change the threshold for normal in a test? If you increase the threshold for what is normal, you will get more negative tests—both true negatives and false negatives. This will decrease the sensitivity and increase the specificity. Why is this? Assume we did this for the previous example. Because the number of people with and without the disease remains the same, the denominators in the sensitivity and specificity equations remain the same. In the sensitivity equation, the numerator decreases (decreased TP due to increased FN), so sensitivity decreases; i.e., fewer of those with the disease are found by the test. In the specificity equation, the numerator increases so specificity increases; i.e., those testing negative are less likely to have the disease.

As a quick trick, think of the threshold for normal in the test as the line in the foursquare that divides the top from the bottom. As the threshold increases, the line rises, indicating a decreased number of TP and FP and an increased number of FN and TN. As the threshold decreases, the line goes lower, indicating an increased number of positives and decreased number of negatives. Because the denominator stays the same, just see what happens to TP and TN. If TP increases, sensitivity increases. If TN increases, specificity increases. You also will see that any time the test normals are redefined, sensitivity will increase at the expense of specificity and vice-versa.

As disease prevalence/incidence decreases, the number of false positives increases while the number of false negatives decreases. So, the ratio of false positives to false negatives increases. This occurs because there is no change in the sensitivity or specificity of the diagnostic test.

P-VALUE

The *P*-value is a way of expressing a study's statistical significance. Suppose a randomized trial compares 2 drugs and concludes that Drug A is better than Drug B. The smaller the *P*-value, the more confident we can be that Drug A really is better than Drug B, and that this is not simply a chance occurrence. Thus, if a study has a *P*-value of .05, the likelihood that the results are due to chance is only 1 in 20 (5%; or $P = .05$). *P*-values of $< .05$—such as .01 or .001—imply even greater statistical significance. For some arbitrary reason, a *P*-value $\leq .05$ is considered statistically significant.

The value $P \leq 0.05$ as statistically significant is probably all you need to know for most questions on *P*-values, but you should know more of the theory. *P*-value is the probability of the result in question occurring, assuming that the distribution of occurrences used for the calculations is correct. Let's do a rough "for instance:" Say you normally see 1 case of giardiasis in your office per week. Then one week, you see 4 cases and wonder if there is an epidemic of giardiasis. How often should you see 4 cases a week, if you normally see only 1 case per week?

What you assume is chance variation results in an average incidence of giardiasis of 1 case per week and that the variation in occurrences is "per" a certain distribution. This is generally called the "null" or "chance" hypothesis. The distribution can be plotted from thousands of cases, or we can further assume it follows a standard distribution, such as the Poisson distribution. Assuming this is correct, what is the probability of 4 cases occurring in one week? Consult a table that displays various values of the Poisson distribution and read the *P*-value off the table. In the case of giardiasis, you'll see $P = .019$.

The way to read this is, "assuming that the average incidence of giardiasis is 1 case per week and further assuming that the incidence of giardiasis follows a normal Poisson distribution, the probability of 4 cases per week occurring by chance is 1.9%." This seems small, and it is, but it does mean that you can expect to see 4 cases per week about once per year (assuming the assumptions are correct). Now, if you see 4 cases again the following week...!

A recent addition to the literature (and ABP) is the use of "95% confidence intervals." This is essentially the same as a $P < .05$, but the Board questions will give you values that will vary. If the "95% confidence interval" does not cross 0, it is considered significant; e.g., if the exam question tells you the

notes

95% confidence interval is 1.5–5.9, that would be a significant result. However, if the question tells you the 95% confidence interval is -0.7–1.6, that is a non-significant result! [Know this!]

TYPE 1 and TYPE 2 ERRORS

Type 1 = concluding there is a difference (reject null hypothesis) when there is no difference. This is typically expressed by the *P*-value. It reflects the willingness of the investigator to declare a benefit when there is none.

Type 2 = concluding there is no difference (fail to reject null hypothesis) when one exists. With Type 2 error, there is the likelihood that the trial will miss a true difference between the two test groups.

META-ANALYSIS

Meta-analysis is the retrospective analysis of many studies concerned with the same topic. There are several methodological flaws and biases involved with these types of analyses, as well as several severe statistical constraints. Compiling studies with differing Type 1 and Type 2 errors is difficult. Other areas of difficulty include ages of participants and assumptions of the magnitude of difference expected between the experimental groups.

Not only will you be asked about all of the above, but you will also see sensitivity, specificity, predictive values, and *P*-values repeatedly in your medical reading.

SCREENING IN CHILDREN

NEWBORN METABOLIC SCREENING

All states (U.S.) currently agree on screening for the following:

Congenital hypothyroidism

Phenylketonuria (PKU)

In addition, 2/3 of states also screen for galactosemia, while an increasing number of states are screening for hemoglobinopathies.

For screening purposes, draw blood before discharge and never later than 7 days of age. PKU requires the "build-up" of metabolites, so if you do a test sooner than 24 hours after birth, repeat it in 1 to 2 weeks. Note: Administration of blood transfusions and dialysis can lead to erroneous results.

VISION AND HEARING SCREENING

Protocols for vision and hearing are dependent on age and developmental factors, particularly findings that suggest a developmental problem.

Here are some general age-based standards and related considerations:

Infancy: Object tracking, red reflex, and conjugate gaze should always be present by 4 months.

Toddler/Preschool: Administer and evaluate unilateral cover test—cover and uncover each eye while the child is looking straight ahead at an object 10 feet away. Movement in the uncovered eye when the opposite is covered or uncovered suggests potential ocular misalignment (strabismus), which requires referral to an ophthalmologist. Refer preschoolers with acuity < 20/40 in either eye.

3–5 years of age: Screen with the Random-dot-E Test. 20% of children will have a refractive error, usually myopia (nearsightedness).

School-aged children, including adolescents: Evaluate these kids annually! Refer children 5–6 years of age who cannot read the majority of the 20/30 line on the vision chart. At all ages, refer a child with a difference of > 1 line in acuity between left and right eyes!

Deafness is a relatively common finding with 1–3/1000 children born deaf. Many more children develop sensorineural deficits during childhood. The AAP has consistently recommended universal screening of infants with the goal of 100% screening of all infants by age 3 months. However, the AAP does not recommend a specific screening modality. Both methods available have problems with sensitivity and specificity. Infants < 6 months have usually been screened with auditory brainstem response testing (ABR). A newer method, known as evoked-otoacoustic-emissions analysis testing (EOEA), is simpler but has more problems with lower specificity (this means it may incorrectly identify more children with problems, resulting in increased costs due to further unnecessary testing.) Regardless of which test you choose, the goal is to identify hearing loss of 35 dB or greater in the 500 Hz to 4000 Hz range. Infants initially screened by neonatal screening should be screened again periodically, depending on the reason for the initial screening; for example, with perinatal CMV, which can result in hearing loss over prolonged periods of time. The AAP additionally recommends formal hearing screening for ALL children at 3, 4, and 5 years of age and every 2–3 years until adolescence! The U.S. Preventative Services Task Force does not recommend routine screening for children after the age of 3 years, so this is controversial. On the Board exam, I advise adhering to the AAP recommendations. Additionally, many states are now mandating newborn hearing screens as well.

Whom should you screen for hearing problems? Screen in all the following situations:

- Parent expresses concerns regarding hearing/language development of a child
- There is a history of bacterial meningitis
- There are confirmed neonatal infections associated with hearing loss (CMV)
- There is a history of significant head trauma (especially temporal bone)
- A syndrome presents that is associated with hearing loss
- There has been exposure to ototoxic medications (gentamicin)
- A neurodegenerative disorder is present
- There is confirmed incidence of infectious diseases, such mumps/measles

notes

Quick Quiz

1) All states (U.S.) screen for which 2 diseases?
2) Name the reasons to screen for hearing loss.
3) At what age is blood pressure screening routinely initiated?
4) Is cholesterol screening universally recommended? If not, for which groups would you consider it?
5) At what blood-lead level cutoff is intervention recommended?
6) True or False: Routine hemoglobin testing is recommended as a screen in 1-year-olds.
7) Name children at risk for iron-deficiency anemia.

BLOOD PRESSURE SCREENING

Conduct routine blood pressure screening for all children on a yearly basis starting at 3 years of age. Also measure blood pressure in children < 3 who may have a coexisting medical condition that predisposes them to hypertension. Measure BP with the child sitting with the arm at heart level. Make sure that the width of the cuff bladder is 40% of the circumference of the upper arm at its midpoint and, when wrapped, covers 80–100% of the circumference of the arm. Inflate the cuff to 20mm Hg above the loss of the radial pulse and then deflate at 2–3 mm Hg/second. The first sound you hear is a tapping sound, known as Korotkoff sound 1, which is recorded as the systolic blood pressure. The level at which all sounds disappear is Korotkoff sound 5, which is the measured diastolic pressure. Normal BP is defined by a systolic and diastolic pressure < the 90th percentile for age and sex. You must determine high-normal (90–95%) and hypertension (> 95%) by 3 separate readings over a period of days to weeks (although depending on the severity of the hypertension and presence of other conditions, you may elect to condense this time frame).

CHOLESTEROL AND LIPID SCREENING

Universal screening of children is not recommended.

In children > 2 years of age whose parents or grandparents have a history of early atherosclerotic disease (MI, angina, + cath, stroke, or sudden cardiac death before the age of 55), the AAP recommends screening with a fasting-serum-lipid profile (total cholesterol, HDL, triglycerides, and LDL). Treatment and other issues are discussed in the chapter on Metabolic Disorders.

LEAD SCREENING

Lead poisoning remains a significant problem in the U.S., and thus, the subject appears on the ABP exam! Lead-based paints were banned in the 1970s, but problems still occur from the exposure to—and/or ingestion of—lead-containing paint chips, as well as dust that occurs with deterioration and remodeling of older homes. Because it is now recognized that even low lead levels can cause significant clinical effects, the CDC recommends a region-selective screening, based on known prevalence of lead in the particular region, or universal blood lead screening if regional prevalence data are not known, for all children from ages 6–72 months. The region-specific measures are for communities where ≥ 12% of 1- and 2-year-olds have blood levels ≥ 10 μg/dL, or if ≥ 27% of houses in the area were built before 1950. The interventional threshold has been lowered to levels > 10 μg/dL.

Risk Factors to assess beginning at 6 months of age:

- Child lives in or regularly visits a house built before 1950
- Child lives in, or regularly visits, a house built before 1978 that is undergoing remodeling
- Child has a sibling or play pal who has had an elevated blood lead level
- The household uses folk remedies that contain lead
- Child emigrated or adopted from a country with high lead levels
- Parental/Caretaker exposed to lead via occupation or vocation (e.g., remodeling, pottery with lead paint, work with lead batteries)
- Some urban environments where lead levels are unknown or known to be high

Venous blood sampling is better than capillary (finger-stick) sampling. If a capillary sample is "positive," get a confirmatory venous sample because of the potential for lead contamination on the surface of the skin.

IRON DEFICIENCY SCREENING

Universal screening for anemia with random hemoglobin/hematocrits is no longer routinely recommended by most organizations, but in their 1999 guidelines, the AAP Committee on Practice and Ambulatory Medicine still recommended hematocrit/hemoglobin testing in children 9–12 months of age.

Screen for the following groups, who are considered to be at increased risk:

- Premature births
- Low birth weight
- Cow's milk feeding before 12 months of age
- Insufficient dietary iron intake
- Low socioeconomic status
- Menstruating adolescents (AAP—annual screening)
- Male and female adolescent athletes

Do not screen children during an episode of acute illness or for several weeks after fever/infection have abated, because mild transient anemia is common in such circumstances. As in lead screening, venous sampling for iron deficiency is more accurate than capillary sampling. Anemia is defined as hemoglobin 2 standard deviations below the mean for similar age and sex.

notes

URINALYSIS SCREENING

Routine screening with urinalysis and urine cultures is not cost-effective. These studies are not recommended by any group (The U.S. Preventative Health Task Force (USPHTF), AAFP, Canadian Task Force on Preventative Health, etc.), except the AAP Committee on Practice and Ambulatory Medicine, which in their 1999 guidelines still recommended routine urinalysis at 5 years of age. The non-AAP groups believe (and it is supported by good evidence) that you should do urine studies only if clinically indicated, or if there is concern for renal disease (i.e., heredity). Whom do you believe? Well, you are taking an examination that is given by the ABP but is written by members of the AAP, so follow the AAP guidelines on the Board Examination!

The AAP also recommends annual dipstick urine testing for leukocytes in sexually active males and females between the ages of 11 and 21 years as a screen for STDs.

TUBERCULOSIS SCREENING

Universal, routine tuberculin testing for all children is no longer recommended. Base initial screening decisions on specific risk factors and do initial screening for children:

- who have contacts with confirmed or suspected infectious TB (includes household contacts who have been in jail/prison in the last 5 years)!
- with x-ray findings consistent with TB.
- emigrating from high-risk countries (Asia, Africa, Latin America, Middle East).
- with significant travel to endemic countries or significant contact with people from those countries.
- who live in areas of high TB prevalence.

Also conduct annual screening for HIV-infected children and adolescents in jail/prison.

Every 2–3 years, screen those exposed to high-risk individuals (HIV-infected adults/adolescents, nursing home residents, illicit drug users, prisoners, etc.), depending on durations of exposure to these individuals. Also periodically screen those children who live in areas with known high levels of TB.

Screen at 4–6 and 11–16 years of age: children who reside in a high-prevalence community, and those whose history regarding risk factors is unknown or incomplete.

Also keep in mind:

Always use the 5 tuberculin units in 0.1 ml intradermal Mantoux test (PPD—purified protein derivative). Do not use multipuncture testing.

Prior vaccination with bacillus Calmette-Guerin (BCG) is not a contraindication. Also, interpret results regardless of BCG vaccination status.

TB testing relies on skin hypersensitivity reactions. It takes 2–10 weeks after infection with tuberculosis for the skin test to become positive. Read the Mantoux test at 48–72 hours by tactile measurement of the margins of induration (not erythema!). If a skin test is positive, do a PA and Lateral CXR.

What is a positive test? It depends on the reaction size and risk factors for possible TB!

Induration ≥ 5 mm is considered positive for children:

- in close contact with a known or suspected infectious case of TB.
- in a household with a person with active or previously active TB who was not adequately treated (or can't confirm completed treatment).
- with suspected active TB disease (CXR positive or clinical evidence of TB).
- receiving immunosuppressive therapy or with immunosuppressive disorders, including HIV.

Induration ≥ 10 mm is considered positive for children:

- < 4 years.
- with accompanying DM, chronic renal failure, malnutrition.
- (or their parents) who were born in a region of the world with high-prevalence.
- who have frequent exposure to adults with HIV, the homeless, illicit-drug users, nursing home residents, prisoners, and/or migrant farm workers.
- who travel to regions of the world with high prevalence.

Induration ≥ 15 mm is considered positive for children ≥ 4 years of age without any risk factors. Treatment and therapy for screening is discussed in the Infectious Disease section.

COMMON TOPICS OF WELL-CHILD VISITS

OVERVIEW

This aspect of health supervision is one of the most important for a pediatrician. However, contemporary time constraints (frequently due to increased overhead, billing and need to generate income) have made this particular part of being a pediatrician more difficult than ever. Just remember for the ABP—you always do counseling and guidance at each child visit, no matter what. Be aware that "more" is not always "better." On the Board exam, if you are given options for counseling in a given visit, be sure you "prioritize" the contextual information provided so it relates clinically to the specific reason for the visit; e.g., if the child is in for his 2-month shots, you really don't need to spend much time on the "drugs, sex, and rock and roll" talk (unless this is the child of a certain band member from an MTV show).

In most cases, the rule to follow is basic "common sense." Most counseling revolves around feeding, injury prevention, developmental/behavioral issues, daily care and medical issues; i.e., during the 2-month visit, counsel on issues such as:

- Bath safety
- Sun exposure
- Breast- vs. bottle-feeding
- Fluoride supplementation, if indicated

notes

Quick Quiz

1) True or False: Universal screening with urinalysis is no longer recommended by the AAP.
2) True or False: Universal tuberculosis screening is mandated by the CDC for all infants 1 year of age.
3) At what age should you make the initial dental referral?
4) At what age should "sex and drugs" be discussed with a child according to the AAP?
5) True or False: Once a mother's milk has "come in," it is acceptable to supplement feedings with bottles.

- Nutrition topics, such as waiting to introduce solids at 4–6 months
- Sleep, crying, and bowel patterns
- Enjoyment of holding, cuddling, talking to baby (cannot spoil)
- Immunizations
- Common cold management, including proper use of bulb syringe and saline nose drops
- Child-care arrangements, etc.

WHEW!! You are supposed to cover all of that and, oh yeah, examine the baby . . . and try to do everything in 15–20 minutes!

An important thing to remember is to be age-appropriate. Notably, the ABP likes to ask about helmets for bicycle riders, initial dental appointment (3-year-olds), discussion about drugs and sex at age 10 (according to AAP guidelines). Carefully review such age-appropriate subjects as a good Board exam prep.

NUTRITION ISSUES

Breastfeeding

Once the mother makes a decision to breastfeed or *not* to breastfeed, it is important that you are supportive and nonjudgmental. Most breastfeeding mothers who wean their infants in the first few weeks postpartum do so because of lack of support or inability to deal with common problems associated with breastfeeding. Questions commonly arise, and it is important that you are available as a resource for the breastfeeding mother. The AAP recently changed their guidelines to strongly support breastfeeding. Data consistently shows that breastfeeding decreases the incidence or severity of bacterial meningitis, otitis media, diarrhea, and urinary tract infections. Some recent evidence suggests that breastfeeding may offer protection against asthma, diabetes, and obesity. Postnatal infection rates are reduced 21% in breastfed infants in the United States. Additionally, breastfeeding has been associated with a slight increase in performance on cognitive developmental tests. There are benefits for the nursing mother as well: breastfeeding may reduce the risk of breast and ovarian cancer, hip fractures, and osteoporosis.

Here's a brief physiology review. The newborn sucking on the nipple stimulates the mother's pituitary to release prolactin and oxytocin. These cause the production (remember PROduction and PROlactin) and "let-down" (oxytocin) of breast milk. Adequate breast drainage maintains prolactin levels. Medications, maternal fatigue, and stress can negatively affect these levels. Oxytocin release and the "milk-ejection reflex" occur in response to the infant suckling, and increase with rest, warmth, a quiet environment, and the sight of the infant. Pain, embarrassment, distraction, or fatigue can inhibit release. The "milk-ejection reflex" also may cause dripping of milk from the opposite breast while nursing, as well as bring relief of nipple discomfort and uterine cramping.

In the first few days of breastfeeding, the baby mainly receives low-volume, antibody-rich colostrum. During this early time, poor feeding or irregular routines rarely impact on future breastfeeding success. However, once milk "has come in" and the mother begins to produce large volumes, poor feeding routines will prevent continued, successful lactation. It is important that mothers do not supplement with a bottle at this point; rather, encourage her to delay the decision for at least several weeks, allowing for a consistent, routine feeding pattern to develop. The infant's motor skills for mouth and tongue movements differ greatly between breastfeeding and bottle-feeding. Current guidelines reject rigid schedules for feeding duration and timing. In the initial few days postpartum, most women can attempt 10–15 minutes per breast with each feed. The infant should take from both breasts at each feeding. Most infants will feed every 2 to 3 hours. Newborns should not go longer than 4–5 hours between feedings. By 2 months of age, most infants will stop one of the middle-of-the-night feedings. However, because protein composition of breast milk results in a more rapid digestion time, breastfed infants generally feed more often than bottle-fed infants.

Sore nipples, engorgement, and maternal fatigue are common. Nipple soreness is most frequently due to not using the correct ventral-to-ventral position, inadequate placement of enough of the areola into the mouth to limit the amount of tension on the nipple itself, and/or forgetting to break the suction before removing the baby from the breast. Discourage use of creams and ointments, which will actually exacerbate the problem. Also, encourage the mother not to decrease the number of feeds or duration because this will lead to engorgement. Inadequate drainage will lead to increased engorgement and involution of the milk supply, which could result in mastitis. If engorgement does occur, increasing the frequency of feedings will alleviate the problem. Use of a pump—or manual milk expression—may also be useful.

The biggest concern generally seems to be whether the baby is "getting enough milk." Remember that infants may lose 10% of birth weight before regaining it in the first 10–14 days of life. Also, during growth spurts, the baby will decrease the interval between feeds to increase milk production.

notes

Formula (Bottle) Feeding

Most commercial formulas for healthy full-term infants are cow's milk-based, formed of reconstituted skim milk or skim milk with added whey protein. The carbohydrate source is lactate. The fat consists of a mixture of vegetable oils and removal of the butterfat. All are essentially the same. Recommend them based on cost and the taste preference of the infant (hmm, ok, it is difficult to ascertain this). Soy-protein formulas today are nutritionally equivalent to cow's milk formulas. But note that recent research has found that soy-based formulas have high aluminum levels. There is also evidence that preterm infants do not grow as well on these formulas. For these reasons, do not recommend soy-protein formulas for infants weighing < 1800 grams. These were once thought to be good "hypo-allergenic" formulas, but we now know that there is a high incidence of cross-reactivity between soy protein and cow's milk protein. The fat content in the soy and cow-milk products is essentially the same. One group of infants who may benefit from soy formulas is that with post-diarrheal, transient-lactase deficiency. Why? Because the carbohydrate is sucrose and/or corn syrup, and thus is digested easily in the face of a lactase deficiency. However, recommend that mothers do not "switch" formulas based on vague GI symptoms or "colic."

Bottle-feeding practices should mimic breastfeeding in that feeding should occur "on demand." This usually means 2–3 ounces every 2–3 hours for newborns with non-feeding intervals lasting no longer than 5 hours. After the first week, most infants will take 2–4 ounces every 2–4 hours. By 2 months of age, most bottle-fed infants won't require the "middle-of-the-night" feeding. The 6-month-old child should be taking in < 30 ounces a day, and calories from formula should not exceed 65% of total caloric intake each day. Encourage mothers to avoid giving infants a "go-to-bed" bottle, because this can lead to a significant problem with dental caries. Most babies can begin weaning from the bottle to cup between 9 and 12 months. Sterilization of bottles and formula is not required. Between uses, bottles simply can be washed with soap and warm water.

Vitamin and Mineral Supplementation

Most physicians do not recommend routine vitamin supplementation, with the exception of vitamin D supplements (200 IU/day) for exclusively breastfed infants, or those receiving < 500 ml/formula per day. Levels of vitamin D in breast milk are relatively low, but most used to believe sunlight exposure made up for any deficiency. However, recent reports show an increased risk of rickets in these babies. Breast milk is itself rich in vitamins A and C. Note also that Vitamin B_{12} deficiency has been reported in breastfed infants whose mothers are strict vegetarians.

Also encourage children and teens to take Vitamin D supplements if they do not drink at least 500 ml of vitamin D-fortified milk per day, do not get regular exposure to sunlight, or do not already take a daily multivitamin with at least 200 IU of vitamin D.

Iron: You must give iron supplements to the full-term infant between 4–6 months of age and to the preterm infant 2 months of age. You can achieve iron supplementation with infant formula, iron-fortified cereal, or ferrous sulfate drops. Elemental iron supplementation of 1 mg/kg/day should be provided for infants who are exclusively breastfed beyond 6 months of age. Begin the preterm, breastfed infant on iron drops at 2 months of age. Introducing whole cow's milk too early can result in occult GI blood loss and worsening of iron deficiency.

Fluoride: This gets a little confusing, depending on the fluoride content of the existing water supply for the household. Note: Do not provide fluoride supplementation to any child under the age of 6 months. If fluoride in the water supply is negligible (< 0.3 PPM), begin supplements at 6 months of age. If the fluoride content is modest (0.3 – 0.6 PPM), begin supplements at 3 years of age. Anytime fluoridation in the water supply is > 0.6 PPM, additional ingestion of fluoride is unnecessary. Excess fluoride can result in fluorosis, a cosmetically disfiguring condition. It is important to counsel parents that children under 6 years of age should only use a "pea-sized" quantity of toothpaste per brushing. Many recommend not using toothpaste until after the age of 2.5 years because the risk of fluorosis is much higher than the risk of caries in children below this age. If fluoride levels are adequate in the community, and assuming the mother drinks the community water, exclusively breastfed infants will not require supplements. What about pregnant women living in areas with non-fluoridated water? Latest guidelines recommend not giving fluoride supplementation to pregnant women, because prenatal fluoride supplementation has been shown not to make a difference in the eventual incidence of caries in the offspring.

What about water filters and bottled water? In general, water filters used in the United States have a negligible effect on the fluoride concentration. Most bottled water, however, does not contain adequate levels of fluoride.

How does fluoride work? It inhibits dental caries formation by 3 mechanisms:

1) Enhancement of tooth mineralization,
2) Reversal of tooth demineralization, and
3) Inhibition of acid-producing bacteria that cause caries.

Fluoride helps calcium and phosphate ions incorporate into enamel as well as itself being incorporated. Fluoride-containing enamel is much harder and less acid soluble.

Advancing the Diet

At 4–6 months of age, most infants are ready to proceed to solid foods. The sequence of beginning such foods is open to debate, and most pediatricians rely on "tradition." This generally means starting with iron-fortified cereals, then strained/pureed vegetables and fruits, followed by meats and poultry products. Most recommend that egg whites, wheat, and fish be introduced later because of concern of GI immaturity and allergic symptomatology commonly associated with these 3 items. Generally, it is best to introduce only one new food at a time and observe for any adverse effect over the next 3–5 days before adding another item.

notes

Quick Quiz

1) True or False: It is a good idea to try different formulas to see what helps alleviate "colic."
2) What vitamin supplement is recommended for all infants who are exclusively breastfed?
3) Which vitamin deficiency is possible in an infant of a mother who is a strict vegetarian?
4) Introduction of cow's milk should be delayed until what age?
5) What has significantly reduced the incidence of SIDS?

Delay whole cow's milk until 12 months of age; but then recommend whole cow's milk instead of skim/2% because of the need for increased dietary fat intake (30–50% of total calories) for optimal growth and development in the first 2 years of life. After age 2 years, children can gradually be transitioned to 2% and skim milk, generally completing such transition by about age 5.

By 6–9 months of age, most infants can begin using a spoon and cup. Babies usually are competent with these items by 15–18 months. Finger foods become popular by 7–9 months of age. Items to avoid because of the risk of aspiration: raw carrots, large pieces of raw apple, whole or coin-shaped pieces of hot dog, whole grapes, large cookies, peanuts, popcorn, and hard candy.

Feeding issues for toddlers: Mealtime routines are very important. Families should sit together and turn the TV off (besides, it seems most shows today have people eating worms or professing their love with a rose—sometimes at the same time). Encourage self-feeding (although very messy). Mealtimes should be of finite duration, such as 20–30 minutes. "Cleaning the plate" should not be a sufficient reason for leaving the table. Discourage "grazing" between meals.

SLEEP (OR THE LACK OF IT)

The first issue with sleep is the importance of reinforcing the "back to sleep" effort. Since implementation of this program, the number of SIDS deaths has been reduced markedly. One consequence of "back to front" is that children tend to achieve slightly slower early motor milestones (raising their head or chest off the bed when in the prone position), but they "catch-up" very quickly once the child is able to roll over to a prone position.

Sleep involves two distinct states:

1) active or REM sleep (rapid eye movements, motor movements, vocalizations, dreaming, and easy awakening), and
2) deeper, quiet or non-REM sleep. In infancy, 50–60% of sleep is spent in REM.

Non-REM intervals last 50 to 60 minutes. In adults, 25% of sleep is in REM with intervals of non-REM sleep lasting 90–100 minutes. Newborns sleep 18 hours/day; 6–15-month-olds sleep 10–12 hours at night with 2 nap periods during the day. After 15 months of age, naps decrease to 1/day, and by 4 years of age, the naps completely disappear (hmm... guess I never reached that stage).

Note: It is important for parents to realize that infants will normally wake up at night and, by 3–4 months of age, they develop the ability to put themselves back to sleep. The problem is usually with the parent, not with the child, when they present with a "she just won't sleep all night" complaint. First, parents will frequently misinterpret the REM sleep as periods of awakening and will attend to the child. In such situations, the parent is actually responsible for the child "waking up." Frequent nighttime feedings with the associated "nocturnal attention" is usually the other culprit. Infants learn nighttime feeding after 6–9 months of age! Infants who always are rocked, fed or soothed to sleep may be unable to return themselves to sleep without these conditions. Numerous experts recommend that parents allow infants to fall asleep on their own and in their own cribs.

Toddlers are a whole 'nother can of worms! Toddlers have an instinctive ability to resist going to bed (that's my philosophy anyway—not proven scientifically). At this age, travel or illness will mess up the best of routines! Normal "separation" issues (i.e., child from parent) also make it more difficult for a 9–18-month-old child to go to sleep. Many recommend the use of a "transition" object, such as a blanket or stuffed toy. Structure in many households is the key for success in this area. Toddlers thrive best on structure, and it is important for them to have a bedtime routine.

CRYING/COLIC/CRAZY PARENT

Reassure parents that Brazelton did a study showing that a 2-week-old infant cries on average 2 hours/day; this increases to 3 hours/day by 6 weeks and then decreases to 1 hour/day by 3 months. Most crying occurs during the evening hours (but of course; that's when you are tired, just getting home from work and ...well ... you get the picture!)

Colic is defined as excessive, unexplained paroxysms of crying in an otherwise well-nourished, normal infant lasting > 3 hours a day and occurring > 3 days a week. 30–50% of kids have this. The crying usually occurs at the same time during the day (usually those dang evenings), and is resistant to everything that attempts to quell it. During these episodes, the infant may have excess flatus and draw the legs up—making some parents interpret this as "gas" or having "bad belly pains." Usually it begins in the 1st week of life and goes away by 3–4 months of age. The cause of colic? No one knows. On the Boards, do not say the answer is to switch formulas if this is the initial presentation for the child with colicky symptoms, and there is nothing else to support lactase deficiency!

Methods to improve colicky symptoms? You know the routine here—each child is different. Some require a quiet environment, some require music, some like to swing at 30 MHz (not 40 or 25 MHz but exactly 30 MHz), some like to ride in a car, some like to just scream their bloody head off. Whatever the preference might be, there is nothing you can do about it.

notes

DENTAL CARE

Primary teeth start to form in utero and permanent teeth start to form soon after birth. At all visits, teeth should be looked for or examined, especially at about the 6-month health supervision. First to emerge are the lower anterior teeth, followed by the upper opposing teeth. Teeth eruption rates and locations can vary significantly but usually the first tooth erupts by 6 months of age with 6 teeth present by 1 year.

Early dentition care usually includes washing the mouth and teeth at bath time with a washcloth (um, usually before you wash the rest of the body). Toothbrushing can begin when the child seems ready and usually is done as an imitation of older siblings or parents. Dental caries risk is increased with more frequent feedings but the most important factor is the amount of time the child has food in their mouth. Therefore, foods should not be allowed to remain in the mouth at bedtime or naps. Bottle caries are very common in children who are allowed to fall asleep with bottles containing milk, flavored drinks, or soft drinks. Usually, the upper anterior and upper/lower posterior teeth are most commonly affected with nursing bottle caries.

Teething is a common concern of parents. Cold items are soothing and many recommend a frozen pacifier. Acetaminophen or other over-the-counter analgesics can be recommended as well.

Dental trauma usually requires evaluation by a dentist, especially if loosening of a secure tooth, chipping or breaking of the crown, lacerating the gingiva, or bleeding around a tooth occurs after trauma. If it is a primary tooth that is broken or damaged it may need to be removed or repaired. Primary teeth that are completely knocked out should not be reimplanted. However, permanent teeth should be reimplanted if possible. The avulsed tooth should not be scrubbed or débrided but rather should be rinsed of visible dirt and material before reinserting. If the tooth cannot be replaced in the mouth immediately, it should be kept in Hank's Balanced Salt Solution® (HBSS), Save-A-Tooth solution®, saline solution, or any available isotonic solution. Teeth left out longer than 1 hour have a poor prognosis for reimplantation but should be attempted anyway.

Dental infections are best treated with penicillins. If the child is allergic to penicillin, clindamycin is a good choice. Most dental infections are actually due to aerobic bacteria, but anaerobes increase in frequency in those with dental abscesses.

DISCIPLINE

This is a difficult one, and we all have our methods, but...I will follow the AAP guidelines here, which should mirror the ABP (which is why you are reading this, right? You don't need an update on the latest from Oprah.) So, for the Boards, corporal punishment is a "No," "NO" and "HECK NO" response. Got it? The ABP likes "time-outs." Parents can use this method as early as 9–12 months, and begin to phase it out by 5–6 years of age. Length of time is generally brief—about 1 minute per year of age (generally to a maximum of 5 minutes—WHEW...I told my wife that 44 minutes was too long for me). If the child leaves the area before time is up, he/she should be escorted back if choosing not to return voluntarily. Minimize conversation with the child, and do not discuss the event. After age 5, most children understand loss of privileges, etc., and this is viewed by the ABP as the most effective. Again, for purposes of Board questions, NEVER choose corporal punishment as an answer!

SAFETY AND INJURY PREVENTION

During a health supervision visit, it is very important to discuss safety and injury prevention. Injuries (both intentional and accidental) are the most common cause of death and morbidity in childhood. 30–75% (depending on age group) of accidental injury-related deaths in children are due to motor vehicle accidents!

Head and facial injuries from bicycle accidents make up a large percentage of emergency department visits and, unfortunately, deaths. Wearing a bicycle helmet is the best way to reduce head and facial injuries.

Additional issues that you frequently need to discuss include:

- Child safety restraints/belts in cars, appropriate for age/height/weight of the child
- Smoke detectors
- Hot-water heater temperature (between 49-55°C or 120-130°F)
- Animal-bite prevention
- Poison prevention
- Choking prevention
- Drowning prevention
- Sports safety (for older children and the adults who supervise)
- Firearm safety
- Alcohol and drug abuse
- Suicide prevention
- Homicide prevention

IMMIGRANT AND INTERNATIONALLY ADOPTED CHILDREN

Immigrant and internationally adopted children are common types of patients seen by pediatricians today. For non-immigrant children, such as tourists or temporary visitors, no medical evaluation is required upon entry into the United States. For those children entering the United States for a permanent residency visa, the medical examination is limited. For permanent visas, active tuberculosis, HIV, syphilis, gonorrhea, lymphogranuloma venereum, chancroid, and leprosy are supposed to be "excluded." However, for children less than 15 years of age, no laboratory testing is required.

Evaluation of the immigrant child depends on several factors. For example, from which country did the child come from? And more specifically, what were the living conditions—was the child living in an orphanage, hospital, or refugee camp?

Common health problems are listed in Table 1-15.

notes

Quick Quiz

1) What types of dental trauma should be referred to a dentist?
2) True or False: Corporal punishment is viewed as an acceptable means of punishment on the ABP examination.
3) What is the safe hot water temperature?
4) Which vaccine(s) is (are) recommended at birth?

Table 1-15

COMMON HEALTH PROBLEMS IN HIGH-RISK IMMIGRANT CHILDREN	
Infections	Immunization Issues Tuberculosis Parasites Hepatitis B Syphilis Malaria
Nutritional/Diet:	Anemia Malnutrition Rickets Iodine deficiency
Toxins	Lead Prenatal alcohol Radioactivity
Growth/Development	Estimated Age Vision and Hearing Dental Caries Congenital defects Developmental delay

For the examination, be particular about the immunization history. An acceptable immunization record documents the date, dose, and name of the vaccine. Be on the look out for these 2 problems:

1) Dose given at too short an interval (4 weeks instead of 6-week minimum), and
2) Dose given at too young an age.

The other thing to be aware of is that children from orphanages in China or the former Soviet Union may not have produced an adequate immunologic response. If the child is under 1 year of age, the "questionable" doses may just be repeated. For older children, it is generally recommended (and more cost-effective) to determine serum immunity for the major antigens.

As far as screening for infectious diseases, most authorities recommend screening for tuberculosis, intestinal parasites, hepatitis B, congenital syphilis, and HIV infection regardless of the test results from a foreign laboratory. Tuberculosis is the most common serious infection encountered. Anemia is very common and children should be retested after treatment of iron-deficiency anemia, since correction may unmask other underlying anemias. Rickets is very common in children from China and the former Soviet Union; iodine deficiency occasionally is noted from these countries as well.

Lead poisoning is also common, especially among children from refugee camps and China. Fetal alcohol syndrome rates are very high in children from eastern Europe and the former Soviet Union.

Vision and hearing screening is recommended early as well. As far as "school" issues, most children should be placed in age-appropriate grades.

"THE SHOTS"

OVERVIEW

WARNING! WARNING!! WARNING!!! KNOW THIS SECTION COLD!

There will be several areas you have to know really well. These include: the immunization schedule, how to get a child caught up on immunizations, the side effects, the contraindications, which vaccines are live vs. inactivated, and the timing of immunizing with certain products (immunoglobulin, PPD).

THE SCHEDULE

The latest on this comes out every year! You can find the latest schedule online at http://www.cdc.gov/mmwr. The schedule will usually be in the first or second January issue of the MMWR for that year. Remember the ABP is "delayed" so for the October certifying exam, you are probably fine with what is presented in the year of, or even up to, 3 years before your exam. If some new vaccine has come out in the past 6 months to a year, don't spend a lot of time on it for the ABP exam, unless there has been a lot of literature on the vaccine and its trials for several preceding years.

Please see the immunization table in the back of this book, taken from the MMWR webpage. Also, the schedule is published in the AAP's journal *Pediatrics*.

By chronological age, then, let's walk through the regimens to be sure you understand them!

Birth: the only vaccine currently recommended at birth is the hepatitis B vaccine! It is mandatory within 12 hours of birth if the mother is Hepatitis B surface antigen-positive (HBsAg+) at birth or the mother's hepatitis B status is unknown!! Don't forget to also give the hepatitis B immune globulin immediately to the infant born to the HBsAg+ mother and ASAP (within 1 week) to the infant, if the mother turns up being HBsAg+ at the time of delivery room screening! Otherwise (i.e., in the HBsAg- mother), you can give the shot anytime within the first 2 months. Give the second dose a minimum of 1 month later than the first dose. Give the third dose at least 4 months after the first dose and at least 2 months after the second dose, but not before 6 months of age

notes

(say that fast 3 times). So, the infant could have any of these regimens for Hepatitis B:

- Birth, 1 month, 6 months, or
- 2 months, 4 months, 6 months, or
- 2 months, 4 months, 1 year

Any of these is acceptable and you don't have to start over if you miss a dose for a year or even several years!

1 month of age: The only vaccine you could give here is the second dose of hepatitis B, if the infant received the first dose at birth.

2–6 months of age: Here is where the fun begins. Now is the appropriate time to give DTaP (D = diphtheria, T = tetanus, aP = acellular pertussis), Hib (Hib = *Haemophilus influenzae* type b conjugate vaccine (the bacterial polysaccharide is "conjugated" to protein), IPV (inactivated polio vaccine), and PCV (pneumococcal conjugate—here pneumococcal polysaccharides are "conjugated" to non-toxic diphtheria toxin). After this multiple immunization, you give all 4 again at 4 months (4 for 4). At 6 months you can give all 4 again, or you may elect to not give the IPV, but instead give that one later, anytime between 6 and 18 months.

You also could give the first or second hepatitis B vaccine, depending on when/if the previous vaccine was given.

Note: all of the vaccines that are given before 12 months of age are non-live vaccines (either killed or recombinant).

So, the majority of practitioners give DTaP, Hib, IPV, and PCV at 2, 4 and 6 months of age with 2–3 of the hepatitis B vaccines interspersed in there at your or the parent's discretion.

12 months of age: A fourth Hib and PCV are due sometime between 12 and 15 months of age. The initial MMR (measles, mumps, and rubella) and varicella vaccines are also due at this time.

15 months of age: The fourth DTaP is due, but you may give as early as 12 months, provided it has been at least 6 months since the third dose.

In summary, by 18 months of age, kids will get:

- 4 DTaP
- 4 Hib (*note for Merck's PedvaxHIB ® or Com Vax ®, a dose at 6 months is not required)
- 3 IPV
- 4 PCV
- 1 MMR
- 1 varicella
- 3 hepatitis B

Also, combination vaccines are being developed to reduce the number of injections an infant/child must receive. Pediarix® is one that contains DTaP, hepatitis B, and IPV.

Note: For children > 24 months, in selected parts of the United States (currently, areas of Oklahoma and at the discretion of local health units), hepatitis A vaccine is recommended.

4–6 years of age: When kids get ready for kindergarten. "Boosters" for DTaP, IPV, and MMR are required.

11–12 years of age: Kids are mostly done with immunizations by this age if they received everything in early childhood. One exception: a booster Td (tetanus and diphtheria only—no pertussis component).

Note: Give a Td booster every 10 years unless a dirty wound has occurred. More on this in the Infectious Disease section.

Note: The areas shaded under 11–12 years in the immunization table (at the end of this section) recognize that hepatitis B, second MMR, and varicella vaccine may not have been either recommended or available when children were initially immunized, so these children need "catching up" at this age.

I'm hoping that you've been over this a million times by now in your residency, practice, or sleep. The ABP will ask you multiple questions about when to give vaccines!

OTHER TIDBITS TO KNOW

All routine childhood immunizations are IM (intramuscular) except for 3 SubQ (subcutaneous): MMR, varicella, and IPV.

Oral polio vaccine, or OPV, is not recommended routinely anywhere in the U.S. However, the Boards still may have an old question about it. Remember, it is a live oral vaccine, so do not give OPV to immunocompromised people or to children who live in a household with an immunocompromised adult (fecal/oral contamination is a concern).

Routinely, give only 2 live vaccines: MMR and varicella (oral typhoid and yellow fever vaccines are also live but rarely given, except for travel). Note: It is acceptable to give the live MMR and in many cases (this changed with the most recent Red Book) varicella vaccine to an HIV-infected person! Note: You can give MMR and varicella vaccine to a child who lives with an immunocompromised person!

For IM injections: use a 20- or 22-gauge 5/8" to 1¼" needle for children; for adults, use a 1½" needle. In infants, use the anterolateral thigh as the injection site; when muscle mass becomes sufficient, you may use the deltoid. Avoid the buttock because of risk of damaging the sciatic nerve and inconsistent intramuscular deposition.

For SubQ injections: use a 25-gauge 5/8"–3/4" needle for all ages.

Anaphylaxis: If a patient has had an anaphylactic reaction to one of the following, perform skin testing to determine safety of the corresponding vaccine:

- Egg antigens: influenza, yellow fever
- Streptomycin, neomycin, polymyxin B: IPV, OPV
- Neomycin: MMR, varicella
- Gelatin: MMR, varicella, yellow fever

Side Effects: Some side effects occur with most vaccine administration, especially local tenderness and low-grade fever.

Other key points (Know!):

- A previous anaphylaxis to the vaccine or one of its components: do not give vaccine
- Previous mild-to-moderate local reaction to a vaccine (soreness, redness, swelling): give vaccine

notes

Quick Quiz

1) Which vaccine should not be given to an infant if he/she is immunocompromised or if someone in the household is immunocompromised?
2) Name 3 subcutaneous vaccines.
3) Which "LIVE" vaccine is it acceptable to give to an asymptomatic HIV-infected child?
4) True of False: It is appropriate to give a vaccine to a child with a cold.
5) True of False: It is appropriate to give a vaccine to a child with a 101 degree fever.
6) True of False: A PPD can be placed on the same day as an MMR vaccine is given.
7) An MMR was given 1 week ago. A 5-year-old presents for TB skin testing due to possible exposure. Is it appropriate to place the PPD today? If not, how long must you wait?
8) True of False: An MMR is considered safe in a child with allergy to eggs.
9) Name the vaccines that should not be given to a pregnant adolescent.
10) True of False: There is good evidence to support the idea that seizures induced by DTaP cause neurologic damage.
11) True or False: If a pregnant woman is inadvertently given MMR vaccine, it is recommended to terminate the pregnancy.

- Concurrent mild, acute illness with or without low-grade fever: give vaccine
- Currently on antibiotics/antivirals: give vaccine
- Recent exposure to an infectious disease: give vaccine
- History of penicillin or other "nonspecific" allergies: give vaccine.
- Family history of seizures: give vaccine
- Family history of previous adverse reaction to vaccine (particularly DTaP): give vaccine
- Active Tuberculosis or PPD-positive: give vaccine
- Simultaneous TB skin testing on day of vaccine: give vaccine (Note: Measles vaccine may suppress tuberculin reactivity. If you don't give the PPD test on the same day as the MMR, wait 4–6 weeks before placing the PPD)

What about the pregnant adolescent?
Hepatitis B and Td are OK! Don't give MMR, varicella, IPV, or OPV.

What about the breastfeeding mother?
All routine vaccines are OK for Mom to receive!

DTaP

DTaP is composed of diphtheria toxoid, tetanus toxoid, and acellular (contains one or more pertussis antigens) pertussis. Note: Do not give children > 7 years of age pertussis-containing products; instead, give Td (which contains only 10% of the concentration of diphtheria toxoid—hence the "little d" as opposed to the Big "D"). Prophylactic use of acetaminophen (15 mg/kg) will diminish side effects.

Specifically for DTaP:

Definitely don't give again if: Hx of encephalopathy within 7 days of dosing.

Probably don't give again if:
- Hx of fever > 40.5 degrees C (105 F) within 48 hours after prior dose.
- Collapse or shock-like state within 48 hours of previous vaccine
- Seizures within 3 days of receiving prior dose
- Persistent, inconsolable crying lasting > 3 hrs within 48 hours

Note: There is no evidence that seizures after DTaP cause neurologic damage or epilepsy.

MMR

MMR is a combination vaccine that contains 3 attenuated live viruses (measles, mumps, and rubella). Single-agent preparations are available but supplies are limited. Measles- and mumps-vaccine strains are grown in chick embryos, while rubella is grown in human diploid cell culture. Of interest is that even though measles and mumps vaccines are grown in chick embryos, the vaccines do not contain significant amounts of cross-reacting egg proteins. So, there is no contraindication to vaccinating someone with severe egg allergy with MMR or its components.

Specifically for MMR:

Definitely don't give if:
- Anaphylactic reaction to neomycin, gelatin
- Pregnancy (but know that no cases of vaccine-associated congential rubella syndrome have been reported to date; and if MMR is inadvertently given to a pregnant women, it is not an indication for termination of pregnancy)
- Immunodeficiency (Exception: non-severely immunocompromised HIV-infected—OK to give to those not severely affected)

Probably should not give MMR if:
- Recent Immunoglobulin (blocks antibody response)— try to give at least 2 weeks before giving immunoglobulin, if possible, or wait at least 3–12 months afterward (dose-dependent)
- History of thrombocytopenia with the first dose of MMR
- History of high dose corticosteroid use for 14 days or more—delay at least 1 month from the termination of corticosteroid therapy

notes

Again Note: MMR is safe in those allergic (even anaphylaxis) to eggs or egg products! Note also that MMR has been proven not to be associated with autism and other neurologic disorders.

IPV and OPV

Because of the risk of paralytic disease in both the recipient and contacts, OPV is no longer recommended for routine use in the United States. This is due mainly to the 8 or 9 cases of vaccine-associated paralysis that occurred in the U.S., with most cases occurring in immunocompetent adults. Since IPV is "inactivated," it does not cause paralytic disease. Of note is that the current "enhanced potency" IPV also does provide some mucosal immunity! The last case of "indigenous" polio appeared in this country in 1979. Since then, over 125 cases of OPV-associated cases of paralysis have occurred—thus, the recommendation to use IPV instead of OPV in the U.S.

Hib

H. influenzae type b vaccines were first marketed in 1985. Since then, the number of cases of invasive *Haemophilus* infections, including meningitis, have plummeted. The current vaccines are Hib capsular polysaccharides, which are conjugated with various carrier proteins. The use of the "conjugate" markedly enhances the efficacy of the vaccine. However, the vaccine is not effective against the "non-type-able" forms of *Haemophilus* that frequently cause otitis media and upper respiratory infections. For this vaccine, there are no major contraindications.

Note also: Do not immunize immunocompetent children > 5 years of age because they are at much lower risk for serious sequelae; and also, they likely have had natural infection by this age. vaccinate children < 24 months of age who have had invasive *H. influenzae* disease because they may fail to develop immunity following natural infection.

Finally, vaccinate those children with functional/anatomical asplenia (patients with sickle cell or AIDS), regardless of age (even > 5 years).

HEPATITIS B VACCINE

Current Hep B vaccines are "recombinant," meaning they use synthetic HBsAg produced in yeast by plasmid gene insertion. The vaccines are now universally recommended for all infants in the U.S., and have been since the early 1990s. Controversy erupted recently with the discovery that this and several other vaccines contained minute amounts of mercury. This led the AAP and ACIP to recommend that mercury-free vaccines be used in newborns. However, until recently, thimerosal-free hepatitis B vaccine was not available to infants before 6 weeks of age.

For purposes of the Boards, the AAP recommends delaying the first hepatitis B vaccine (previously given at birth) until 6 weeks of age in healthy term infants born to HBsAg-negative mothers—but this is only if the question tells you the vaccine contains mercury! If it is mercury-free, give it at birth.

Note: If the mother is HBsAg+ or her status is unknown, give the vaccine at birth, or within 12 hours! If mom is HBsAg+, also give HBIG (hepatitis B immune globulin) within 12 hours of delivery at a different injection site. If the mother's status is initially "unknown" and turns out to be positive on testing, give HBIG within 1 week of birth—but preferably as soon as testing is confirmed positive!

Don't forget to immunize older children and adolescents born after universal early-life immunization began! Be sure you discern if children > 10 years of age were immunized as babies!

VARICELLA VACCINE

Varicella vaccine was first marketed in the U.S. in 1995. Before its availability, over 10,000 hospitalizations and 100 deaths occurred yearly from chicken pox. Varicella vaccine is made from a live, attenuated virus and contains miniscule amounts of neomycin and gelatin.

For kids < 12 years of age, a single dose is sufficient. For older children and adults, 2 doses are required, administered 1–2 months apart. Usually, give the vaccine between 12 and 18 months of age. You can give it with the MMR on the same day, but if they are not administered simultaneously, give 1 month or more apart. Immunity evaluated to date appears to be long-lasting (> 20 years).

Note: 3–5% of children receiving the vaccine will develop a varicella-like rash about 1 month after immunization. If a vaccine-related rash develops, ensure the child avoids contact with immunocompromised individuals until the rash resolves.

Remember: This is a live-virus vaccine, so do not give to immunocompromised children (except now you may vaccinate children with HIV, hypogammaglobulinemia, and dysgammaglobulinemia)! Also, it is OK to give this vaccine to a child who lives with an immunocompromised adult or other child!

You also can safely immunize children with asthma and other conditions when they are on inhaled or oral steroids in doses < 2 mg/kg/day (or < 20 mg/day for those children over 10 kg)!

Do not give the vaccine to pregnant women! But children of pregnant women can receive the vaccine safely.

PNEUMOCOCCAL CONJUGATE VACCINE

Until February 2000, only a 23-valent polysaccharide pneumococcal vaccine (23PS) was available in the United States for prevention of invasive pneumococcal disease. It was mainly given to children with functional/anatomical asplenia, immunodeficiencies, and chronic diseases. In February 2000, a new 7-valent pneumococcal conjugate vaccine (PCV7) was marketed for use for all children < 24 months of age. This vaccine also contains aluminum in small quantities. These 7

notes

Quick Quiz

1) Is it safe to give MMR to a child with egg allergy?
2) Which 2 vaccines are recommended for patients with sickle cell disease to prevent disease with encapsulated organisms?
3) If a mother is known to be hepatitis B surface antigen positive, what should the infant receive soon after delivery?
4) What are the contraindications to receiving varicella vaccine?
5) Why was rotavirus vaccine pulled from the market?

serotypes are responsible for 80% of the invasive pneumococcal disease in the U.S. The vaccine has been shown to markedly reduce severe invasive pneumococcal disease. It is also associated with a modest but important decrease in acute otitis media, pneumonia, and nasopharyngeal carriage of vaccine serotypes.

Currently, it is recommended at 2, 4, 6 and 12–15 months of age. For children 24–59 months of age, the vaccine is also recommended for those who are at high risk (sickle cell disease, asplenia, HIV, chronic cardiac/pulmonary disease, diabetes etc.) and for those at "moderate" risk—those children age 24–59 months who are in day care and children of Native American/Alaska Native/African American descent. For those children in the "high risk" groups, give the old 23-valent vaccine after they have finished the 7-valent dosing!

MENINGOCOCCAL VACCINE

In January 2005, a tetravalent meningococcal polysaccharide-protein conjugate vaccine, MCV4 (Menactra™) was licensed for use among persons aged between 11 and 55 years of age. The ACIP recommends vaccination before high school entry as an effective strategy to reduce meningococcal disease incidence. By 2008, the goal will be routine vaccination of all adolescents beginning at age 11 years. Routine vaccination is also recommended currently for all college freshmen living in dormitories and for other populations at increased risk (e.g. military recruits, asplenic, terminal complement deficiency, etc.)

As of October 2005, the Food and Drug Administration (FDA) and Centers for Disease Control and Prevention (CDC) have posted an alert about a possible connection between the quadrivalent meningococcal conjugate vaccine and Guillain-Barré syndrome (GBS). Five teens in 4 states developed GBS symptoms 2–4 weeks after receiving Menactra™. Although the rate is similar to that expected without vaccination, the timing is of concern and requires further investigation, according to the FDA. At the time of publication the vaccine remains recommended by the ACIP.

ROTAVIRUS VACCINE

This vaccine became available in the late 1990s. However, with widespread use, increasing numbers of children developed intussusception, leading to the removal of the vaccine from the market. Newer vaccines for rotavirus are currently in development.

notes

FIGURE. Recommended childhood and adolescent immunization schedule,[1] by vaccine and age — United States, 2005

<table>
<tr><th>Vaccine</th><th>Birth</th><th>1 mo</th><th>2 mos</th><th>4 mos</th><th>6 mos</th><th>12 mos</th><th>15 mos</th><th>18 mos</th><th>24 mos</th><th>4–6 yrs</th><th>11–12 yrs</th><th>13–18 yrs</th></tr>
<tr><td rowspan="2">Hepatitis B[2]</td><td>HepB #1</td><td colspan="2">only if mother HBsAg (-)</td><td></td><td colspan="4" rowspan="2">HepB #3</td><td colspan="4" rowspan="2">HepB series</td></tr>
<tr><td></td><td colspan="3">HepB #2</td></tr>
<tr><td>Diphtheria, tetanus, pertussis[3]</td><td></td><td></td><td>DTaP</td><td>DTaP</td><td>DTaP</td><td></td><td colspan="2">DTaP</td><td></td><td>DTaP</td><td>Td</td><td>Td</td></tr>
<tr><td>Haemophilus influenzae type b[4]</td><td></td><td></td><td>Hib</td><td>Hib</td><td>Hib[4]</td><td colspan="2">Hib</td><td></td><td></td><td></td><td></td><td></td></tr>
<tr><td>Inactivated poliovirus</td><td></td><td></td><td>IPV</td><td>IPV</td><td colspan="4">IPV</td><td></td><td>IPV</td><td></td><td></td></tr>
<tr><td>Measles, mumps, rubella[5]</td><td></td><td></td><td></td><td></td><td></td><td colspan="2">MMR #1</td><td></td><td></td><td>MMR #2</td><td colspan="2">MMR #2</td></tr>
<tr><td>Varicella[6]</td><td></td><td></td><td></td><td></td><td></td><td colspan="3">Varicella</td><td colspan="4">Varicella</td></tr>
<tr><td>Pneumococcal[7]</td><td></td><td></td><td>PCV</td><td>PCV</td><td>PCV</td><td colspan="2">PCV</td><td></td><td>PCV</td><td colspan="3">PPV</td></tr>
<tr><td>Influenza[8]</td><td></td><td></td><td></td><td></td><td colspan="4">Influenza (yearly)</td><td colspan="4">Influenza (yearly)</td></tr>
<tr><td colspan="13">Vaccines below red line are for selected populations</td></tr>
<tr><td>Hepatitis A[9]</td><td></td><td></td><td></td><td></td><td></td><td></td><td></td><td></td><td colspan="4">Hepatitis A series</td></tr>
</table>

Range of recommended ages | Catch-up immunization | Preadolescent assessment

1. This schedule indicates the recommended ages for routine administration of currently licensed childhood vaccines, as of December 1, 2004, for children aged ≤18 years. Any dose not administered at the recommended age should be administered at any subsequent visit when indicated and feasible. [green box] Indicates age groups that warrant special effort to administer those vaccines not previously administered. Additional vaccines might be licensed and recommended during the year. Licensed combination vaccines may be used whenever any components of the combination are indicated and other components of the vaccine are not contraindicated. Providers should consult package inserts for detailed recommendations. Clinically significant adverse events that follow immunization should be reported to the Vaccine Adverse Event Reporting System; guidance is available at http://www.vaers.org or by telephone, 800-822-7967.

2. Hepatitis B (HepB) vaccine. All infants should receive the first dose of HepB vaccine soon after birth and before hospital discharge; the first dose may also be administered by age 2 months if the mother is hepatitis B surface antigen (HBsAg) negative. Only monovalent HepB may be used for the birth dose. Monovalent or combination vaccine containing HepB may be used to complete the series. Four doses of vaccine may be administered when a birth dose is administered. The second dose should be administered at least 4 weeks after the first dose, except for combination vaccines, which cannot be administered before age 6 weeks. The third dose should be administered at least 16 weeks after the first dose and at least 8 weeks after the second dose. The final dose in the vaccination series (third or fourth dose) should not be administered before age 24 weeks. ***Infants born to HBsAg-positive mothers*** should receive HepB and 0.5 mL of hepatitis B immune globulin (HBIG) at separate sites within 12 hours of birth. The second dose is recommended at age 1–2 months. The final dose in the immunization series should not be administered before age 24 weeks. These infants should be tested for HBsAg and antibody to HBsAg at age 9–15 months. ***Infants born to mothers whose HBsAg status is unknown*** should receive the first dose of the HepB series within 12 hours of birth. Maternal blood should be drawn as soon as possible to determine the mother's HBsAg status; if the HBsAg test is positive, the infant should receive HBIG as soon as possible (no later than age 1 week). The second dose is recommended at age 1–2 months. The last dose in the immunization series should not be administered before age 24 weeks.

3. Diphtheria and tetanus toxoids and acellular pertussis (DTaP) vaccine. The fourth dose of DTaP may be administered as early as age 12 months, provided 6 months have elapsed since the third dose and the child is unlikely to return at age 15–18 months. The final dose in the series should be administered at age ≥4 years. **Tetanus and diphtheria toxoids (Td)** is recommended at age 11–12 years if at least 5 years have elapsed since the last dose of tetanus and diphtheria toxoid-containing vaccine. Subsequent routine Td boosters are recommended every 10 years.

4. *Haemophilus influenzae* type b (Hib) conjugate vaccine. Three Hib conjugate vaccines are licensed for infant use. If PRP-OMP (PedvaxHIB® or ComVax® [Merck]) is administered at ages 2 and 4 months, a dose at age 6 months is not required. DTaP/Hib combination products should not be used for primary immunization in infants at ages 2, 4, or 6 months but can be used as boosters after any Hib vaccine. The final dose in the series should be administered at age ≥12 months.

5. Measles, mumps, and rubella (MMR) vaccine. The second dose of MMR is recommended routinely at age 4–6 years but may be administered during any visit, provided at least 4 weeks have elapsed since the first dose and both doses are administered beginning at or after age 12 months. Those who have not previously received the second dose should complete the schedule by age 11–12 years.

6. Varicella vaccine. Varicella vaccine is recommended at any visit at or after age 12 months for susceptible children (i.e., those who lack a reliable history of chickenpox). Susceptible persons aged ≥13 years should receive 2 doses administered at least 4 weeks apart.

7. Pneumococcal vaccine. The heptavalent **pneumococcal conjugate vaccine (PCV)** is recommended for all children aged 2–23 months and for certain children aged 24–59 months. The final dose in the series should be administered at age ≥12 months. **Pneumococcal polysaccharide vaccine (PPV)** is recommended in addition to PCV for certain groups at high risk. See *MMWR* 2000;49(No. RR-9).

8. Influenza vaccine. Influenza vaccine is recommended annually for children aged ≥6 months with certain risk factors (including, but not limited to, asthma, cardiac disease, sickle cell disease, human immunodeficiency virus [HIV], and diabetes), health-care workers, and other persons (including household members) in close contact with persons in groups at high risk (see *MMWR* 2004;53[No. RR-6]). In addition, healthy children aged 6–23 months and close contacts of healthy children aged 0–23 months are recommended to receive influenza vaccine because children in this age group are at substantially increased risk for influenza-related hospitalizations. For healthy persons aged 5–49 years, the intranasally administered, live, attenuated influenza vaccine (LAIV) is an acceptable alternative to the intramuscular trivalent inactivated influenza vaccine (TIV). See *MMWR* 2004;53(No. RR-6). Children receiving TIV should be administered a dosage appropriate for their age (0.25 mL if aged 6–35 months or 0.5 mL if aged ≥3 years). Children aged ≤8 years who are receiving influenza vaccine for the first time should receive 2 doses (separated by at least 4 weeks for TIV and at least 6 weeks for LAIV).

9. Hepatitis A vaccine. Hepatitis A vaccine is recommended for children and adolescents in selected states and regions and for certain groups at high risk; consult your local public health authority. Children and adolescents in these states, regions, and groups who have not been immunized against hepatitis A can begin the hepatitis A immunization series during any visit. The 2 doses in the series should be administered at least 6 months apart. See *MMWR* 1999;48(No. RR-12).

Approved by the **Advisory Committee on Immunization Practices** (http://www.cdc.gov/nip/acip), the **American Academy of Pediatrics** (http://www.aap.org), and the **American Academy of Family Physicians** (http://www.aafp.org). Additional information about vaccines, including precautions and contraindications for vaccination and vaccine shortages, is available at http://www.cdc.gov/nip or from the National Immunization Information Hotline, 800-232-2522 (English) or 800-232-0233 (Spanish).

TABLE. Catch-up immunization schedule for children and adolescents who start late or who are >1 month behind, by age group, vaccine, and dosage interval — United States, 2005

Catch-up schedule for children aged 4 months–6 years

Vaccine	Minimum age for dose 1	Minimum interval between doses			
		Dose 1 to dose 2	Dose 2 to dose 3	Dose 3 to dose 4	Dose 4 to dose 5
DTaP[1]	6 wks	4 wks	4 wks	6 mos	6 mos[1]
IPV[2]	6 wks	4 wks	4 wks	4 wks[2]	
HepB[3]	Birth	4 wks	8 wks (and 16 wks after first dose)		
MMR[4]	12 mos	4 wks[4]			
Varicella	12 mos				
Hib[5]	6 wks	4 wks: if first dose administered at age <12 mos 8 wks (as final dose): if first dose administered at age 12–14 mos No further doses needed if first dose administered at age ≥15 mos	4 wks[6]: if current age <12 mos 8 wks (as final dose)[6]: if current age ≥12 mos and second dose administered at age <15 mos No further doses needed if previous dose administered at age ≥15 mos	8 wks (as final dose): This dose only necessary for children aged 12 mos–5 yrs who received 3 doses before age 12 mos	
PCV[7]	6 wks	4 wks: if first dose administered at age <12 mos and current age <24 mos 8 wks (as final dose): if first dose administered at age ≥12 mos or current age 24–59 mos No further doses needed for healthy children if first dose administered at age ≥24 mos	4 wks: if current age <12 mos 8 wks (as final dose): if current age ≥12 mos No further doses needed for healthy children if previous dose administered at age ≥24 mos	8 wks (as final dose): This dose only necessary for children aged 12 mos–5 yrs who received 3 doses before age 12 mos	

Catch-up schedule for children aged 7–18 years

Vaccine	Minimum interval between doses		
	Dose 1 to dose 2	Dose 2 to dose 3	Dose 3 to booster dose
Td[8]	4 wks	6 mos	6 mos[8]: if first dose administered at age <12 mos and current age <11 yrs 5 yrs[8]: if first dose administered at age ≥12 mos and third dose administered at age <7 yrs and current age ≥11 yrs 10 yrs[8]: if third dose administered at age ≥7 yrs
IPV[9]	4 wks	4 wks	IPV[2,9]
HepB	4 wks	8 wks (and 16 wks after first dose)	
MMR	4 wks[4]		
Varicella[10]	4 wks		

Note: A vaccine series does not require restarting, regardless of the time that has elapsed between doses.

1. Diphtheria and tetanus toxoids and acellular pertussis (DTaP) vaccine. The fifth dose is not necessary if the fourth dose was administered after the fourth birthday.

2. Inactivated poliovirus (IPV) vaccine. For children who received an all-IPV or all-oral poliovirus (OPV) series, a fourth dose is not necessary if the third dose was administered at age ≥4 years. If both OPV and IPV were administered as part of a series, a total of 4 doses should be administered, regardless of the child's current age.

3. Hepatitis B (HepB) vaccine. All children and adolescents who have not been immunized against hepatitis B should begin the HepB immunization series during any visit. Providers should make special efforts to immunize children who were born in, or whose parents were born in, areas of the world where hepatitis B virus infection is moderately or highly endemic.

4. Measles, mumps, and rubella (MMR) vaccine. The second dose of MMR is recommended routinely at age 4–6 years but may be administered earlier if desired.

5. *Haemophilus influenzae* type b (Hib) vaccine. Vaccine is not generally recommended for children aged ≥5 years.

6. Hib vaccine. If current age is <12 months and the first 2 doses were PRP-OMP (PedvaxHIB® or ComVax® [Merck]), the third (and final) dose should be administered at age 12–15 months and at least 8 weeks after the second dose.

7. Pneumococcal conjugate (PCV) vaccine. Vaccine is not generally recommended for children aged ≥5 years.

8. Tetanus and diphtheria toxoids (Td). For children aged 7–10 years, the interval between the third and booster dose is determined by the age when the first dose was administered. For adolescents aged 11–18 years, the interval is determined by the age when the third dose was administered.

9. IPV. Vaccine is not generally recommended for persons aged ≥18 years.

10. Varicella vaccine. Administer the 2-dose series to all susceptible adolescents aged ≥13 years.

MedStudy

2nd Edition
Pediatrics Board Review
Core Curriculum

Childhood Development and Common Pediatric Disorders

Authored by J. Thomas Cross, Jr., MD, MPH, FAAP

Many thanks to

Keith Boyd, MD
Associate Chair of Education
Department of Pediatrics
Rush University Medical Center
Chicago, IL

and

Thomas Krzmarzick, MD
Medical Director, Emergency Department
The Children's Medical Center
Dayton, OH

Childhood Development and
Common Pediatric Disorders

Table of Contents

Childhood Development and Common Pediatric Disorders

COMMON CONCERNS OF PARENTS

COLIC

Colic is a syndrome of findings believed to be a specific condition, but this condition has yet to be fully understood. Clues to colic are:

- Crying in the later afternoon/evening that peaks in the 2nd month and wanes in the 3rd–4th month
- Physical findings—legs over abdomen, clenched fists, pained facies, gas, spitting up, and lack of response to soothing
- Crying bouts that are prolonged and paroxysmal—begin and end without warning and are unrelated to the environment

A simple way to diagnose colic is through Wessel's rules of 3's: Crying > 3 hours/day for > 3 days a week for > 3 weeks. It is estimated that colic occurs in 30–50% of infants.

The difficulty is determining if the crying is due to colic or an organic cause. For infants < 1 month, you must rule out other causes of irritability. If the child is > 4 months, it is not colic. Other criteria that point more toward organic causes are:

- A high-pitched cry that is not diurnal
- On physical exam and history, there are findings besides crying
- Later onset (starts in the 3rd month) and follows switching from breast to formula feeds—indicating that cow's milk protein intolerance is likely

Treatment for colic is difficult. Most resolve by age 3 months, but about 1/3 will persist to 4 months, and then resolve. If it does not resolve after 4 months, search for organic causes. Provide parents with information about the typical pattern and the characteristic lack of response to soothing. Reassure them of both the typical excellent outcome, and the fact that colic is not due to being "bad parents." Environmental factors, such as music or car rides, help some infants. Caution parents against the idea of using washer/dryer vibrations to alleviate colic symptoms because of the risk that the child could fall off the appliance (or inadvertently be left in the dryer—Just a joke to see if you are still awake). It is essential that caretakers have someone to relieve them of dealing with the colicky infant on a periodic basis.

SLEEPING PROBLEMS

Normal Sleep Development

By age 3 months, 50–70% of children will sleep from midnight to 5 a.m. without parental intervention. This percentage increases to 80% by age 5–7 months, and to 85–90% by 1 year. Between ages 6 and 12 months, about 1/2 of those who have been sleeping during the night will have periods of wakefulness and crying—thought to be related to "separation anxiety" (a new cognition) and object permanence. Persistent, disruptive sleeping occurs when children are not allowed or able to handle the normal arousals (end of sleep cycle, REM sleep, and non-REM sleep).

Sleep Associations

Sleep associations are behaviors/expectations the child develops based on relationships created in his world, most often by parents. A common sleep association is when a parent holds, rocks, or sings to the child at bedtime. The child associates falling asleep with this behavior. When the behavior does not occur, the child has difficulty falling asleep. It is particularly a problem if the child wakes up during the night—she cannot soothe herself to sleep, because she is accustomed to the stimulation/reinforcement provided by her parents.

Feeding during the night after 6 months of age is another learned association. It is not physiologically dictated, but infants learn it through reinforced behavior.

Other sleep associations—more correctly, child-waking associations—occur when parents take the infant from the crib, watch television, play with the child, or do other activities in the child's room as a response to the child waking during the night.

Psychosocial factors can aggravate poor sleep patterns. Family stressors, such as changes in jobs, moves, marital discord, etc., can manifest as sleep disturbances—likely due to the parents' preoccupation with the life stressors instead of carrying through the usual child-management strategies.

Co-sleeping (sleeping in a parental bed) occurs with 35–55% of children < age 4 years. Cultural and ethnic differences are common; the prevalence is much higher in Latino and African-American families.

Nightmares

Nightmares are disturbing dreams that occur during REM sleep. They are usually followed by awakening and distress about the dream. Peak age of onset is between years 3 and 5, and nightmares are common. Parental reassurance is the best response. Recurrent nightmares with frequent night waking usually indicate significant distress in a child's daytime life. (Note: Nightmares concurrent with studying for the boards are also common, especially those "showing up for the test naked" dreams).

Night Terrors

Night terrors differ from nightmares. Night terrors produce a distinct non-REM parasomnia—an abrupt arousal from stage 4 non-REM sleep to near arousal. Most occur during the first third of the night. The child appears to be awake but is unresponsive. Later, the child doesn't remember the episode (Hmm...reminds me of sitting in anatomy class). Night terrors are more common in males and occur in ~ 1–6% of children. Again, parental reassurance is the best therapy. These can persist into adolescence. Frequently, you will find a family history of night terrors in your evaluation.

notes

Sleepwalking (Somnambulism)

Sleepwalking is another phenomenon where the child appears to be awake but isn't. It also occurs during stage 4 non-REM sleep. It tends to occur in children between ages 4 and 8 years, with a prevalence of about 15%.

Sleeptalking (Somniloquy)

Sleeptalking can occur during any stage of sleep, from partial arousal to REM sleep. It is common and can persist throughout adulthood.

Treatment and Management of Sleep Problems

As parents and practitioners, we vary on treatment approaches, but what you need to know is what the books say to do, because that is what the ABP expects you to know and do (even though your "real world" may be different).

First, a regular daily routine is very important. Infants should be in a crib that is not located in the parents' room. A baby should be put down when he/she is drowsy, and not yet asleep. Middle-of-the-night feedings should stop by age 4–6 months.

Older children (toddler to preschoolers) should have a regular pre-sleep routine—bathing, changing clothes, brushing teeth, reading books, etc. Night-lights are helpful for those afraid of the dark. Meet attempts by the child at bedtime to "get this" or "do that" with a gentle but firm "No, it is bedtime." Younger, school-aged kids generally enjoy this time to get special attention from the parent—to hear a story, read together, or to talk about the activities for the next day. Adolescents generally want to be left alone, and arrange their own bedtime activities.

Parents can best handle night waking in older infants by ignoring it. It often resolves after a week, with the infant falling back to sleep without intervention. Occasional, verbal reassurance can be useful, but encourage parents to not pick up and hold the infant, unless there are unusual circumstances.

Children with nightmares need to be reassured that the dream is over, and that they are safe in their bed. Also, talking about the dream the next day may be helpful. Frequent nightmares may be a reaction to a serious stressor occurring in the household; you should take care to consider if this is the case, and what you can do to lessen the stressor.

Parents should just observe night terrors without awakening the child. In fact, awakening a child with a night terror will prolong the attack. Some have noted that recurrent night terrors occur at about the same time of the night, and a "preemptive awakening" before the usual time of the night terror can actually break the cycle and prevent further terrors from occurring.

For sleepwalkers, encourage parents to ensure the environment is safe, to observe the child, and to gently lead him/her back to bed. The same process of "preemptive awakening" prior to the usual sleepwalking event can be successful in stopping the behavior.

Sleeptalkers require no specific intervention (although my wife seems to prefer a strong kick to my back.)

LANGUAGE DEVELOPMENT

Language development is obviously very important—and the ABP thinks so too—so plan to memorize and/or understand when appropriate language ability is supposed to occur. Definitely plan on a few questions about this on the Board exam.

Table 2-1 lists the "Expressive" Language development.

On the exam, the ABP will ask you what is "normal" and what is "abnormal." It is a pain to remember these. If you are a recent new parent, you may be able to remember these developmental things first-hand. If not, up to the time you take your exam, pay special attention to the developmental history when you see children. Get it straight in your mind what is normal for a 2-year-old, a 3-year-old, etc. It will help you tremendously on the ABP exam! Table 2-2 lists observations to be concerned about for Speech and Language Development as these relate to specific age groups.

From the table, know that a **2**-year-old should be using **2**-syllable words, and that a 4-year-old should be able to tell a simple story. These standards are easy for you to use in practice too.

"Late talking" generally defines any set of circumstances in which the verbal abilities of a child are noticeably behind the

Table 2-1

EXPRESSIVE LANGUAGE DEVELOPMENT	
6 months	Babbles, different cries noted
12 months	Points, shakes head "Mama" or "Dada"
18 months	Uses gestures well Has about a 15-20 word vocabulary Uses 2-3 word phrases Speaks in a way that immediate household family members can understand
24 months	Expanding vocabulary More fluency--less stuttering About 25% of words are intelligible to strangers
3 years	Can use complete sentences Talks in short paragraphs Most words are intelligible to strangers Uses plurals, pronouns, prepositions
4 years	Can use past tense 4-5 word sentences Short paragraphs Able to tell a story or explain a recent event

notes

Quick Quiz

1) For colic, what is the upper age limit of "normal?"
2) Do nightmares occur during REM or non-REM sleep? What about night terrors?
3) Know Table 2-1!
4) Would you be concerned if a 2-year-old pointed at a ball without also saying the word "ball" in order to receive the ball? Why or why not?
5) True or False: You should be concerned if a 5-year-old cannot pronounce the letter "d" correctly in words.
6) What is the most common cause of conductive hearing loss in children?
7) What is the most likely etiology for severe or profound hearing loss?

norm. What are its probable causes? A common cause is hearing impairment—which dictates a formal assessment by an audiologist. This is not something to be done in a pediatrician's office, where the conditions are less than ideal. Another common cause is developmental delay, which could be due to a variety of etiologies. Other causes of "late talking" include mental retardation, specific language disorders, autism, dysarthria, dyspraxia, maturation delay, and neglect.

Table 2-2

CLUES TO ABNORMAL SPEECH AND LANGUAGE DEVELOPMENT BY AGE	
12-15 months	Child is not babbling or using different sounds
18-24 months	Child only uses a few words, hardly any phrases
2 years	Child cannot follow simple directions Child points instead of speaking Child is not using 2-syllable words or combining words
2½ years	Child cannot be understood most of the time Child frequently omits first or last consonant of a word Child cannot understand 2-step directions Child cannot pronounce: b, h, m, n, p, w
3 years	Child cannot repeat a 4- or 5-word sentence
3½ years	Child cannot name specific objects easily Child omits words in sentences Child cannot pronounce d, f, g, k, t
4 years	Child cannot tell a simple story
5 years	Child cannot pronounce l, j, v, ch, sh
6 years	Child cannot pronounce r, s, z, st, th

HEARING PROBLEMS

Deafness is defined as hearing loss > 90 dB. This results in the inability to distinguish between elements of spoken language. "Mild" hearing loss = 25 dB loss, but even a 15 dB loss can result in problems with speech perception, especially during early childhood.

Conductive hearing loss (more common) is due to disruption of mechanical components required for the transduction of sound wave energy. The most common cause of conductive hearing loss is fluid in the middle ear. Children with this type of loss can hear speech, but fluid-caused distortions can lead to problems in early language discrimination. About 2/3 children have some degree of intermittent conductive hearing loss. This hearing loss is limited to sounds at 50 dB or lower, because sounds louder than this can be conducted directly by bone to the cochlea.

Sensorineural hearing loss (less common) is a problem due to dysfunction of the sensory epithelium, the cochlea, or the neural pathways to the auditory cortex, using the 8th cranial nerve and other connections. Severe or profound hearing loss is always sensorineural, and most often affects high frequencies. Severe and profound hearing loss affects about 1–2/1000 children at birth; an additional 2–3/1000 experience an acquired, severe hearing loss in childhood.

Cortical hearing problems can also occur. These result in the inability, or impaired ability, to perceive or process sounds.

Deafness can be due to either an isolated event or a syndrome. It is inherited in ~ 50% of cases. 80% are inherited as autosomal recessive, 18% autosomal dominant, and 2% are X-linked recessive. Infectious etiologies are the other significant factor in deafness. Today, CMV and toxoplasmosis account for the majority of infectious causes, in contrast to decades ago, when rubella was one of the most common causes (Rubella as a cause is now rare because of an effective preventive vaccine). Bacterial meningitis is still a common cause of deafness, and occurs in about 10% of those affected. Immunizations (both *Haemophilus* and pneumococcus) have reduced this in recent years. Prolonged exposure to loud noise is a common cause of high-pitched hearing loss in adolescents.

Table 2-3 lists factors identified by the Joint Committee on Infant Hearing as risk factors for neonatal hearing loss.

~ 50% of infants with sensorineural hearing loss will have one of the risk factors listed in Table 2-3. But since this also leaves 50% of infants not exhibiting these risk factors, many states have initiated universal screening for infants.

Screening is done with either Evoked Otoacoustic Emissions (EOAE), most commonly done first, or automated Auditory Brainstem Response (ABR) systems if the baby fails EOAE testing.

Other children who should be screened are those with a persistent, middle-ear effusion that has lasted > 2 months.

notes

Table 2-3
FACTORS ASSOCIATED WITH HEARING LOSS IN NEONATES
Family history of sensorineural hearing loss
Congenital infection
Presence of craniofacial anomalies
Birth weight under 1500 grams
Neonatal jaundice resulting in exchange transfusion
Ototoxic medications (furosemide, aminoglycosides)
Bacterial meningitis
Apgar Scores of 3 or less at 5 minutes
Physical findings consistent with a syndrome associated with hearing loss

Key to success in treating hearing loss is early diagnosis and intervention.

VISION PROBLEMS

Overview

The most prevalent vision disorders are: amblyopia, strabismus, significant refractive error, color-vision defects, and ocular disease. In the U.S., the leading causes of blindness in children are cortical visual impairment, retinopathy of prematurity, and optic nerve hypoplasia. The leading cause of "acquired" blindness is ocular trauma. The #1 cause of such trauma is accidental or intentional injury by another child. The next most common cause is sports-related injuries.

Normal Visual Development

In formal terminology, here are some important basics:

1) *Visual fixation* occurs in the newborn and achieves accuracy by 6–9 weeks.
2) *Optokinetic nystagmus* and *vestibular ocular reflex* are involuntary eye movements that provide stability of visual images.
3) *Accommodation* is the ability to focus the intraocular lens for near-viewing, and is present at birth; however, it is inaccurate until age 2–3 months.
4) Most term infants are *hyperopic* (farsighted) at birth, while premature infants are *myopic* (nearsighted).
5) *Color discrimination* occurs by 2 weeks of age, and improves over the next 3 months.
6) *Fine-depth perception* occurs at ~ 3 months and is near adult functionality by 6 months.

Strabismus

Strabismus is the misalignment of the eyes (visual axes), in which one and/or the other eye is turned in (esotropia), out (exotropia), up (hypertrophia), or down (hypotropia). The misalignment can occur continuously or intermittently. The most common forms in childhood are the infantile and accommodative esotropia. Amblyopia commonly occurs with esotropia.

Amblyopia

Amblyopia occurs at a rate of 75,000 new cases each year in 3-year-olds. Amblyopia causes more vision loss than any other disease in individuals < 45 years. Amblyopia is loss of visual acuity that is not due to ocular pathology, and is not correctable with glasses or contact lenses. Amblyopia may result from early childhood refractive disorders, strabismus, cataracts, or corneal opacities. The most common causes of amblyopia are strabismus and anisometropia, an unequal refractive error between the eyes.

Color-Vision Defects

The ability to match colors is present by age 2 years (hmm… some of us never get that, I guess). Abnormal color vision occurs in ~ 8–10% of boys and < 0.5% of girls, and is due to X-linked inheritance protan and deutan deficits (blue-green). Other rare defects that affect color vision include retinal or optic nerve disorders.

Cortical Visual Impairment

Cortical visual impairment is vision loss due to damage to the geniculostriate pathway, which is composed of the visual cortex and optic radiations. It presents as reduced vision, absence of optokinetic nystagmus, and intact pupillary light responses. Its causes are numerous, including hypoxia, meningitis, encephalitis, metabolic disease, head trauma, and hydrocephalus. The most common cause is hypoxia. Usually, these children have other, associated abnormalities, including cerebral palsy, seizures, or paralysis.

Retinopathy of Prematurity (ROP)

Retinopathy of prematurity is a disorder of immature retinal vasculature, and is provoked by excess oxygen use in premature infants. Today, severe ROP occurs mainly in infants < 30 weeks and with birth weights < 1250 grams. More on this is discussed in the Newborn chapter.

Optic Nerve Hypoplasia

Optic nerve hypoplasia is a nonspecific finding due to damage of the visual system before it is fully developed. It is associated with maternal diabetes, alcohol abuse, and maternal exposure to toxins. You might also see optic nerve hypoplasia with hypothyroidism, growth hormone deficiency, and neonatal hypoglycemia.

notes

Quick Quiz

1) Are most term infants near- or far-sighted at birth? What about premature infants?
2) Define strabismus.
3) What is the most common cause of amblyopia?
4) How common are color-vision abnormalities in boys compared to girls?
5) What is the most common reason for retinopathy of prematurity?
6) What is the most common malignant ocular tumor in childhood? How does it usually present?
7) When a new sibling is about to arrive, what should the father do?
8) What are the brain injury risks of breath-holding spells?
9) Does the ABP examination encourage spanking as a form of punishment?

Retinoblastoma

Retinoblastoma is the leading malignant ocular tumor of childhood. It occurs at a rate of 1/20,000. ~ 50% of cases are familial. The tumor comes from the primitive retinal cells, and you will see them most in children < age 4 years. With treatment, survival is > 90%. The most common symptom/sign is a white pupil, known as leukokoria. Strabismus, glaucoma, and poor vision can also occur, but are less common presentations.

BIRTH OF A SIBLING—RESPONSES

Birth of a sibling almost always invokes some feelings of hostility by the older sibling toward the new baby. Some children will exhibit signs of developmental regression, such as thumb sucking or regressive toilet training. Others may become sad or withdrawn, and still others may develop aggressive behaviors at home or at day care. Some note that boys are more likely to be aggressive; girls are more likely to be anxious or depressed.

Some parents ask "when is the best time to have another child?" Experts disagree, but a 2-year interval appears to be optimal in some anecdotal data. Note: There is no definitive data on this question at this point.

It is important to encourage parents to be open with the older child about the pregnancy, and prepare him/her for its impacts. Allow the older child to participate in the planning before the delivery, and to be involved in taking care of the newborn when he/she arrives at home. If changes in bedrooms or beds are necessary because of the birth, carry these out well in advance of the delivery. Be sure to not associate the changes with the arrival of the new baby.

If he is present, encourage the father to increase his attention and involvement with the older child. Studies show that this involvement provides the best intervention to ensure comfort and reassurance for the older child. If no father is present, suggest that another male relative assume the role of providing the older child with extra attention and encouragement.

TEMPER TANTRUMS

Temper tantrums occur in nearly all 2-to-4-year olds. Occurrences may be daily in ~ 20% of 2-year-olds, and 10% of 4-year-olds. These can manifest in many ways. Breath holding is common in infants and children, and usually occurs just prior to a temper tantrum caused by an environmental event. It appears to be autosomal dominant with reduced penetrance! Therefore, family history is frequently positive for a history of breath holding or fainting. Temper tantrums usually begin in the 2nd year, but may appear as early as 7 months! They usually resolve by age 5 years.

There are 2 types of breath-holding temper tantrums: 1) A cyanotic form, in which the face turns blue until breathing returns, and 2) A pale form, in which the face turns pale due to vasovagal syncope. In either case, the child will stop breathing, followed by a period of profound crying. Syncope may occur, especially with the pale form, at the onset of crying. The period of not breathing is brief, and the child will then have spontaneous respiration. With the syncope, tonic-clonic movements can occasionally occur.

Breath-holding spells are benign—there are no long-term effects or brain injury. But they scare the heck out of the parents! Aim treatment at preventing situations that may induce an attack; reassure parents that these spells are not life-threatening or dangerous. (Recently, limited data—disputed by many—show that iron therapy may be effective in reducing the frequency of breath holding in some children—even if they don't have iron deficiency, though the mechanism is unknown).

DISCIPLINE

Effective discipline is a difficult and common subject of query to pediatricians! Discipline is very important for normal development, and central to the emotional stability of a child. Modeling positive behaviors is the most effective means of discipline. Parents do this with positive language and actions. Punishments should be consistent from one family member to another, and from one similar episode of misbehavior to another. Discipline should occur as quickly as possible after the event that triggers it.

For the ABP exam, any type of physical punishment, such as spanking, is unacceptable. However common and acceptable corporal punishment is in certain cultures and among certain ethnic groups, for the Board exam, spanking is an unacceptable punishment! "Time-outs" are a favorite, and many consider loss of privileges (no television, no sleep-overs, etc.) as sending a strong message — so go with these types of options on the Boards!

notes

SEPARATION ANXIETY

Separation anxiety—often exhibited as "clingy" behavior toward the mother—usually becomes noticeable at > age 6 months. It is especially prominent at ~ 9–18 months, and begins to lessen by age 3 years. These children are afraid to leave their mothers, be with strangers, and/or are fearful of new situations. Many children > age 3 years will continue to have uneasiness about unknown or new situations, but most children can handle the feelings internally or verbally without crying or other symptoms.

A majority of children are considered "secure"—they will protest the mother leaving, but be consoled and distracted with toys, etc., in the room, and then seek contact with the mother on her return to the room. ~ 20% of children are termed "avoidant"—they don't notice the mother coming or going and, when she returns, they move away from the mother and continue to play. About 10% are "ambivalent"—these kids suffer great distress when the mother leaves the room, cannot be consoled while the mother is gone, and cannot easily be consoled on the mother's return. The final 10% are considered "disorganized"—they exhibit both the avoidant and ambivalent behaviors.

SCHOOL REFUSAL

School refusal is not to be confused or equated with truancy. In truancy, the child is not at home or at school, and the parent is unaware. With school refusal, the parent is aware because the child is home. School refusal usually occurs in association with somatic complaints—headache, stomachache, etc. School refusal is defined as missing at least 2 weeks of school for 2–3 days/week. You may find anxiety, phobias, and behavior disorders in these children.

School refusal occurs in about 3–5/1000 children overall, with an increased prevalence in high school of 1–2/100.

School refusal is most common in the early teen years and more common in boys than girls. There is no difference between races or socioeconomic statuses.

Encourage parents to set strong expectations that children attend school. Although a parent should never dismiss physical complaints, the focus should be on getting the child to school *in spite of* the physical complaints. Parents can enroll the help of teachers and the school social worker (if available) to facilitate school attendance, while reducing the child's anxiety.

"BAD" HABITS AND UNDESIRABLE BEHAVIORS

Body Rocking

Body rocking occurs at ~ age 6 months in 5–20% of children. The rocking occurs in either the sitting or crawling position, and can be quite vigorous. Some kids have been known to rock their cribs across the room or damage walls/cribs with the banging. It is most common around bedtime and lasts ~ 1/2 hour. Body rocking usually stops by age 2–3 years—It rarely continues into adolescence.

Head Banging

Head banging occurs in 5–15% of "normal" children. The onset of head banging is usually ~ ages 8–9 months and stops by age 4 (unless they join a rock-and-roll band in high school). It occurs much more frequently in males, and most commonly at bedtime or in the middle of the night. The episodes can be very short, or may persist for 3–4 hours!

Multiple studies have been done on these kids, but no EEG or other neurologic abnormalities have been noted. Reassure parents that this is normal behavior and that no permanent damage will occur. Padding areas of favorite banging is useful to minimize bruising or callus formation. Children with mental retardation or autism who head bang may require helmets or medications to lessen the head-banging activity and prevent injury.

Thumb Sucking

Thumb sucking has been described in utero as early as 28 weeks gestation, and can continue until age 5 years or so. Peak thumb sucking age is 18–21 months; most stop by age 4. Thumb sucking occurs in anywhere from 1/10 to 1/3 of children. Thumb sucking that persists into adolescence is more common in girls than boys, and may indicate underlying psychological problems. Prevalence of thumb sucking in breastfed infants is higher than bottle-fed infants, but the duration of thumb sucking is lower in the breastfed group.

Thumb sucking beyond age 4 years merits referral for dental evaluation, because of the significant potential for dental problems. Before the child turns 4, reassure parents that thumb sucking is natural and usually resolves spontaneously. Attempts by parents to stop the behavior may actually reinforce it. Positive feedback when the child is not sucking his/her thumb is helpful. Some recommend hypnotherapy, or adversive therapy, such as applying bitter nail polish to discourage sucking, which has also been successful. Older children may require a dental appliance to prevent any comfortable insertion of the thumb.

Nail Biting (Onychophagia)

Nail biting (fancy name: onychophagia) is a common habit of children and adults. It includes biting of the nail itself, the cuticles, and/or soft tissue, and frequently leads to irritation, bleeding, and infection. Nail biting is most common between ages 10–18 years. About 50% of children have the habit at some time in their childhood. Between ages 5–10 years, boys and girls are equally affected, but after age 10, boys are more commonly affected. About 10–20% of men > 25 persist in biting their nails.

Again, aim treatment at positive reinforcement. Encourage parents to praise children during the periods in which they don't bite their nails.

notes

Quick Quiz

1) At what age does separation anxiety become noticeable? When does it begin to lessen?
2) What behaviors are commonly associated with school refusal?
3) At what age(s) does body rocking occur?
4) At what age(s) does head banging occur?
5) True or False: In most children with head banging, radiologic and neurologic studies are required to evaluate the condition.
6) At what age do most children stop sucking their thumbs?
7) True or False: You should be concerned about an adolescent female who sucks her thumb.
8) Do boys or girls > 10 years of age more commonly bite their fingernails?
9) Differentiate early- from late-onset trichotillomania.
10) True or False: Tics usually are suppressed during sleep.
11) A child with ADHD is placed on stimulant medication. What is a possible side effect of this medication?

Clinching/Grinding of Teeth (Bruxism)

Grinding or clinching of the teeth produces a high-pitched, annoying sound that is typically nocturnal, during REM sleep. Prolonged grinding can cause tenderness in the muscles of the mouth, temporomandibular joint pain, tooth damage, tension headaches, face pain, and neck stiffness. Bruxism is most common in boys and appears to be familial. Teeth and supporting structures can be damaged over time. Recommend the use of a splint or bite guards.

Trichotillomania (Pulling Hair)

Less common than the other habits we have discussed so far, trichotillomania is the inability to resist pulling out one's own hair. The child usually removes hair from the scalp and creates bald spots, but some pull eyelashes, eyebrows, and pubic hair. Some children will chew the hair and then swallow it—called trichophagy—and over time large amounts can result in a hair bezoar—trichobezoar. Most believe this behavior to be within the obsessive-compulsive disorders.

Most affected are girls. There are 2 categories within this disorder:

1) Early onset—which presents < age 5 and then with a long history of hair pulling. These children pull hair when bored or tense.
2) Late onset—presents in later childhood, adolescence, or adulthood. Other pathologies, such as depression, anxiety, bipolar disorders, substance abuse, and personality disorders are commonly associated with the late-onset group.

Alopecia is common and must be differentiated from alopecia areata, tinea capitis, syphilis, and traumatic/traction alopecia.

Treat early-onset trichotillomania with positive-reinforcement techniques, and use time-outs for episodes. The late-onset disorder is difficult to treat, and usually involves dealing with the underlying psychiatric disorder. Note: Iron deficiency anemia has been associated with trichotillomania and trichophagia, so consider screening for iron deficiency.

Tics

Tics are involuntary, purposeless movements, gestures, or utterances. The areas most commonly affected are the muscle groups of the eyes, mouth, face, and neck. Variants of these disorders include copropraxia—obscene gestures, self-injury, and vocal tics—which can range from simple throat-clearing to vocalizing obscene words (coprolalia). Tics usually are suppressed during sleep, and become more prominent during times of stress.

About 1/10 adults and children experience a tic that persists for at least a month. Tics most commonly affect school-aged males.

Tourette Syndrome

Tourette syndrome is the most severe of the tic disorders. It usually starts in early childhood with simple motor tics, such as eye blinking or twitching of the face. From there, the character of the tic can vary—from touching, squatting, and twirling to development of *vocal* tics after a year or two. The vocal tics begin as simple sounds, but frequently progress to barks, sniffs, echolalia, or coprolalia. There is an association between this syndrome and obsessive thoughts and compulsions. ADHD and OCD also commonly display vocal tics. One thing to look out for is a child on stimulant medication for ADHD. It may unmask the tic disorder; thus, stop the medication. However, a recent trial showed that stimulant medications may not be a major concern.

Age of onset on average is ~ 7 years, with males predominating. Those in late adolescence and early adulthood usually see a period of less frequency and intensity of the tics. Tourette syndrome is familial and suggests an autosomal dominant inheritance pattern.

Historically, the best treatment of the tics themselves is haloperidol—which relieves symptoms in ~ 80% of patients, but unfortunately has serious side effects. Today many use fluphenazine, pimozide, and tetrabenazine instead as first-line therapy. You can also use clonidine in those who cannot tolerate the side effects of haloperidol. Many times, treating an underlying obsessive compulsive or other disorder will result in resolution or improvement of the tics.

Transient Tic Disorder

Transient tic disorder occurs in children under age 18 and is defined as lasting at least 4 weeks for less than 12 consecutive months. Tics typically will show up many times a day, on an everyday basis. Most commonly, eye blinking or facial tics occur; sometimes, vocal-transient tics also occur. Boys are more commonly affected between ages 3–10. Treatment is generally parental assurance, but diagnosis is really one of

notes

exclusion. Obviously, the end point of this disorder is its transient nature, so you have to wait it out to see if it goes away to make the diagnosis.

SEXUAL DEVELOPMENT AND PARENTAL CONCERNS

OVERVIEW

Note: for all of the following touchy issues to be discussed, we're going with the presumed standard of care, as published by the AAP, major textbooks of Pediatrics, and/or "expert" opinion. For the ABP Board exam, know that these are what you will likely be asked about; in other words, follow the standard guidelines of management and treatment as outlined here. I realize that everyone has his/her own opinion about these difficult issues. However, put your opinions aside for the exam, and answer the way the ABP wants you to. After all, passing the exam is your goal. There are very different views regarding these subjects, based on religion, ethnicity, and culture, but the key is to always remember to put the child first. Keep your primary concerns for them, and you'll get these types of Board questions right☺!

MASTURBATION

Masturbation, or self-stimulation of the genitals, is universal from infancy to adulthood. It peaks at age 4 years and again at adolescence. Vulvovaginitis, tight clothing, or urethral irritation can trigger masturbation. Counsel children to keep this behavior private. In families with religious prohibition, encourage parents to provide simple teaching and redirecting behavior. Avoid negative reactions or punishments. Masturbation with auxiliary objects is very unusual in childhood, and should raise concerns about sexual abuse.

Masturbation does not cause any physical or mental difficulties, and is common behavior. Parents with conservative beliefs, religious or otherwise, may be upset to find a child masturbating. Encourage parents to avoid use of phrases such as "it will make you go blind" or other invalid threats.

SEXUAL EXPLORATION

Overview

Sexual exploration is common in the first 3 years of life. This includes the handling of one's own or a playmate's genitals. Typically, children may participate in "nude parading," showing one's genitals, or observing others as they toilet or bathe. Between ages 3–6, exhibitionism is common, but becomes noticeably uncommon after this.

Clues to abnormalities include: imitation of sexual intercourse, asking to have sexual intercourse, doll play that includes oral, anal, or vaginal penetration, or putting one's mouth on another's genitals. These behaviors are red flags, and should alert you to either sexual abuse or the possibility that the child has witnessed numerous sexual acts. Usually, children do not adopt these behaviors from television or movies alone; but, rather, they have witnessed them personally.

Children with behavioral problems also are more likely to act out in a sexual way. Additionally, children with developmental delay will generally follow their developmental age rather than their chronologic age; so, a grade-school-aged child with developmental delay may still be preoccupied with genital touching of themselves or others.

Refer adolescents who repeatedly perform exhibitionistic behavior to a mental health specialist. The "consistent" exhibitionist will usually surface at around age 15.

Anatomically Correct Drawings

Children ages 3½–5 years will frequently include genitals in their drawings. After age 4 years, the drawings become more gender-specific, especially with regard to clothing and hair on the drawings. It is unusual for older, grade-school-age children to draw genitals on figures; this requires further inquiry if and when it occurs. Consider sexual abuse when an older child includes genitals in a drawing, but know that such a drawing is not diagnostic for abuse.

Interest in Pornography

Older children and adolescents frequently show interest in pornography. Today, especially with Internet availability, it is quite easy for minors to have intentional or unintentional access. A couple of episodes of "exploring" pornography are normal, but if it becomes persistent, or is associated with other abnormal behaviors, pursue further investigation.

Children's exposure to sexually explicit movies and videos has the potential for harm. For the most part, experts agree that the separation of sex from genuine affection and commitment, and/or erroneous or incomplete depiction of the consequences of certain sexual activity, are the wrong messages for teenagers. Parents must stay involved in their children's viewing choices across all media, and have open discussions about limits and acceptable content. Sexual interest is a developmental issue, but acceptable norms are a family-driven issue.

Cross-Dressing

Cross-dressing (the dressing up in the outer clothes of the opposite sex) is entirely normal for children < age 5 years. Use of the opposite sex's undergarments, however, by a kindergartner or older child is abnormal. Older children and adolescents who experience sexual pleasure from cross-dressing—known as transvestitism—do so with great guilt and stress. For the most part, these kids are heterosexual, but some may be homosexual. Some recommend behavioral modification techniques for the child who cross-dresses, if the child is motivated and there are no other underlying psychological problems. Do not encourage punishment for cross-dressing due to any etiology, but conduct further investigation to determine the overall well-being of the child.

notes

Quick Quiz

1) You are told that a 4-year-old child is masturbating in the bathtub. What reactions or punishments are appropriate for this behavior?
2) A 5-year-old girl shows her mother how her two dolls "Barb" and "Kyle" kiss each other. The mother is upset that the child shows "Barb" kissing "Kyle's" genital area. True or False: This is normal behavior for a 5-year-old.
3) What is gender-identity disorder?
4) True or False: Most tomboys (aggressive-acting girls) have gender-identity disorder.
5) True or False. Homosexual youth make up a large percentage of youth who are homeless.

"Sissies" and "Tomboys"

The term "sissy" is used to describe ~ 5% of boys, and "tomboy" ~ 10% of girls. For the most part, this is just a normal variation, but it can lead to gender identity disorder, atypical sexual orientation, or other sexual issues.

Gender identity disorder (GID) applies to children who truly believe they are the opposite of their genetic sex. It occurs in about 1/25,000 males and 1/125,000 females. It presents clinically between ages 2½–5. These kids are distressed about every aspect of their gender, including their genitals, clothes, sports, and friends. Girls with GID will claim they are growing penises and refuse to sit down to urinate. Boys with GID claim their penises will disappear, and they will grow up to be a woman.

Evidence suggests that GID is not due to behavior of the parents, although there is a higher incidence of parental psychopathology and depression in families of affected children. These children are usually unhappy. Affected boys avoid all sports and many other male-associated activities. The boys are often shy and anxious. About 2/3 have separation anxiety disorder. Girls tend to participate in boy-type activities.

Most effeminate boys and most tomboys do not have GID. Usually, these groups like being their sex and have no desire to change it. This is very different from the child with GID, who literally abhors his/her own sex, and wants to desperately change to the opposite sex.

Current evidence indicates that therapy will not change children with GID. About 3/4 will be homosexual, bisexual, or have "indeterminate" sexual orientation. Note: Most homosexuals and lesbians do not have GID. They like being males and females, but are attracted to others of the same sex.

Note also that some adolescents and adults continue to get sexual pleasure from cross-dressing, but do not have GID. These adolescents/adults have transvestitism only—they wish to remain their sex, but like to dress up in the clothing of the opposite sex.

Gay and Lesbian Parents

It is estimated that 10–14 million children in the U.S. have a homosexual parent. No data indicate that having a homosexual parent results in an abnormal effect on social functioning, psychological well-being, increased risk of the child being homosexual, or increased risk of gender identity problems among their children. Data do show that two parents, no matter what the gender(s), improve the child's developmental outcome over one parent. The key is likely the consistency of love and affection for the child.

Homosexuality

Homosexuality is defined as having persistent same-sex arousal, with a minimal or absent opposite-sex arousal. Prevalence reports vary, but many suggest that 1–10% of men, and 1–6% of women, are homosexual. Adolescents frequently engage in activities with or fantasize about the same sex, but these isolated events do not indicate a sustained homosexual predilection. Biological and genetic factors are gaining prominence as the etiology for homosexuality. Homosexuality, per se, most likely is not a "choice;" but sexual behaviors and life styles are choices all people make, based on their sexual orientations.

Many children become aware of their homosexuality during adolescence and struggle with "coming out." The accompanying issues of guilt and self-doubt lead to academic problems, truancy, peer problems, potential parental rejection, and homelessness. Physical attacks against adolescent males who have "come out" are well documented in the media. The homelessness issue cannot be overstressed: 25–40% of homeless youth are homosexual. Males are more at risk to be homeless than females. Eating disorders are prominent in the men. Therapy to "convert" the homosexual into a heterosexual is *contraindicated.* The key is to encourage parents to be supportive, and to persuade the individuals to accept themselves, be responsible for their actions, and develop a strong life plan in line with their future goals and objectives.

COMMON PAIN SYNDROMES OF CHILDHOOD

HEADACHE

Overview

Headaches are the most common recurrent pain syndrome in children. Headaches can be divided into 3 main groups: 1) migraine, 2) tension, and 3) organic. Tension headaches are the most common, followed by migraines. The average age of onset for headaches is ~ age 7 years. Girls are more commonly affected than boys. More specific information on headaches is in the Neurology chapter.

notes

Migraines

Migraines were once thought to be due to vascular disturbances, but recent data suggest that they may actually be due to abnormalities with serotonin and other brain receptors. To meet the adult definition, migraines must occur at least 5 times and last 2–72 hours without an identifiable etiology.

Two of the following criteria are mandatory to diagnose migraine headaches:

- Pain on one side
- Pulsating/throbbing character
- Moderate-to-severe intensity
- Increasing severity with activity

Additionally, the pain is associated with nausea, photophobia, or phonophobia. Migraines can be spontaneous, or induced by psychological stress or other factors.

Tension Headaches

Tension headaches are due to muscle contraction, and tend to become more severe as the day goes on. They present as a pressing, dull, persistent tightness—often described as a band around the head.

Organic Headaches

Organic headaches are due to structural abnormalities, metabolic diseases, or infectious etiologies. Severity and frequency usually increase, and they are not relieved with mild, over-the-counter pain relievers. Further physical examination, laboratory, and/or radiologic studies are critical to revealing the etiology. Headaches due to tumors commonly occur in the morning on awakening. Again, more on headaches in the Neurology section.

ABDOMINAL PAIN

Abdominal pain is a common complaint in childhood. Peak incidences are ~ ages 7–10, and these occur more commonly in girls than boys. ~ 1/3 of children will report abdominal pain lasting 2 weeks or longer.

Most define recurrent abdominal pain as occurring at least 3 times in 3 or more months. It can be dull, crampy, or sharp in character, and usually involves the periumbilical area. The pain may affect daily living, but growth and development are normal; the latter is the key! Environmental stress (school, sports, social, family), a relative with an ulcer, temperament of the child, and secondary gain from having the abdominal pain (e.g., extra attention, getting out of school early, etc.) can all influence the rapidity and duration of the pain.

Note: Only ~ 5% of children with recurrent abdominal pain have a true organic etiology. These include constipation, cholelithiasis, inflammatory bowel disease, celiac sprue, pregnancy, UTI, and lactase deficiency. It is important in the initial evaluation of recurrent abdominal pain to consider the non-organic etiologies so they can simultaneously be explored with the organic etiologies.

LIMB PAIN

Limb pain, also known as "growing pains," is the most common musculoskeletal problem of children. Anywhere from 10–20% of children have it during the school-age years. The most common peak is ages 7–12 years, with girls twice as likely as boys to be affected.

"Growing pains" are benign limb pains that are not due to growing. Usually, they are bilateral and the child describes them as a deep, aching pain in the muscles of the legs. Most of the pain occurs late in the day or in the middle of the night and resolves by morning. There is no joint involvement, and no inflammation is present.

Specific etiologies to exclude or consider include:

- Trauma (stress fracture, myositis ossificans)
- Bone problems (chondromalacia, Osgood-Schlatter disease)
- Collagen vascular disease (JRA, fibromyalgia)
- Infections
- Cancers
- Endocrine disorders
- Some storage diseases

Psychosomatic pain also can occur similar to "growing" pains, and may be due to school phobia or conversion reactions.

Osgood-Schlatter Disease is a repetitive stress injury to the patellar tendon at its insertion into the tibial tubercle. You see it most commonly in children ages 10–15 years. Look for a swollen tibial tubercle. Besides mild antiinflammatory agents, no specific therapy is necessary.

Legg-Calve-Perthes Disease is a partial or complete idiopathic avascular necrosis of the femoral head. Look for this in a boy between the ages of 4 and 8 years. It resolves with time and no treatment seems to speed the return of blood flow to the femoral head. See Figure 2-1, note the misshapen and "ratty" appearance to the left femoral head.

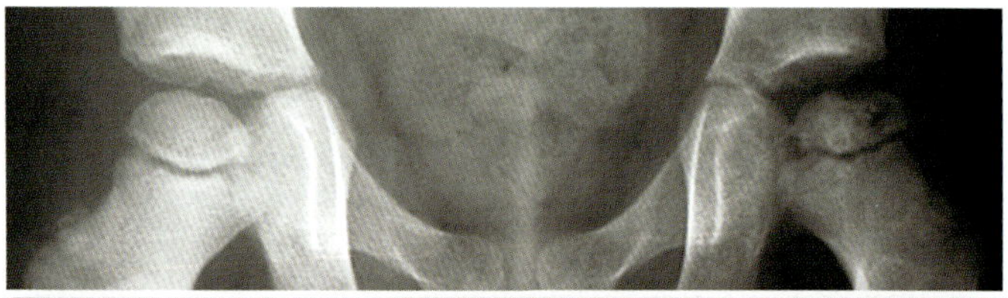

Figure 2-1: Legg-Calve-Perthes Disease

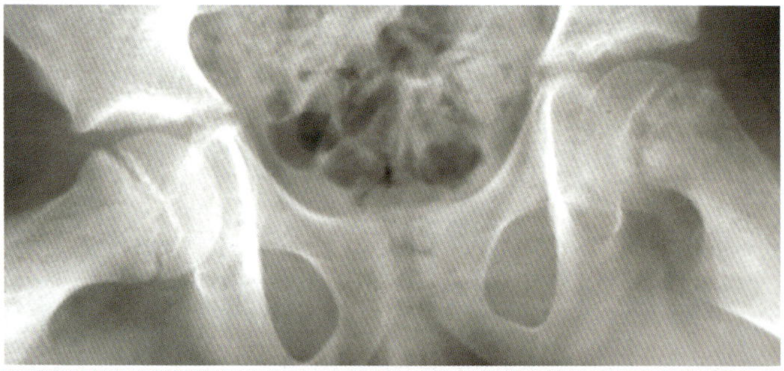

Figure 2-2: Slipped Capital Femoral Epiphysis

notes

Quick Quiz

1) Differentiate a migraine from a tension headache.
2) True or False: Abdominal pain that is non-organic in nature will present with growth and development problems in the child.
3) Are growing pains actually due to "growing"?
4) Describe a typical child with ADHD.
5) True or False: Sugars or artificial flavorings increase the risk of developing ADHD.

Slipped capital femoral epiphysis is the slipping of the epiphysis off the metaphysis. Look for an obese, eunuchoid adolescent, although some patients are thin. Get an AP and frog-leg view. Treat with surgery. See Figure 2-2, note the slippage on the left side.

CHEST PAIN

Chest pain is very common, and is the second most common reason for referral to a pediatric cardiologist (heart murmur is #1). In children, it is very rare that these pains are cardiac in origin. Most are idiopathic. In children > 13, which is the average age for presentation, the etiology is usually psychogenic.

History and physical examination guide the need for further studies. More in the Cardiology section.

ATTENTION DEFICIT DISORDER (ADD, ADHD)

OVERVIEW

Attention deficit disorder and attention deficit hyperactivity disorder (ADD, ADHD) are controversial in both diagnosis and treatment. The problem is that presentation variability is so broad. Generally, short attention span, impulsivity, and overactivity characterize this disorder. Average children occasionally have these same traits, which adds to the difficulty of defining who has the syndrome, and who is just an average, everyday kid.

Some estimate that 2–4% of school-aged children meet the definition for ADHD. DSM-IV lists behaviors that comprise the diagnostic criteria for ADHD. Look for them in Table 2-4. Boys are much more likely to be affected.

ETIOLOGY

For most children, no etiology can be found. Genetic factors are possible in some children, and there is an increased frequency of alcoholism, sociopathy, and hysteria among parents of children with ADHD. Toxin exposure both prenatally and postnatally has been implicated. And it is well known that fetal exposure to alcohol or lead may result in attention and hyperactivity problems. Controlled studies have failed to consistently implicate sugars, artificial flavorings, and salicylates as etiologies.

Recent theories report that ADHD is actually an inhibitory control problem and/or a difficulty with goal persistence. The theory is still controversial and not widely accepted.

One thing we do know—attention deficit disorder does not have a single cause.

CLINICAL FINDINGS

The clinical findings center on 5 main areas:

1. Easy distractibility
2. Impulsivity
3. Hyperactivity and inability to sit still
4. Inability to organize or plan tasks
5. Emotional lability

LABORATORY

Generally, laboratory is unnecessary, but consider lead screening, especially if history dictates—and know that thyroid abnormalities are more common in children with ADHD than the unaffected population. Routine use of EEG, MRI, etc., is not indicated.

Table 2-4

BEHAVIORS SUGGESTIVE OF ADHD
Inattentive Behaviors
Easily distracted by extraneous stimuli
Makes careless mistakes in schoolwork or other activities
Has difficulty maintaining attention to task
Does not seem to listen to what is being said to them
Fails to finish schoolwork, chores, or other duties
Loses things necessary for tasks or activities
Has difficulty organizing tasks and activities
Forgetful in daily activities
Hyperactive/Impulsive Behaviors
Runs about or climbs excessively in inappropriate situations
Fidgets with hands or feet or squirms
Has difficulty awaiting turn in games or groups
Blurts out answers to questions

notes

TREATMENT

Treatment is multifactorial. Behavior management is important, and can include positive reinforcement, strategies such as "time outs," and "extinction" techniques—systematically ignoring undesirable behaviors.

Drug therapy is beneficial for a majority of children affected with ADHD. Most commonly use stimulant medications: methylphenidate, dextroamphetamine, and Adderall® (a single entity amphetamine product combining the neutral sulfate salts of dextroamphetamine and amphetamine, with the dextroisomer of amphetamine saccharate and 6, I-amphetamine aspartate). They all increase the release and inhibit the reuptake of dopamine and norepinephrine. Side effects include the potential for growth suppression, weight loss due to appetite suppression, and exacerbation of tic disorders. Other agents include tricyclic antidepressants and clonidine—helpful for those with aggressive or hyperaroused behavior.

Non-conventional treatments, such as mineral therapy, diet restriction, or other dietary manipulations have failed to show improvement in controlled trials.

PROGNOSIS

Children with ADD/ADHD persist into adulthood with the disorder, although the hyperactivity symptoms tend to diminish over time.

DISRUPTIVE BEHAVIORS

OPPOSITIONAL DEFIANT DISORDER

Oppositional defiant disorder occurs in otherwise average children during the school-age and adolescent stages of development. Boys are much more commonly affected than girls. Key to the behaviors is a duration of at least 6 months. Table 2-5 summarizes DSM-IV diagnostic criteria.

CONDUCT DISORDER

Conduct disorder is a complex, multifactorial disorder. Generally, think of it in kids who have repetitive, persistent (> 6 months) behaviors that violate the rights or property of others. These children lack guilt or remorse about their behavior. These are the kids who have been caught repeatedly stealing, lying, fighting, setting fires, using drugs, or instigating sexual abuse.

There are 2 groups in Conduct Disorder:

1) The undersocialized group comprises kids who are unpopular, lack any close friends, and tend to be socially isolated. They lack any empathy for their age group and despise adults. The behaviors occur at home, at school, and in the community
2) The socialized group participates with a peer group in their behaviors—they have strong interpersonal ties, but are confrontational with adults.

Table 2-5

FOUR CRITERIA FOR THE DIAGNOSIS OF OPPOSITIONAL DEFIANT DISORDER
1. Behavior has to last at least 6 months, and 4 or more of the following must occur more frequently than is commonly seen for that age group:
Often loses temper
Often argues with adults
Actively defies or refuses to comply with adults' rules/requests
Annoys people on purpose
Blames others for his/her misbehavior
Easily annoyed by other people
Often angry or resentful
Often spiteful or vindictive
2. The behavior must cause clinically significant deviation in social, academic, or occupational functioning
3. The behaviors do not always occur in association with a Psychotic or Mood Disorder
4. Criteria are not met for Conduct Disorder and if older than 18 years of age, subjects don't meet criteria for Antisocial Personality Disorder.

Refer children and adolescents with Conduct Disorder for behavioral and psychotherapeutic intervention.

PERVASIVE DEVELOPMENTAL DISORDERS

OVERVIEW

Pervasive developmental disorders comprise a wide group and occur at a rate of ~ 5–7/100,000. Males are much more commonly affected, except with the incidence of Rett Syndrome. Etiologies for these conditions are unknown, but some evidence indicates that genetics may be a factor. In autism, you will see elevated levels of serotonin in platelets in ~1/3 of affected individuals—although the significance of this finding is unknown. Generally, prognosis is poor among most children with these disorders, and you will need assistance from other health care providers (psychologists, social workers, therapists, etc.)

notes

Quick Quiz

1) How long must a behavior occur for it to be classified as oppositional defiant behavior?
2) Do children with conduct disorder have guilt or remorse over their actions?
3) Which pervasive developmental disorder is usually only seen in girls?
4) How does Asperger syndrome differ from autism?
5) Define the terms "obsession" and "compulsion" as they relate to obsessive-compulsive disorder.
6) What is the most common OCD "ritual" in childhood?
7) What is the most common obsession in children?
8) Describe the usual perpetrator in Munchausen-by-Proxy syndrome.

AUTISM

Autism is now a subset of "pervasive developmental disorders," and is the most common one. There are multiple diagnostic criteria for autism that spread over 3 areas:

1) social interactions,
2) verbal and nonverbal communications, and
3) behaviors and activities.

To meet the definition, the developmental problems of autism must begin < age 3.

RETT SYNDROME

Children with Rett syndrome have many of the features of a child with autism. With Rett syndrome, early development up until age 5 months is normal; but then rapid developmental deterioration follows. It occurs almost exclusively in girls.

ASPERGER SYNDROME

Asperger syndrome is a newly described disorder. It is similar to autism in that these children have severe and pervasive impairment in social interactions, and also have restrictive, repetitive, stereotypic behaviors. The difference is that these children develop normal language and cognitive development skills.

PSYCHIATRIC DISORDERS

OBSESSIVE-COMPULSIVE DISORDER

Obsessive-compulsive disorder is a complex syndrome that may border on "normal areas" at some point. Generally, consider OCD when rituals or superstitions lose their age appropriateness, cause excessive actions (hand washing, etc.), impede socialization, or detract from normal duties and experiences. Obsessions must be persistent and recurrent, and involve senseless ideas, images, or impulses that intrude on normal activities. The obsessions must be involuntary. Compulsions are repetitive, purposeful behaviors that are performed in response to an obsession, and are often done in an attempt to stop the obsession. Those affected do not deem the compulsions as pleasurable, but believe them to be necessities. An example: the compulsion to check the alarm clock every 15 minutes to be sure it is set.

Recent data support OCD as a neurobiological disorder; there also is an increased familial nature to the disorder. Boys are more commonly affected, and tend to have an earlier age of onset than girls.

The most common OCD "ritual" in childhood is repetitive cleaning and washing. This includes showering, hand washing, or tooth brushing. Other common OCD rituals include going in and out of doors, rereading, rechecking doors to be sure they are locked, rechecking the alarm clock, and counting, ordering or arranging objects. However, the most common obsessions in children concern dirt and germs. Other obsessions include the feeling that something hasn't been done correctly or that something terrible is going to happen.

The differential for OCD is extensive. Tourette syndrome can involve complex tics that can resemble the rituals of OCD. Excessive rumination on gloomy thoughts is a common feature of depression; but the depressed person views these thoughts as making sense while the person with OCD views them as abnormal. Note: Eating disorders, by definition, are excluded from the diagnosis of OCD.

Also remember that almost all children experience some superstitions or rituals at age-appropriate levels. For example, children may collect POKEMON cards, elaborately store them, and categorize them. For most kids, this is an enjoyable activity and provides them time to socialize with friends who have similar interests. In contrast, a child who collects the cards but keeps them wrapped in plastic to prevent germs from getting on them, or refuses to let friends see or handle the cards, and who does not seem to have any enjoyment in sharing or discussing the cards with another child, actually may be exhibiting OCD-type behavior.

Direct treatment for OCD behavior is expressive and supportive psychotherapy. Behavioral therapies are also helpful, as are pharmacologic therapies, such as serotonin reuptake inhibitors (SSRIs), although recent overuse has brought these drugs into question. Any of the agents work, including fluoxetine, sertraline, fluvoxamine, and paroxetine. Clomipramine, a tricyclic, may also be helpful.

Studies show that ~ 50% of children with OCD continue to have OCD as adults.

MUNCHAUSEN-BY-PROXY SYNDROME

Munchausen-by-Proxy syndrome is a bizarre disorder in which the caregiver-child relationship is "disturbed." The mother almost always is the one involved, is deliberately dishonest about a history of illness in her child, and/or harms the child to create an illness. Children may be at risk at any age, but this most commonly affects infants and school-aged children.

notes

Frequently, no father is present, and the mother is socially isolated, appears to be extremely devoted to her child, and is very knowledgeable about the child's "illness."

Interestingly, the mother is frequently a member of the health care profession.

Clues that Munchausen-by-Proxy may be occurring:

1) Recurrent, serious illness that cannot be satisfactorily explained
2) Failure of routine management of an illness
3) Symptoms do not match with scientific evidence
4) History of illnesses in the past are inconsistent
5) History of an unexplained illness or death of a sibling
6) A mother who appears inappropriately calm or even euphoric when her child is in the hospital
7) She seems inappropriately excited that her child is going to be admitted
8) You get a creepy feeling just being around the mother
9) She requests for specific diagnostic studies or procedures of the child

This is difficult to sort out, because many inborn errors of metabolism or unusual diseases may "not respond to routine management" or may not "be satisfactorily explained." In the real world, be sure you have ruled out just about everything before you consider this diagnosis. Diagnosis is very tricky and involves a multidisciplinary approach, including referral to mental health workers familiar with this disorder. Long-term prognosis and outcomes are guarded and usually not good for these families. Usually, on the Board examination, you can pick these questions out because the mother's history notes she is a nurse or physician (clue—why are they telling me this?) and you begin to get a creepy feeling (2nd clue) while reading the question that something is "just not right."

Note: Depression is covered in the Adolescent section.

CHILD MALTREATMENT SYNDROMES

OVERVIEW

Child maltreatment syndromes include physical abuse, neglect, sexual abuse, and emotional maltreatment. Overall, there are 3–4 million reports of child maltreatment in the U.S. each year, with ~ 1200 deaths. The most commonly reported are: neglect (> 1/2), physical abuse, sexual abuse (~ 1/10), and emotional abuse. Males and females are equally affected, except for sexual abuse, where 75% of cases affect females. 40% of affected children are < 6. Of the reported cases, only 1/3 are substantiated by an investigative agency. However, this does not mean that the abuse did not occur, just that evidence to support it was lacking. In fact, some studies indicate that abuse may actually be underreported.

Abuse and neglect are reported more commonly in families who are poor and less educated (although abuse occurs in families at all income levels and educational statuses). Other factors associated with increased risk of abuse are young maternal age, single-parent households, ethnic minority status, and parental alcohol/drug abuse. Almost all cases occur in the child's home. Sexual perpetrators are almost always male, and about 1/5 of the perpetrators are < 18. A majority of the abused children know the sexual perpetrators. Recent studies estimate that 15–20% of adult women and 5–10% of adult men were sexually abused as children.

For all types of abuse, it is paramount that communication exists between the parents and the clinician; but of utmost concern is the safety and well-being of the child. Generally, child protection agencies are available to assist the clinician, but frequently it may fall to you to provide relevant information (or actually decide) on whether it is appropriate for the child to return to the home environment, or if the child requires alternate shelter, including possibly hospitalization.

PHYSICAL ABUSE

The classic definition of physical abuse is "an act against a child that results in harm or intended harm to the child." Many prefer to limit this to "deformation or leaving a lasting mark on the child's body." The intention here is to separate "physical abuse" from common practices, such as "spanking," which many consider harmful to a child, but it would not necessarily qualify as "physical abuse," per se (Note: Some experts feel that spanking also should be considered physical abuse). So, the bottom line is the definition can be controversial; but generally for the Boards, think of physical abuse as harm that may cause bruises, broken bones, or even death.

Note the following histories: They should raise your suspicion for physical abuse in real life and on the ABP exam!

1) Serious injury (fracture) with no history of preceding trauma ("I don't know how it happened; her leg is just limp"), or the history is inconsistent with the findings
2) A delay in seeking medical advice for a significant injury
3) "The story keeps changing" as to how the injury occurred
4) History of recurrent injuries—especially those with poor explanations
5) Physical findings, such as burns, bruises around the eyes, etc.
6) Unexplained death of a sibling

Soft tissue injuries (hand marks from slapping; bruises; linear marks from belts or cords; and bite or burn marks) are the most common manifestation of physical abuse. You must take into account developmental characteristics. A 1-year-old just learning to walk will frequently have bruises on the face or shins from falling. However, it is very unusual to see bruising on a child who is not cruising or crawling yet. Be very suspicious of black eyes, bruises around the ears, injury in the genital area or on the posterior surfaces of the body; e.g., "she fell forward and bruised herself"—hmm, how did the back of her leg get bruised falling forward?

Burns are a very common injury of abuse. These can range from scald injuries to cigarette burns. Patients with immersion burns present with bilateral burns to the buttocks or back, and will usually have a sharp area of demarcation between normal and burned skin, the so-called "stocking glove" distribution. Non-abusive burns will usually be asymmetric—e.g., only on one foot due to stepping on a burn source

notes

Quick Quiz

1) Who are more commonly sexually abused—boys or girls?
2) A 1-year-old presents with a broken left femur. The mother says the child was with his father for most of the day, while the mother was out shopping. The mother says she found the child in his crib refusing to bear weight on the leg. The mother says she doesn't know how the child was injured. True or false: You should be suspicious of physical abuse.
3) A 1-year-old boy presents for an otitis media follow-up appointment. You note a bruise to the child's left cheek. His father says that the child fell against the edge of the coffee table when attempting to walk 2 days ago. A few scrapes also are noted on the child's shins. True or False: You should be suspicious of physical abuse.
4) What is the most common cause of death due to child abuse?
5) What eye finding is important to look for in a child you suspect may have been "shaken" violently?
6) True or False: Rib fractures should make you suspect child abuse.
7) What radiologic test is useful for detecting acute rib fractures?

by accident or otherwise uneven, such as a hot liquid that was accidentally spilled on them.

Multiple cigarette burns are strong evidence for abuse, while a single burn could be an accident (unless it is in an unlikely area, such as the back, buttocks, or genital area).

Head injuries are the most common causes of death due to child abuse. In children < 1 year, shaking the child can cause intracranial bleeding due to repeated accelerations and decelerations of the brain, producing shearing of the bridging vessels. This results in subdural or subarachnoid hemorrhages and retinal hemorrhages. Many of these shaken babies also have injury due to impact with the floor, crib, or other surface. These children can present with seizures, coma, apnea, or arrhythmias. Parents may only complain "the baby is not acting right." Frequently, there are other signs of abuse, such as bruising, etc. Rib fractures are common with the Shaken Baby syndrome, but may not show up on x-ray until 10–14 days out—at the beginning of callus formation. Rib fractures on x-ray usually indicate prior abuse.

Bone fractures also are a common indication of abuse in children. In one study of injured children < 3, officials believed 25% of injuries were due to abuse. Skull fractures are the most common fracture seen in abuse—specifically the linear fracture of the parietal bone. Humerus and femur fractures (especially if < age 1 year) should raise the suspicion of abuse. Note: It is common for a 2–3-year-old to have a fracture of the supracondylar area of the humerus from a fall to the elbow, or a spiral fracture of the femur or tibia from falling and twisting. Spiral fractures by themselves are not diagnostic of abuse.

Two fractures more specific for abuse are:

1) Bucket handle (metaphyseal) fractures
2) Rib fractures—particularly those posterior and near the spine

Other injuries to raise suspicion of abuse are lacerations to the liver or spleen and suspicious poisonings.

An extreme type of abuse is Munchausen syndrome by Proxy, discussed earlier in this section. In this syndrome, the mother (rarely the father) makes up symptoms of an illness for the child, and takes internal pleasure in the child undergoing multiple tests/procedures. Additionally, she may cause the child to be ill by poisoning or injecting the child with contaminated feces or other material.

Recently, multiple SIDS deaths in a family have been linked to abuse by suffocation. When more than 1 infant in a family dies of SIDS, investigate both child abuse and other causes, such as metabolic diseases.

For children with serious head injuries, perform an ophthalmologic exam to look for retinal hemorrhages; CT/MRI scans also are usually indicated. If abuse has occurred in a child < age 3, a skeletal survey is usually indicated. Bone scans are useful for detecting acute rib fractures and other older fractures. Laboratory tests include CBC, lead level (children < 6), and U/A. If bleeding or bruising is present, PT, PTT, and platelet counts are appropriate. Liver transaminases may be helpful if you suspect abdominal trauma.

NEGLECT

Neglect is defined as an "act of omission," such as failure to provide adequate food, shelter, clothing, or supervision. It includes abandonment or failure to provide the child with adequate health care and/or education.

A common manifestation of neglect is poor growth and developmental delay of the child. Older, neglected children may seem "emotionally needy," or can be very adult-like in their behaviors.

SEXUAL ABUSE

Sexual abuse is defined as adult or adolescent sexual involvement with a child or younger adolescent in which the latter do not fully understand or comprehend. These children cannot give informed consent. Such sexual abuse includes the act of sexual intercourse, genital fondling, and exposure to pornography.

Generally, you will see victims of sexual abuse because the child/young adolescent confided in a relative or other adult, or, you notice signs of genital or anal abnormality on physical examination. After the disclosure, the child may retract the story or change it because of the turmoil that will occur in the family after the event is known. Assessing the truthfulness of the child's statements makes this diagnosis very

notes

complex, especially if it occurs in the setting of custody or other issues.

Sexually abused children demonstrate variable behaviors. Many are non-specific and can manifest as poor school performance, anxiety, encopresis, or suicidal gestures. Others are more specific—such as excessive masturbation, sexually overt behaviors, vaginal discharge/bleeding, or rectal bleeding. Note: Vaginal discharge alone represents a low risk (< 5% of the time) of indicating sexual abuse. Of those children who are sexually abused, only ~ 1/5 will have evidence of a suspicious, abnormal genital or rectal finding. A normal exam, obviously, does not rule out abuse. Acute abrasions, lacerations, or hematomas of the female genitals should raise your suspicions about a recent abuse incident. Other suspicious findings include U- or V-shaped clefts in the posterior rim of the hymen or decreased hymenal tissue posteriorly. These findings are especially suspicious if they persist when you examine the child in the prone, knee-chest position. An enlarged hymenal opening does not by itself indicate abuse. For males, findings are rare, except for acute anal fissures or thickened rugae.

Obviously, a diagnosis of STDs or pregnancy is definitive evidence that sex has occurred. Gonorrhea, chlamydia, and human papillomavirus are the most commonly found STDs.

Most cities and hospitals have protocols for the evaluation of sexual abuse. Appropriate law enforcement authorities are contacted, and the clinician takes appropriate forensic evidence, along with necessary laboratory tests.

EMOTIONAL MALTREATMENT

Emotional maltreatment is probably one of the most common forms of abuse, but difficult to define or identify. It includes repeated verbal denigration, belittling, "making fun of," and scapegoating for problems that have nothing to do with the child. These attacks result in a child with low self-esteem and feelings of worthlessness.

OBESITY

Obesity is defined as having a weight > 120% of the median weight for height, or a triceps skinfold thickness or body mass index (BMI) > the 85th–95th percentile. A strong risk factor for obesity in a child is having an obese parent (no difference which one), and there is even more risk if both parents are obese. By age 10–14, the risk of being an obese adult is more likely associated simply with being obese at 10–14 (in other words, not related so much to the parent's obesity status).

Recently, we discovered "obesity genes," but there is still considerable controversy about whether they are completely responsible for the condition. Most likely, heredity plays a role in the susceptibility of a person to become obese, but it is the behavior and environment of the individual that determines if the obesity will be phenotypically expressed.

We know there are 3 critical periods in childhood that result in an increased likelihood of persistent obesity:
1) prenatal period,
2) age 5–7 years, and
3) early adolescent years.

The more common problems with adolescent obesity include dyslipidemia, hyperinsulinemia, and a markedly increased risk of obesity in adulthood. Obese adults are at increased risk due to complications from diabetes, hypertension, heart disease, cancer, joint problems, and digestive disorders.

Treatment of obesity must be family and behavior oriented. Family support is most critical. Parents must be invested (better yet, involved themselves) in the program if weight loss is to occur. Results are still disappointing, but better than those seen in adult programs. About 1/3 of children who actively participate in a state-of-the-art program will be obesity-free at 10 years. The family and the child both must be ready and willing for intervention to succeed.

DRUG POISONINGS

OVERVIEW

In the U.S., over 2 million poisoning events occur and over 60% of these occur in children under the age of 6. The peak age for ingestions is 18 months to 3 years. 92% of the events occur in the home and involve only 1 substance. Luckily, 75% can be managed in the home.

85% of poisonings are unintentional and generally occur in children less than 5 years of age. Boys are more commonly affected than girls and > ½ are non-pharmaceutical ingestions, with the most common being cosmetics, cleaning products, plants, and foreign bodies. For the pharmaceuticals, the most common unintentional ingestions are acetaminophen, cough and cold preparations, vitamins, and antibiotics.

Of the 15% of poisonings that are intentional, a majority occur in adolescents and adults. Girls are more commonly affected and the pharmaceuticals make up a majority of the cases, including acetaminophen, barbiturates, stimulants, antidepressants, and alcohol.

INITIAL MANAGEMENT

Overview

Initial management for all poisoning follows the ABCDs and stabilization management rules. Airway and antidotes, breathing, circulation, and disability/decontamination.

The physical exam can be a clue to what the potential toxin is. Pay close attention on the examination for miosis or mydriasis.

Causes of miosis include (COPS):
- Cholinergics, Clonidine
- Opiates, Organophosphates
- Phenothiazine, Pilocarpine
- Sedatives (barbiturates)

Causes of mydriasis include:
- Antihistamine

notes

Quick Quiz

1) True or False: In a child who you suspect has been sexually abused, a normal genital and rectal examination rules out sexual abuse as a possibility.
2) What is a major risk factor for obesity in a child?
3) What are some of the medical complications of obesity?
4) What are the common causes of miosis and mydriasis?
5) What are the contraindications for using ipecac? Gastric lavage?
6) Name some products that activated charcoal would NOT be useful in absorbing.
7) KNOW Acetaminophen poisoning!!!!!

- Antidepressant
- Anticholinergics (morphine)
- Sympathomimetics (amphetamine, cocaine, PCP)

Other clues include laboratory findings:

- ECG—look for prolonged QRS in tricyclic ingestions
- Osmolar gap—look for in unknown alcohol ingestions
- Anion gap—look for in MUDPILES (Methanol, uremia, DKA, phenols, iron, INH, lactate, ethanol, ethylene glycol, and salicylates)
- X-rays—May pick up pill fragments (CHIPS: Chloral hydrate, heavy metals, iron, phenothiazines, sustained-release tablets)

In the management of poisoning, you'll want to prevent agents from being further absorbed, depending on the type of exposure:

- Dermal—remove clothing, wash skin with water and then soap and water
- Ocular—irrigate eyes with copious (1000 cc) NS
- Respiratory—remove patient to fresh air
- GI—see the more extensive discussion next.

GI Decontamination

Most liquids are absorbed in 30 minutes and most solids are absorbed in 1–2 hours. There are four choices available for decreasing or inhibiting absorption:

1) Ipecac
2) Gastric lavage
3) Activated charcoal
4) Cathartics

Ipecac is an over-the-counter, chemo-trigger zone stimulant; in other words, it causes vomiting. Vomiting usually occurs 20–30 minutes after dosing and will continue for 1–2 hours. Indications are now very limited (iron ingestion within 1 hour). It is no longer recommended for home use and is rarely used anymore. Absolute contraindications include: altered mental state, hematemesis, seizure, hydrocarbon ingestion, and corrosive ingestion. Also you don't use the agent in infants < 6 months of age. Once given, follow with 8 ounces of water.

Gastric lavage is also not routine anymore. It can be considered when a life-threatening ingestion has occurred within 30–60 minutes. It is only recommended for older children and adults (the tube is too small in younger children to be effective). The worrisome complication is pulmonary aspiration. Contraindications for gastric lavage include caustic, hydrocarbon, and sharp item ingestions. If no pill fragments are seen, this does not rule out toxic ingestion.

Activated charcoal is used to absorb substances and decrease bioavailability. In vitro, 10 grams of charcoal will generally absorb 1 gram of toxin. For a 1–12-year-old, generally give between 10 and 30 grams of activated charcoal; for adolescents and adults, give 30 to 100 grams. There is some benefit if the offending substance has been absorbed in the last hour. Complications include pulmonary aspiration, emesis, and constipation. Contraindications include ingestion of hydrocarbons or corrosives, or having an ileus or compromised airway. Charcoal is used today with acetaminophen ingestions.

Activated charcoal is ineffective in the following:
(think CHEMICaL CamP)

- Cyanide
- Hydrocarbon
- Ethanol
- Metals
- Iron
- Caustics
- Lithium
- Camphor
- Phosphorus

Cathartics are thought to decrease GI transit time, but no clinical studies to date have shown improved outcomes. Sorbitol is the most commonly used agent and is frequently fixed with charcoal. Cathartics alone are never recommended. Routine use is not common.

ACETAMINOPHEN INGESTION

Acetaminophen is the most commonly used analgesic in the U.S. It is rapidly absorbed and reaches peak levels 1 hour after ingestion. It is metabolized in the liver to non-toxic metabolites using glutathione. This is the problem; with toxic levels, glutathione stores are overwhelmed and toxic metabolites accumulate.

An acute toxic dose in a child < 12 years of age is about 200 mg/kg, and in adolescents and adults it is ~7.5 grams. Note: Chronic, repeated large doses may lead to toxicity as well.

The symptoms of acetaminophen overdose occur as follows:

- 0–24 hours: nausea, vomiting, normal liver function tests (LFTs)
- 24–48 hours: asymptomatic, maybe RUQ pain, LFTs may begin to increase
- 48–96 hours: peak of symptoms, AST > 20,000, prolonged PT, death from hepatic failure

notes

When a child/adolescent presents with acetaminophen overdose, begin the ABCs first; and then to prevent further absorption, give activated charcoal. Next, check acetaminophen levels at least 4 hours after ingestion and use the Rumack-Matthew nomogram to determine if toxicity is likely. If toxicity is possible or probable using the nomogram, start IV N-acetylcysteine (NAC or Mucomyst) within 8–10 hours of ingestion. Continue a full course of treatment if started. The IV form is just as effective as the oral form. Don't forget to consider co-ingestions. There is no need to follow acetaminophen levels after toxicity has been determined. You do need to follow AST, ALT, PT, and PTT.

ANTICHOLINERGIC INGESTION

These agents include diphenhydramine, atropine, antispasmodics, mushrooms, jimson weed, and deadly nightshade. The symptoms are the key for these!

Dry as a bone	↓ sweating, ↓ urine output
Red as a beet	Flushing
Blind as a bat	Mydriasis
Mad as a hatter	Agitation, seizures
Hot as a hare	Hyperthermia

Treatment is with activated charcoal. Use of physostigmine is currently controversial.

CARBAMAZEPINE INGESTION

Carbamazepine ingestion (even though it seems rare, it is listed in the content specifications for the Board Exam!) results in CNS depression, and symptoms usually occur within 6 to 24 hours. Mild ingestions may just result in drowsiness, vomiting, ataxia, slurred speech, and nystagmus. Severe intoxications can result in coma, seizures, and respiratory depression. Follow carbamazepine levels (there will be a delayed peak for 24–72 hours) and renal function. Treat with activated charcoal and supportive measures. Charcoal hemoperfusion can be effective for severe intoxications.

CLONIDINE INGESTION

Clonidine is an antihypertensive agent with α-2 adrenergic receptor blocking ability. Children are very sensitive (a dose as small as 0.1 mg can cause toxicity). Symptoms occur within an hour of ingestion and include lethargy, miosis, bradycardia, hypotension, apnea, and coma. Paradoxically, it may also cause hypertension. Gastric decontamination is not helpful. Supportive care is necessary with serial ECG and blood gases. Naloxone has had mixed success in some studies. Toxicity usually resolves within 24 hours.

ETHANOL INGESTION

Ethanol is found in many products in the home, including mouthwash, perfume, over-the-counter medications, etc. Symptoms of acute ethanol toxicity include nausea, vomiting, stupor, and ataxia. Apnea may occur and result in coma and death. In infants and toddlers, a level of 50–100 mg/dl can result in coma, hypothermia, hypoglycemia, and metabolic acidosis. For adolescents, a level of 100–150 mg/dl will cause neurologic findings, but levels > 500 mg/dl can result in death.

Diagnose by checking drug levels and also noting an osmolal gap. Note: Ethanol intoxication may mask toxicities from co-ingestions—be especially careful on the Boards with an adolescent with just presumed alcohol intoxication, who may also have ingested other items.

Treat with ABCs initially. Check glucose levels and treat any hypoglycemia. Activated charcoal is not used for ethanol ingestion alone, but you may consider it if you think the patient has a co-ingestion. In rare life-threatening cases, hemodialysis can be used.

IBUPROFEN INGESTION

Ibuprofen inhibits prostaglandin synthesis and may result in GI irritation, reduced renal blood flow, and platelet dysfunction. A dose of 100 mg/kg does not cause toxicity, while a dose of 400 mg/kg can cause seizures and coma. Symptoms generally occur within 4 hours of ingestion and resolve in 24 hours. Commonly nausea, vomiting, epigastric pain, drowsiness, lethargy, and ataxia occur. Serious complications are rare but can include anion gap acidosis, renal failure, coma, and seizures—but are all rare. Use of activated charcoal and supportive care are recommended.

IRON INGESTION

Iron is a common cause of pediatric poisoning, because iron is common in vitamins, especially those that look and taste like "candy." Iron is corrosive to gastric and intestinal mucosa. It also causes mitochondrial dysfunction, which results in cell dysfunction and capillary leak. Hypotension then results. A toxic dose is considered to be > 60 mg of elemental iron/kg.

There are 4 phases of iron toxicity:

1) GI stage (30 mins to 6 hours)
   - Nausea, vomiting, diarrhea, abdominal pain
   - Hematemesis and bloody diarrhea in severe cases
   - Due to the direct damage to the GI and intestinal mucosa
2) Stability (6–24 hours)
3) Hepatotoxicity (within 48 hours)
   - Severe metabolic acidosis
   - Hypotension, hypo/hyperglycemia, GI bleeding, hepatic and renal failure
4) GI/Pyloric scarring (2–4 weeks post-ingestion)

X-ray may show pill fragments. Obtain a serum iron level at 4 hours: A nontoxic ingestion is < 500 mcg/dl 4–8 hours post-ingestion; a toxic ingestion is > 500 mcg/dl.

Treatment includes supportive care. Chelation with IV deferoxamine is recommended if the serum iron level is > 500 mcg/dl or if the patient has moderate or severe symptoms regardless of the iron level. You can consider ipecac if the ingestion oc-

notes

Quick Quiz

1) What are the symptoms of an anticholinergic ingestion?
2) KNOW Iron poisoning!!!
3) What is the classic triad of opiate ingestion?
4) What drug is useful in treating dystonic reactions in phenothiazine ingestion?
5) What are the acute findings of salicylate ingestion?
6) Why is bicarbonate given during therapy for treatment of salicylate ingestion?
7) Name the common electrolyte abnormalities found in theophylline toxicity.
8) Name the cardiac findings associated with tricyclic antidepressant ingestion?

curred within an hour, whole bowel irrigation, or endoscopic gastric removal. Do not use gastric lavage (tablets too large), activated charcoal (does not bind iron), oral bicarbonate, magnesium hydroxide, or oral deferoxamine.

OPIATE INGESTION

Common opiates include morphine, heroin, methadone, propoxyphene, codeine, and meperidine. Most cases present from drug abuse.

Physical findings include:

- Miosis
- Respiratory depression
- Coma
- Decreased GI motility
- Hypotension (from histamine release)
- No changes in heart rate

Treatment consists of ABCs, intubation if necessary, and naloxone as needed.

Note: The triad of coma, pinpoint pupils, and respiratory depression suggests opioid poisoning.

PHENOTHIAZINE INGESTION

Phenothiazines include the drugs promethazine, prochlorperazine, and chlorpromazine. Symptoms are much like those with the anticholinergics, and the prominent finding may be hypertension! Patients can have cogwheel rigidity, dystonic reactions (spasms of the neck, tongue thrusting, oculogyric crisis), and CNS depression. Treat with charcoal and also treat the hypertension (or occasional hypo-). Diphenhydramine is useful for treating dystonic reactions.

SALICYLATE INGESTION

Salicylate ingestions are much less common, but they are still sometimes seen in children because of ingestion of oil of wintergreen or antidiarrheal products. Salicylate uncouples oxidative phosphorylation. An acute toxic dose is > 150 mg/kg.

Know the acute signs, symptoms, and laboratory findings:

- Nausea, vomiting, tinnitus, fever
- Hyperventilation, respiratory alkalosis
- Dehydration; metabolic acidosis

With severe intoxication, you can get agitation, confusion, and coma. Death occurs from pulmonary edema, electrolyte imbalances, and cardiovascular collapse.

Diagnosis requires checking salicylate levels:

> 20 mg/kg are potentially toxic—follow the patient

> 70 mg/kg gives serious toxicity

Monitor levels every 2–3 hours. The Done nomogram is no longer used. Activated charcoal is given, but be careful that bezoar formation with the drug can occur. Rehydrate and replace bicarbonate and potassium. Give bicarbonate to raise urine pH, which results in enhanced excretion of the drug. Hemodialysis may be helpful in serious cases.

THEOPHYLLINE INGESTION

Theophylline is used less and less, but still is a common ingestion to appear on the Boards. Remember that the therapeutic level for theophylline is in a small window and upper normal levels can cause symptoms of toxicity. Normal therapeutic levels are usually between 10–20 mcg/dL. With between 20–50 mcg/dL, nausea, vomiting, and muscle tremor can occur. > 60–70 mcg/dL can result in seizures and arrhythmias. Electrolyte abnormalities are common with high levels including:

↑ Glucose
↑ Calcium
↓ Potassium
Metabolic acidosis

Management centers on correcting the electrolyte abnormalities and ABCs. Repeated doses of activated charcoal are effective. Hemoperfusion is effective in serious overdoses.

TRICYCLIC ANTIDEPRESSANT INGESTION

Tricyclic antidepressants work by blocking norepinephrine, serotonin, and dopamine. They also inhibit cardiac fast sodium channels. On the Boards, look out for ingestion of tricyclics by a younger sibling. Symptoms occur within 30 mins to 6 hours. In children, CNS effects are more prominent including drowsiness, lethargy, seizures, and coma.

Cardiac effects are usually asked about on Board exams:

- Tachycardia
- Hypertension or hypotension
- Widened QRS
- Prolonged QT

notes

Be aware of **CCCA** in **TRI-C** cyclic **A**ntidepressants:

- **C**oma
- **C**onvulsions
- **C**ardiac dysrhythmias
- **A**cidosis

For treatment, it is important not to induce emesis because of the increased risk of aspiration. Give activated charcoal and add sodium bicarbonate to alkalize the serum to prevent dysrhythmias. Most dysrhythmias that occur with tricyclic overdose will respond to lidocaine. ECG monitoring is obviously important. Physostigmine is not given.

ENVIRONMENTAL INGESTIONS

OVERVIEW

These include the non-pharmaceuticals and will be discussed in further detail with each ingestion. As noted previously, 60% of the unintentional poisonings are with non-pharmaceuticals in the < 5 years age group.

CARBON MONOXIDE

Carbon monoxide binds to hemoglobin preferentially and displaces oxygen. It also impairs oxygen release (shifts the curve to the left) and impedes oxygen utilization. Carbon monoxide is colorless and odorless.

Children and adults will present with headache, malaise, nausea, and in many cases may appear to have "the flu." With further exposure, severe headache, dizziness, visual changes, syncope, vomiting, and ataxia may occur. Then eventually, coma, seizures, and death result. "Cherry red skin" may be helpful on the Boards, but really is not of diagnostic value.

To diagnose carbon monoxide poisoning, check CO concentration on a blood gas. If it is > 20%, most patients will have symptoms.

Treatment is with oxygen! Correct any underlying anemia and treat metabolic acidosis if it has occurred. Severely affected patients may benefit from hyperbaric oxygen. In addition to CO poisoning, consider cyanide poisoning in those from a house fire.

CAUSTIC SUBSTANCE INGESTION

Generally, these fall into either alkali or acidic agents.

Alkali Agent Characteristics:

- Drain cleaners, lye, dishwasher detergent
- Tasteless
- Severe, deep, liquefaction necrosis
- Household bleach (5%) is only an irritant

Acidic Agent Characteristics:

- Toilet bowl cleaner, grout cleaner, gun bluing
- Bitter taste
- Coagulation necrosis (superficial)
- Thick eschar formation
- Severe gastritis

Caustic ingestions cause major problems with esophageal and gastric inflammation and can potentially cause perforation. Note: Acids can cause severe gastritis, perforation, or late stricture even without severe mouth/esophageal burns! Stricture formation probably occurs in 20% of caustic ingestions. Symptoms with both alkali and acidic ingestions include vomiting, drooling, refusal to drink, oral burns, dysphagia, abdominal pain, and stridor.

The absence of symptoms usually implies little or no injury; however, remember that absence of oral lesions does not preclude severe esophageal or stomach injury.

Upper endoscopy is recommended in all symptomatic children.

Treatment includes diluting with water or milk (the current Nelson's says this, but most ER people disagree). Remove contaminated clothing and rinse. Check chest and abdominal film, and start an IV if necessary. Analgesia may be needed as well. After endoscopy, consider use of steroids if indicated. Strictures require treatment with dilatation and possible surgical resection. Do not neutralize or induce emesis. Do not do gastric lavage. More in the GI section.

HYDROCARBON INGESTION

Hydrocarbons are low viscosity compounds and can lead to pulmonary aspiration. The most common ones listed on Boards are mineral spirits, kerosene, gasoline, and lamp oil. Other agents include toluene, propellants, and refrigerants; these are known to sensitize to cardiac arrhythmias. Commonly, they are vehicles as well for pesticides.

Clinical findings include mild CNS depression, coughing, severe respiratory distress, and fever. They may have a leukocytosis, and it is important to remember that the CXR may be normal for 8–12 hours after the exposure!

Generally, for these types of exposures in the asymptomatic child, you will observe for 6–8 hours. These children can be discharged if still asymptomatic and the CXR is normal. If symptomatic, start supportive care with airway control and the other ABCs. ARDS is likely in severe cases. Do not give ipecac, gastric lavage (except in very special circumstances), activated charcoal, steroids, prophylactic antibiotics, or epinephrine (will induce ventricular fibrillation).

METHANOL INGESTION

Methanol is found in windshield washer fluid and as a fuel additive. If ingested, it is metabolized and forms a metabolite, formic acid, which inhibits mitochondrial respiration. Initially, the child will have malaise, headache, nausea, and vomiting.

24 hours later the child will develop:

- Visual disturbances (described as a snowstorm)
- Optic nerve damage leading to blindness
- CNS depression
- Severe Metabolic acidosis (high anion gap!)

Gastric decontamination and activated charcoal do not work. Treat the metabolic acidosis with bicarbonate and give IV

notes

Quick Quiz

1) What agent is used in treating tricyclic antidepressant overdose that will help prevent dysrhythmias?
2) What lab test is useful in diagnosing carbon monoxide poisoning?
3) True or False: Acid ingestions can cause severe gastritis, perforation, or late stricture even without severe mouth/esophageal burns.
4) Know methanol ingestion!
5) Know ethylene glycol ingestion!
6) What are the symptoms of organophosphate ingestion? Treatment?
7) Explain the differences between first-, second-, and third-degree burns.
8) Be able to determine burn surface area in an adolescent and a child.

ethanol or fomepizole as an antidote. Hemodialysis is effective in removing the agent and will help correct the metabolic acidosis.

ETHYLENE GLYCOL INGESTION

Ethylene glycol is found in antifreeze. When ingested, it causes the development of glycolic and oxalic acid, which are both toxic. Calcium oxalate crystals will be found in the urine, as well as an osmolal gap! Urine will fluoresce with a Woods lamp.

In the initial 1–12 hours, the child will have nausea, vomiting, drowsiness, and appear inebriated.

In the next 12–24 hours, cardiac dysrhythmias, muscle pain, and tetany develop due to hypocalcemia.

Later, cardiac failure, seizures, cerebral edema, and renal failure occur.

As with methanol ingestion, do not give gastric decontamination or activated charcoal. Treat the metabolic acidosis with bicarbonate and give IV ethanol and fomepizole; hemodialysis is effective as well.

ORGANOPHOSPHATE INGESTION

Organophosphates are found in pesticides. They inhibit cholinesterase enzymes and can have permanent bonds over 2–3 days. The result is inability of an impulse to transmit across a nerve synapse. It can take weeks to months for regeneration of these enzymes.

Classic findings seen with organophosphate poisoning are (SLUDGE):

- **S**alivation
- **L**acrimation
- **U**rination
- **D**iarrhea, **D**iaphoresis
- **GI** symptoms
- **E**mesis

As the child worsens, delirium, seizures, and coma occur.

For treatment, it is important for health care workers involved to wear gloves! Decontaminate the child's clothing and skin. Activated charcoal is recommended. Begin ABCs and give 2 antidotes:

1) Atropine—may need large doses
2) Pralidoxime (2-PAM)—only effective before the bond becomes permanent! Always use with atropine.

Diazepam can be used for CNS symptoms. Symptoms can persist for weeks without treatment.

PLANT EXPOSURES

For the Board exam, you need to know a few plants that can cause problems:

- Digitalis effects: Foxglove, lily of the valley
- Atropine effects: Jimson weed, deadly nightshade
- Cyanide effects: Pear and apple seeds, peach pit, bitter almond
- Liver toxicity: mushrooms (lethal ones will have symptoms > 6 hours after ingestion)

BURNS

OVERVIEW

Burns are the second leading cause of unintentional pediatric death. 18% of burns are due to abuse. Burn first aid includes ABCs, removal of clothing, washing off chemicals, covering the burn with a clean dry sheet. For small burns, cold wet compresses may be applied; for large burns do not use cold/wet compresses as this will lead to hypothermia. no grease, butter, or ointments!

First degree burns are classified by superficial redness, minor swelling, and pain. They generally resolve in 3–5 days.

Second degree burns cause blisters or blebs, have redness, and are painful. The tissue underneath is still well perfused. It may take 4–5 weeks for these to heal.

Third degree burns are dry, leathery, waxy, and have no pain associated with them. They require grafting in large areas or healing from the edges in smaller burn areas.

Burn surface area follows the Rule of Nines (> 14 years old):

- Head and neck: 9%
- Each upper limb: 9%
- Thorax and abdomen, front: 18%
- Thorax and abdomen, back: 18%
- Perineum: 1%
- Each lower limb: 18%

notes

Rule of Palm (< 10 years of age)
- Useful in smaller burns
- Child's palm not including fingers = 1% body surface area

MINOR BURN CARE

First degree burns require no therapy
Partial thickness burns:
- Clean with soap and water daily
- Leave blisters intact, débride when ruptured
- Antibiotic ointment (Silver sulfadiazine (Silvadene®) or bacitracin)
- Dressing changes once daily
- Facial burns may be left open
- Pain control
- Td if needed
- Re-evaluate every 2–3 days as the burn may progress

MAJOR BURN CARE

ABCs and don't forget to also consider carbon monoxide.
IVF for burns > 15% body surface area
Parkland Formula:
- Four cc/kg in the first 24 hours, with ½ of the volume in the first 8 hours, the rest over the next 16 hours
- Add maintenance rate to this volume for smaller children

Refer to a burn center for:
- Burns > 15% of body surface area
- Larger burns of hands, feet, face, perineum
- Concern for abuse

ELECTRICAL BURNS

Minor electrical burns are usually asymptomatic and do not require evaluation. Use minor cleansing and antibiotic cream. If the burn is an "extension cord bite" with burns to the oral commissure, refer to a burn surgeon.

High tension, electrical wire burns are serious and require admission. Deep tissue injury is common in this type of burn.

DROWNING

Drowning is a major cause of pediatric injury and death. 40% occur in those < 5 years of age and is more common in boys. With the initial swallowing of water, laryngospasm occurs. Loss of consciousness follows with vomiting and aspiration in 90%. Hypoxia occurs and results in loss of circulation in 3–4 minutes with CNS injury in 3–5 minutes. CNS injury is the most frequent cause of death. Pulmonary aspiration is usually very small, but ARDS or pulmonary edema may develop. Hyponatremia is uncommon.

Hypothermia can be protective. Documented survivors with good outcomes have occurred in those with time underwater of 10–150 minutes in icy water (< 5° C) and had a core temperature of < 30° C. Cold water above this temperature is not protective. Freshwater and saltwater drowning are not managed differently.

Treatment includes the ABCs. Protect the spine if appropriate (abuse, diving injury). Vomiting is common, so apply cricoid pressure or a nasogastric tube if available. Use warmed IVF and oxygen as well as warmed gastric and bladder lavage. You do not have to completely rewarm the patient in most drownings. For freezing-water drowning, do resuscitative efforts until the core temperature is 32° C. Hospitalize all near-drownings for at least 12 hours; respiratory symptoms will develop by 8 hours.

HEAD INJURY

OVERVIEW

Head injuries are a common pediatric complaint. Most are not serious and only require observation. Symptoms to be on the look-out for include vomiting, lethargy, headache, irritability, or behavioral changes.

Physical findings to steer you towards more serious injury:

1) Scalp swelling or stepoff
2) Basilar skull fracture:
   - Raccoon eyes (see Figure 2-3)
   - Battles sign (see Figure 2-4)
   - Hemotympanum
3) Temporal bone fracture:
   - Bleeding from the external auditory canal
   - Hearing loss
   - Facial paralysis
   - CSF otorrhea

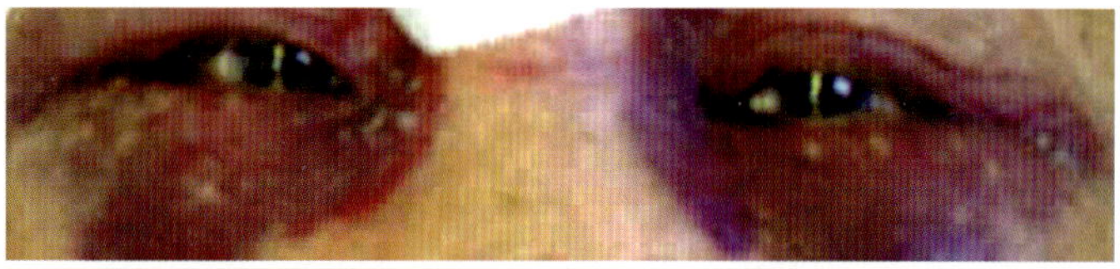

Figure 2-3: Raccoon Eyes

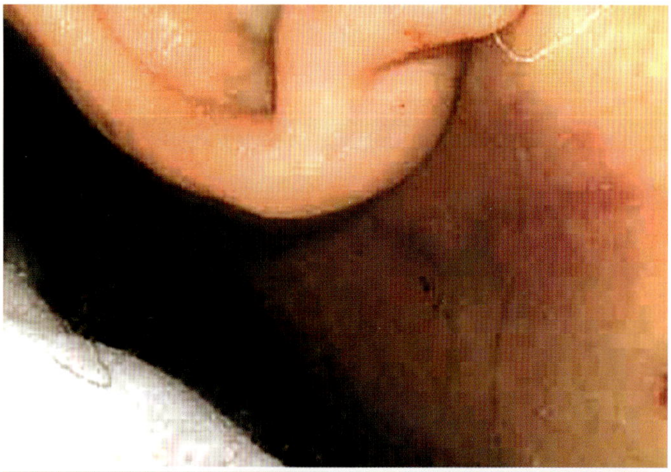

Figure 2-4: Battles Sign

notes

Quick Quiz

1) How do you manage a near-drowning victim?
2) Describe findings in a basilar skull fracture.
3) Describe findings in a temporal bone fracture.
4) What do retinal hemorrhages in an infant indicate?
5) Which is better for diagnosing a skull fracture: a CT scan of the head or x-rays?
6) In a head injury case, when should you definitely order a CT scan of the head?
7) In a head injury case, when is it OK to send the patient home for observation?

Pupillary changes—Note that papilledema does not develop immediately!

Infants:

- Retinal hemorrhages (abuse!)
- Other bruises

There does not have to be significant signs of external head trauma to have a significant brain injury!

SKULL X-RAYS

The best study to diagnose a skull fracture is skull x-rays!

But a few caveats:

- Positive skull films do not mean there is a significant intracranial injury
- Negative skull films do not mean there is not a significant intracranial injury
- Routine skull films are not necessary in children with scalp hematomas, unless there are other findings suggestive of a skull fracture (such as a stepoff)
- Most children with minor head trauma and without symptoms do not need skull films

CT SCAN OF THE HEAD

These are best for looking at intracranial contents, not for skull fractures—it will sometimes miss those parallel to the CT cuts.

When to definitely order a CT scan: (high risk):

- Depressed mental status
- Focal neurological signs
- Signs of basilar skull fracture
- Seizures
- Irritability
- Acute skull fracture
- Bulging fontanelle
- Vomiting more than 5 times in 6 hours
- Loss of consciousness > 1 minute

When to Order a CT scan or Observe for 4–6 hours (High-intermediate risk):

- Vomiting 3–4 times
- Behavioral changes
- Nonacute skull fracture

When to do a CT scan, Skull Films, or Observe 4–6 hours (Intermediate risk):

- Patients with concerning history
- Unknown mechanism of injury
- Physical exam with sign of skull fracture
- In children < 1 year and especially in those < 6 months, probably proceed to CT scan anyway

When to Discharge with Instructions (Low Risk):

- Normal mental status
- Normal neurologic exam(s)
- No loss of consciousness
- No vomiting
- No sign of head trauma
- Mechanism of injury is unequivocally trivial
- No patients involved in MVA or with unwitnessed head trauma are placed in this category!

Notice that I only highlighted the high risk and the low risk groups; the others are controversial and less likely to appear on your Board exam.

CONCUSSIONS

Concussion injury questions on the Boards usually are sports-related. A concussion is defined as a traumatic alteration in mental status and can result in any or all of the following: disturbance of vision, loss of equilibrium, amnesia, headache, cognitive dysfunction, and loss of consciousness.

In the "game" situation, ask the player about the game (e.g. what period is it, the score, the team they are playing) instead of asking for name and phone number. A major concern with second-impact syndrome is head injury occurring again before full recovery from a previous concussion. This can result in loss of autoregulation of cerebral blood flow, with rapid development of increased intracranial pressure.

Many systems exist for grading concussion, but I'll give you a simplified version here to remember:

See Table 2-6. So to make it easy, just remember that for grade I, there is no amnesia and for Grade II, there is no loss of consciousness.

Table 2-6

CONCUSSION GRADES			
Grade	Confusion	Amnesia	Loss of Consciousness
I	Yes	No	No
II	Yes	Yes	No
III	Yes	Yes	Yes

notes

Table 2-7		
CONCUSSION AND TIME TO RETURN TO CONTACT SPORT		
Grade	Minimum Time to Return To Play	Time Asymptomatic
I	20 minutes	At the initial Exam
II	1 week	1 week
III	1 month	1 week

The other big question is "when can the kid return to the game?" See Table 2-7.

After 2 Grade I concussions, 2 weeks is required to return. Any repeat Grade III, or 3rd time of a Grade I or II, means the season is over.

LACERATIONS

Irrigation is the best way to clean a laceration. Make sure that tetanus immunization is up-to-date. On the scalp, do not use Dermabond. Do not use LET (lidocaine, epinephrine, tetracaine) gel on fingers, nose, toes, or penis. Eyelid lacerations require an ophthalmologist for tear duct repair. If the vermillion border needs to be lined up, call a plastic surgeon. A clenched fist hand laceration is at high risk of infection and should be referred to a hand surgeon.

- Complications of lacerations include:
- Tendon laceration with loss of function
- Arterial or vascular compromise
- Infection
- Limited flexibility
- Cosmetic considerations: (Keloid, scarring)

FRACTURES

OVERVIEW

Fractures are common in pediatrics. Most follow the classic Salter Harris classification (see Figure 2-5).

Types I (the epiphysis slips or separates from the metaphysis) and II (a fracture through the epiphyseal plate leaves a fragment of metaphysis attached to the epiphysis) are common and have an excellent prognosis because, although they extend through the growth plate, the germinal layer is usually left intact—so that growth disturbance is uncommon. Undisplaced fractures simply require immobilization in a cast. Types III (a fracture through the epiphysis extending to the epiphyseal plate) and IV (a fracture extends from the articular surface, through the epiphysis, and through the metaphysis) are uncommon, and a precise reduction is required with orthopedic consultant. Involvement of the articular surface and germinal layer make growth disturbance and functional impairment more likely if not managed correctly. This manipulation will usually involve a general anesthetic. Type V is a crushing injury to the epiphysis, not originally described by Salter and Harris. It is rare and has a poor prognosis due to disruption of the blood supply to the epiphysis.

Unfortunately, this is usually diagnosed retrospectively when limb deformity becomes apparent.

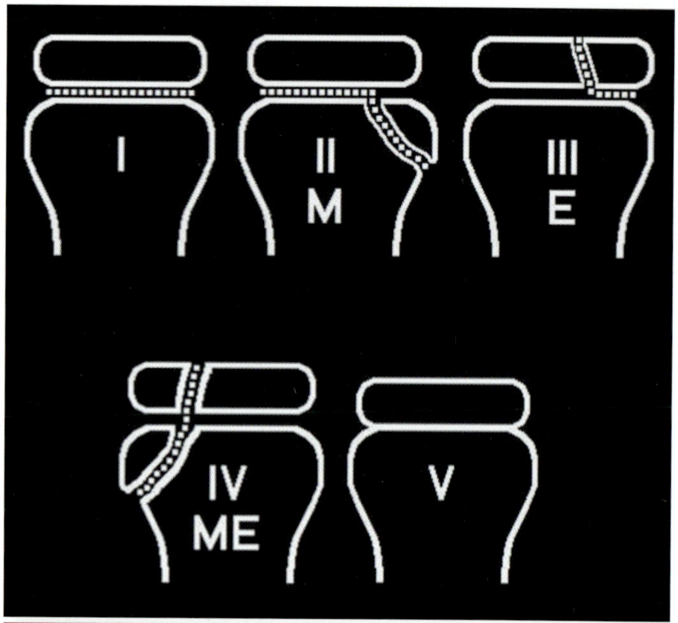

Figure 2-5: Salter Harris Classification of Fractures

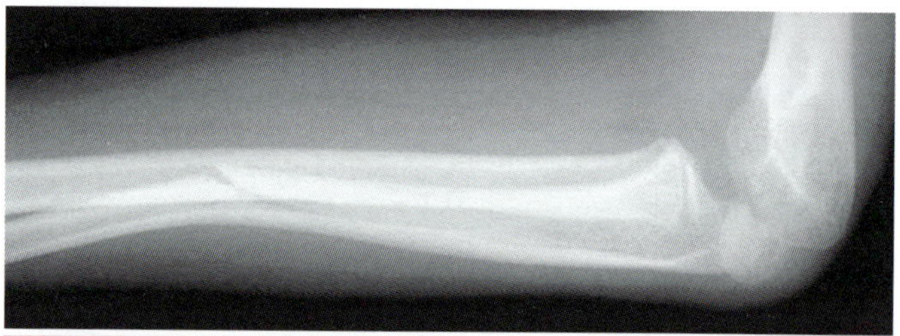
Figure 2-6: Greenstick Fracture

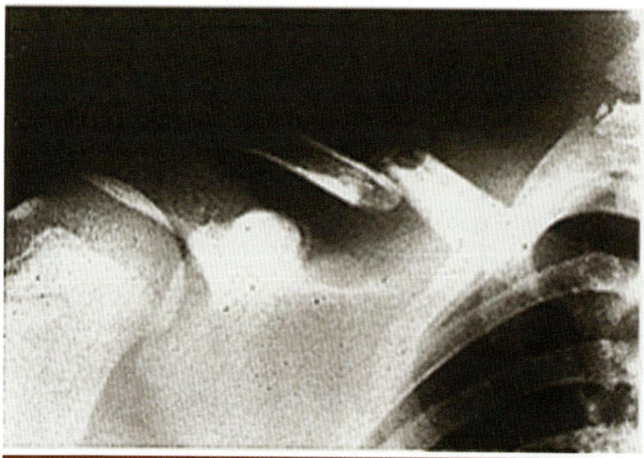
Figure 2-7: Clavicle Fracture

notes

Quick Quiz

1) Explain the Salter Harris classification of fractures.
2) What is the treatment for a greenstick fracture?
3) How do you treat a clavicle fracture?

GREENSTICK FRACTURE

This is a fractured cortex on the tension side and plastic deformity on the compression side. It is not a complete fracture. Immobilization alone is effective therapy. See Figure 2-6.

CLAVICLE FRACTURE

This is the most common fracture in children < 10 years of age. Usually, it affects the middle and lateral portion of the clavicle. Most cases occur as a result of falling on an outstretched arm or direct trauma. Neurovascular injury is uncommon. Diagnosis is usually made by physical exam and/or radiograph (see Figure 2-7).

Treatment is with figure-of-eight clavicle strap, or a simple sling is also often effective. Usually, it heals in 3–6 weeks.

TORUS (BUCKLE) FRACTURE

This is compression of the bone and produces a "torus" or "buckle" fracture. It is most common in the distal radial metaphysis. It usually heals with 3 weeks of immobilization. (see Figure 2-8)

SPIRAL FRACTURE

This sounds just like its name, with a fracture having a curvilinear course. It is most common in toddlers. Think abuse in a child who is not walking yet, especially if it is the femur! (see Figure 2-9)

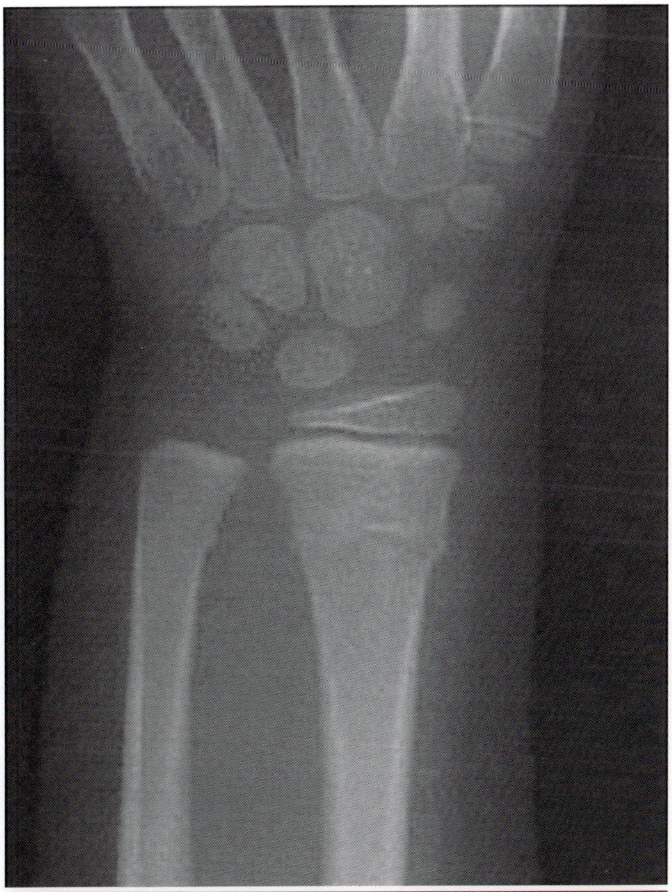

Figure 2-8: Buckle Fracture

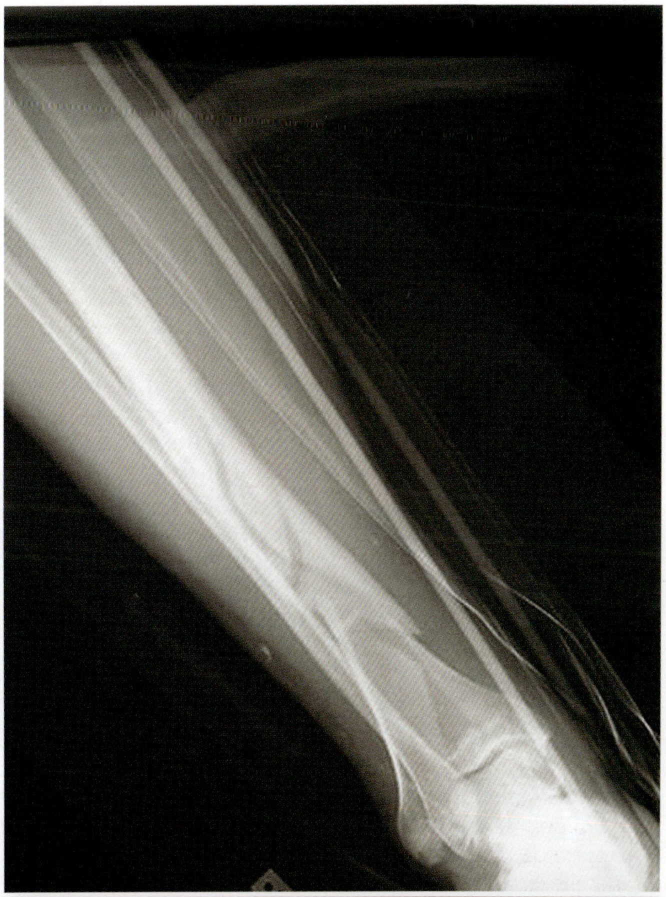

Figure 2-9: Spiral Fracture

notes

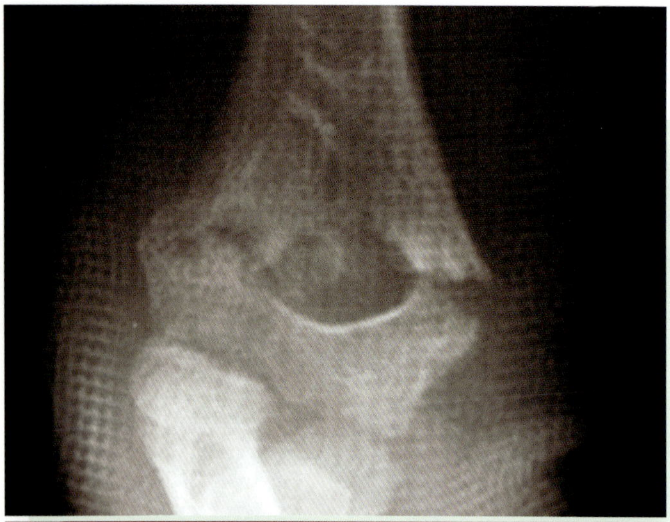

Figure 2-10: Distal Humerus Fracture

DISTAL HUMERUS (ELBOW) FRACTURE

The most common elbow fracture is the supracondylar fracture and occurs usually after a fall on an outstretched hand or elbow. Look for the posterior fat pad sign! These fractures have a high risk of complication. If the fracture is displaced, evaluate for brachial artery, median nerve, or radial nerve damage. Neurovascular status must be monitored carefully! (see Figure 2-10)

FRACTURE COMPLICATIONS

We already mentioned that you should be on the look-out for neurovascular compromise with the supracondylar fracture.

Compartment syndrome is another concern and is most common with tibial and supracondylar fractures. The fracture results in swelling; then vascular injury results leading to ischemia. Tissue blood flow can become compromised. Pulses may be normal! The clue is pain out of proportion to the fracture, especially pain remote to the fracture site. Compartment syndrome requires an emergent orthopedic consult!

Occult fractures are those not evident on x-rays. Clues can include:

- Clinical exam is consistent with a fracture but no fracture seen on x-ray
- Persistent pain
- Gait disturbances, especially in younger children!
- Treat as if fractured and follow x-rays

SUBLUXATION OF THE RADIAL HEAD

This is also known as "nursemaid's elbow." Usually, it occurs in children between the ages of 6 months and 5 years. What happens is that traction occurs on the child's pronated wrist and the annular ligament slides over the radial head. The child then holds the arm limply to the side. X-rays are not necessary. To fix the problem, supinate the forearm and flex the elbow or, alternatively, you can pronate the forearm. Sometimes you hear a "click." After reduction, the child will return to normal functioning of the arm within 15 minutes.

Table 2-8

GRADE OF ANKLE SPRAINS			
	Grade I (Mild)	Grade II (Moderate)	Grade III (Severe)
Swelling	Mild	Moderate	Severe
Tenderness	Mild	Moderate	Severe
Loss of Function	Minimal	Difficult to ambulate	Unable to bear weight
Treatment	7-10 days rest	2-4 weeks rest	5-10 weeks rest

SPRAINS

A sprain is an injury to the ligament around a joint when it is forced to move in an unnatural position. Sprains are rare in prepubescent children because the ligament is stronger than the growth plate; thus, these children more often get fractures than sprains. The most common sprains are of the ankle and fingers. On physical examination, the key thing to look for is tenderness. Swelling and bruising are common as well. Ankle sprains are graded based on the findings in Table 2-8.

In general, you need to obtain x-rays of the ankle to rule out a fracture. Treat with RICE (Rest, Ice, Compression, and Elevation). Ice for 20 minutes every 2 hours for 48 hour—to prevent swelling. The patient should remove the ice if the contact area numbness develops, and protect the skin with a towel if using a plastic bag! Severe strains require a splint for protection and comfort.

EYE ABNORMALITIES

CORNEAL ABRASION

Symptoms of corneal abrasions include pain, tearing, photophobia, and decreased vision. Diagnosis is best made with fluorescein dye and a Slit/Woods lamp (see Figure 2-11). An abrasion is transparent, whereas an ulcer is opaque; both light up under fluorescein. Treat with a topical antibiotic. Do not send the patient home with a topical anesthetic to apply; only use these in the office! Do not use a semi-pressure patch.

HYPHEMA

Hyphema is the presence of blood in the anterior chamber of the eye. Usually, it occurs after blunt or perforating injury, and appears as a bright or dark red fluid level between the

notes

Quick Quiz

1) What is the concern with distal humerus fractures?
2) What is a compartment syndrome?
3) KNOW subluxation of the radial head!
4) Name the common physical findings in a sprain of the ankle.
5) How do you treat an ankle sprain?
6) What are the symptoms of corneal abrasions? How do you diagnose it?
7) What is a hyphema?
8) Explain how to do rescue breaths in an infant and a child. How are they different for each?
9) Explain how to do chest compressions in an infant, younger child, and older child.
10) How do you manage symptomatic bradycardia?
11) How do you manage pulseless vtach?

cornea and iris, or a diffuse murkiness of the aqueous humor. Eye pain is common, as is somnolence. Ophthalmologic consult is required.

Treatment is bed rest, with the head elevated 30–45 degrees and close monitoring of the intraocular pressure. (see Figure 2-12)

PALS

OVERVIEW

Just a few brief things to review, but make sure you know everything on these last few pages about PALS (Pediatric Advanced Life Support). I don't include all of the protocols for you, but mainly the areas that would likely appear on the Board exam.

Always start with your ABCs. For A, remember head tilt/chin lift, jaw thrust, etc. For B, don't forget oxygen (if available); for infants, use mouth-to-mouth/nose breathing and for children you pinch the nose and use mouth to mouth breathing. Breaths are delivered slowly over 1–1 ½ seconds.

CIRCULATION

Overview

Remember: For infants, check the brachial pulse; children and older, the carotid pulse. Start compressions for HR < 60 with poor perfusion.

For infants < 1 year:

- Hands encircle the chest, or 2 fingers over the lower half of sternum
- ½-to-1-inch deep compressions
- 100 times a minute
- 5:1 ratio breaths to compressions

Child 1 to 8 years:

- Heel of one hand over the lower ½ of the sternum
- 1-to-1½-inch deep compressions
- 100 times a minute
- 5:1 ratio breaths to compressions

Child > 8 years:

- Heel of one hand over the lower half of the sternum with heel of the other hand on top
- 1½-to-2-inch deep compressions
- 100 times a minute
- 15:2 ratio breaths to compressions—unless 2 rescuers with a protected airway, then 5:1

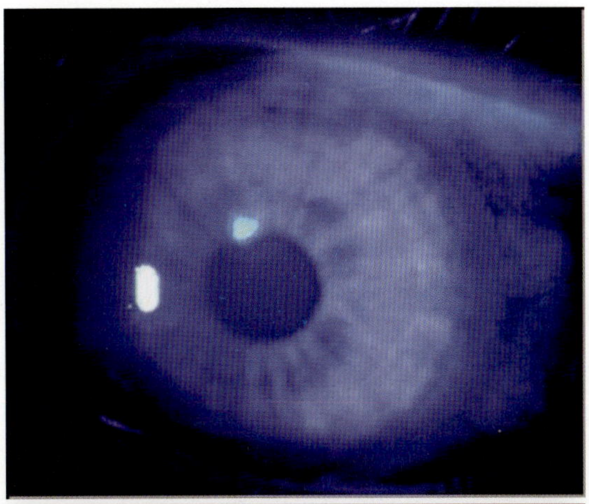

Figure 2-11: Corneal Abrasion with Ulceration

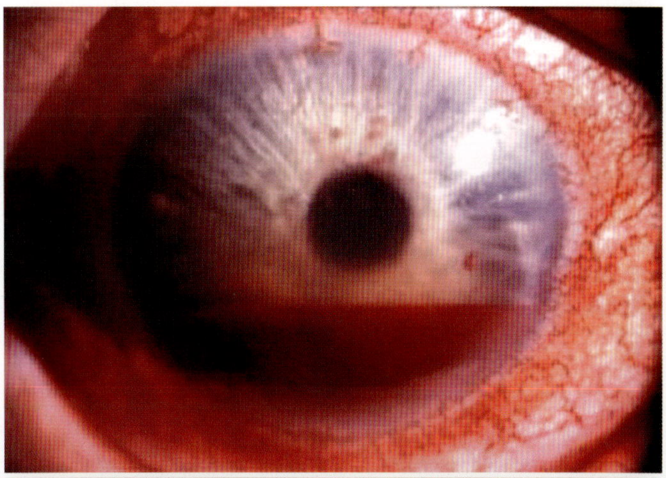

Figure 2-12: Hyphema

notes

Pediatric Bradycardia

If no cardiovascular compromise, just observe!
Cardiovascular compromise and HR < 60:

- CPR
- Epinephrine
  - 0.01 mg/kg (1:10,000, 0.1 ml/kg) IV/IO
  - 0.1 mg/kg (1:1000, 0.1 ml/kg) endotracheal
- Atropine (0.02 mg/kg, minimum of 0.1 mg) (give atropine first if you suspect increased vagal tone or primary AV block!)
- Consider pacing

Pediatric Tachycardia

Covered in cardiology section.

Pediatric Pulseless Algorithm

Vfib or Vtach

- Start CPR
- Defibrillation up to 3 times
  - 2 J/kg, 2-4 J/kg, 4 J/kg
- Epinephrine
  - 0.01 mg/kg (1:10,000, 0.1 ml/kg) IV/IO
  - 0.1 mg/kg (1:1000, 0.1 ml) endotracheal
- Repeat defibrillation after every epi dose
- Lidocaine
- Repeat defibrillation
- Then drug-shock-drug-shock

Not Vfib or Vtach

- CPR
- Epinephrine as above

notes

MedStudy

2nd Edition
Pediatrics Board Review
Core Curriculum

Adolescent Health

Authored by J. Thomas Cross, Jr., MD, MPH, FAAP
and Robert A. Hannaman, MD

Many thanks to

Keith Boyd, MD
Associate Chair of Education
Department of Pediatrics
Rush University Medical Center
Chicago, IL

Adolescent Health

Table of Contents

Adolescent Health

SPECIAL ISSUES OF ADOLESCENTS

Adolescents are a distinctive group of individuals and, unfortunately, the Boards like to ask about them because of the ways they differ from younger children. The definition of an adolescent varies, but most consider them to be 10–21 years of age. Things to note:

1. Adolescents receive much of their care in emergency rooms, and much of this is "non-urgent" care. Injuries are the leading diagnosis category; females present frequently with abdominal pain or sore throat as their main complaint.
2. In the general outpatient clinic, health supervision is the most common diagnostic code for 10–14-year-olds; for 15–24-year-olds, the most common diagnostic code is pregnancy!!!
3. Acne is the 3rd most common problem presented.
4. The reasons for hospitalizations for adolescents (10–21-year-olds—in order of incidence):
   - #1 pregnancy
   - #2 mental disorders
   - #3 injuries
   - #4 digestive tract disorders
   - #5 respiratory tract diseases
5. Smoking, alcohol, and illicit drug use are a continuing problem, and obesity is an emerging issue.
6. Automobile and motorcycle accidents are the leading cause of adolescent morbidity and mortality. Homicides are the 2nd leading cause of death, and the #1 cause of death in African-American adolescents. HIV ranks as #1 in mortality for 24–44-year-old Hispanics and African-Americans, many of whom became infected in adolescence or young adulthood.

Remember these items when a Board question refers to an adolescent. Such questions are likely to involve sex, drugs (even rock and roll if hearing loss is an issue!), injuries, mental illness, pregnancy, emancipation rights, or supervisory guidance.

THE DEVELOPING ADOLESCENT

GENERAL CONSIDERATIONS

Many define the beginning of puberty as the beginning of adolescence. However, in the U.S., pubescence frequently occurs in Caucasian girls at a mean age of 9.7 years (7.8–11.6) and for African-American girls at a mean age of 8.1 years (6.1–10.1)! Puberty for girls generally lasts an average of 4 years (1.5–8 years). In boys, the mean age has remained relatively stable at 11.4 years (9.5–13.5 years), and usually lasts an average of 3 years (2–5 years). Puberty affects everything! Skeletal growth, body composition, cardiorespiratory, hematologic, neuroendocrine, and reproductive changes all occur at varying rates and stages. Chronological age frequently does not correlate with biological maturity. Because of this, most use sexual maturation ratings (our old friend Tanner) to provide us with guidance regarding the "biological" maturation of adolescent patients.

Skeletal growth: During adolescence, skeletal growth accounts for ~ 25% of final adult height. The growth spurt for girls occurs earlier than for boys (Tanner 2–3 for girls vs. Tanner 4 for boys). Girls also reach their final adult height earlier than boys (average: 16 years for girls and 18 years for boys). Hint: Just think of the tall high school girl with the short high school boy!

Body Composition: 40% of adult weight is gained during adolescence. In boys, lean body mass actually increases from 80 to 90%, but girls see a decrease from 80 to 75%. Body fat changes also differ between girls and boys. Body fat increases in girls throughout puberty, up to 26.7%. Body fat increases in boys, up to 11.2%, occurring very early in puberty and remaining stable thereafter. (Well, until they get desk jobs for medical publishing companies.) Visualize the chubby 12-year-old boy at the beach who, at 17, is lean and mean. During puberty, girls keep adding adipose to appropriate areas for curves to occur. Muscle mass generally peaks after the growth spurt.

Hematologic Changes: In boys, blood volume, RBC mass and hematocrit all increase during puberty. No corresponding increases occur in girls.

Cardiorespiratory Development: The heart doubles in weight and systolic blood pressure increases for boys, but these remain stable for girls. For both boys and girls, vital capacity increases markedly as lung size increases; additionally, respiratory rates fall while heart rates increase.

Neuroendocrine Changes: As any parent can tell you, the structure and mass of the brain do not change during adolescence, but there are definite changes in brain activity! It appears that adolescents gradually develop the α rhythm of the adult brain.

Reproductive System Changes: These will be discussed in greater detail in the endocrine section. Girls usually show signs of sexual maturation with breast development (thelarche), which occurs anywhere between ages 6 and 11.5 years. The mean age for the beginning of menses is 12.75 years (10–16.5 years).

SURVIVING ADOLESCENCE

Here we get into those "difficult" years and their attendant issues. Androgens are probably responsible for many of the behavioral changes we see in adolescents. Boys have increasing conflict with their parents, particularly with their mothers, and especially during the growth spurt. Also, all of the extra testosterone causes them to behave more impatiently, aggressively, and irritably. Girls have increased conflicts with their mothers and less contact with their fathers.

On the Board exam (and in the real world), look for a girl maturing early, who likely has greater dissatisfaction with her looks, lower self-esteem and a greater degree of unhappiness. These girls tend to manifest problems in school as their academic interests wane. The opposite is true for boys—it's the "late bloomers" who tend to have a more negative self-concept and body image.

There is a behavioral spectrum that all adolescents go through that we need to examine a little more closely.

notes

Early Adolescence (10–13 Years): Lots of questions about physical maturation; occasional masturbation; increasing emphasis on relationships with peers; cognition is concrete! (For the Boards, if a health issue is presented relative to this age period, look for an answer option favoring the use of simple, explicit discussions using visual and verbal cues.) Kids in this age group tend to be impulsive without cognition.

Middle Adolescence (14–16 Years): Pubertal development is nearing completion, and these kids explore relationships with the opposite (and same) sex. Masturbation frequency increases. Their peers are the most important group for effecting change/support. Cognition begins to develop, but there is noticeable immaturity in ability to interact with the real world. These teens are still very impulsive.

Late Adolescence (17–21 Years): Body image and gender role defined. Individual relationships become more important than peer group. Idealistic! Cognitive development is complete. "Life goals" become the center point of discussion. You will still see impulsiveness, but now with the cognition to understand their actions. (Well, sometimes!)

EMANCIPATION and HEALTH CARE

This is a difficult one for the Boards. In the U.S., the right of an adolescent (minor < age 18) to seek and receive treatment without parental consent varies from state to state. Usually, the right to self-consent for treatment is specified through public health statutes when there is clinical suspicion of a sexually transmitted disease. Many states allow minors to seek help for pregnancy, contraception, drug and other substance abuse, and mental health issues—without parental consent. This is the problem with the Boards—each state is different, so it is difficult to ask these questions. However, there are some "absolutes," or "almosts:"

Emancipated minors: These kids have moved outside of the home and pay their own bills, etc. They are no longer subject to parental authority. Also, this category includes those who are married or members of the military. Being a parent in most states also makes you an emancipated minor.

Emergencies: The physician's judgment to treat may occur without explicit consent of the parent (or the patient, for that matter) if he/she is unconscious or unable to give consent.

Mature-minor rule: This rule is relatively recent. There is a trend to recognize minors who have the ability to comprehend the risks and benefits of a specified treatment/therapy, and they may provide their own consent. Usually, this occurs in cases where the care is "low risk" and will clearly benefit the minor.

Confidentiality is a whole "nuther can of worms." Generally, if you have the ability to self-consent on an issue, you have the right to confidentiality. Exceptions to remember (especially for the Boards) are: child abuse and cases where the minor may cause damage to self or someone else, unless the physician acts or notifies appropriate public/private officials. Some states require legal disclosure to parents, depending on the diagnosis, and this requirement must be conveyed to the minor. The best choice is to encourage the minor to agree to bring the parents into the decision-making process, with you acting as facilitator.

THE ADOLESCENT HEALTH VISIT

This is an important issue, but we'll be brief in our discussion. The key here is to allow the adolescent to become autonomous, and involve the parents only as much as the adolescent wishes. For matters involving sex and substance use, interview the adolescent alone, but inform your patient that in areas of life-threatening behavior (suicide, management of chronic disease, etc.), you have the right to (or by law, must) involve a parent or other guardian. Psychosocial assessment is very important in this age group, but frequently difficult to ascertain. Ask questions about peer and family relationships; depression; sexual relationships, if they have occurred; substance use; and eating disorders. Understand that a minor chief complaint at presentation may not be the real reason for the patient's visit, and it may require a return follow-up to get to the heart of the matter.

Recommend that adolescents have an annual preventive services visit to address the biomedical and psychosocial aspects of health.

Focus physical examination on these important areas:

- Hearing testing, especially if the adolescent admits to listening to loud music
- Vision testing, because the growth spurt also affects the globe, possibly resulting in myopia
- Screening for hypertension
- Scoliosis, which occurs in 5% of boys and 10–15% of girls (the cutoff for referral to orthopedics is generally a 10° curvature or greater)
- Breast examination (most recommend teaching about self-breast examination in this age group, even though the risk of breast cancer is near zero, because of the potential to start "good habits" early)
- Pelvic examination, primarily if the girl is sexually active or is having menstrual problems/abdominal pain
- Scrotum examination (it is very important to instruct boys in self-examination since testicular cancer does occur in this age group!)

Laboratory screening is much more controversial, and not well documented as necessary. However, screen any sexually active adolescent for STDs; conduct a pelvic exam with Pap smear on sexually active girls or those > age 18. Newer recommendations specifically recommend screening all asymptomatic sexually active females for *Chlamydia*. Most recommend tuberculin skin tests for youth who are at risk, but not for general screening. All menstruating girls are at risk for anemia; thus, consider performing a screening HCT, especially in those with heavy menses. Also, consider cholesterol screening for those youth with a family history for early cardiovascular disease or hyperlipidemia. In addition, consider dipstick urinalysis for leukocytes for all sexually active males and females.

notes

Quick Quiz

1) What is the most common reason for 10–14-year-olds to visit outpatient clinics? 15–24-year-olds?
2) What is the #1 reason for hospitalizing adolescents?
3) What is the mean age for puberty in Caucasian girls? African-American girls?
4) True or False: Boys have their pubescence growth spurt before girls.
5) Define an emancipated minor.
6) What are the medical exceptions for notifying parents against an adolescent's wishes?
7) What parts of the physical examination are important to focus on in an adolescent boy or girl?
8) How many MMR inoculations should adolescents have by the time they are 12?
9) How often should adolescents see a medical professional for health supervision and guidance?
10) Who is more likely to smoke, a boy or girl? Drink?

Immunizations (Know): If the adolescent has not had two MMRs, give the second one in early adolescence by age 12 years. Usually, Td boosters are due at age 11–12 years, then every 10 years thereafter. Also, give the Hepatitis B immunization in early adolescence if the teen hasn't already received it. Consider giving the varicella vaccine if there is no reliable history of chickenpox, although some recommend checking titers before giving the required 2 immunizations. Hepatitis A vaccine is indicated in some areas of the U.S., and particularly for youth who are high risk or already have chronic liver disease.

It is very important that you give parents or other adult caregivers health guidance at least once during their child's early, middle, and late adolescence.

Include in this information:

- Normal adolescent development
- Signs and symptoms of disease and emotional distress
- Parenting behaviors that promote healthy adolescent adjustment
- Ways to be role models for adolescent behaviors in the household
- How to monitor/manage new drivers
- Adequate weapon control in the house
- Removing weapons and lethal medications in a house where an adolescent has suicidal intent
- Ways to monitor adolescent social and recreational use of tobacco, alcohol and other drugs, and sex

A key point that the Boards might ask about: Give adolescents health guidance annually to promote injury prevention (including seat-belt use, alcohol/substance use, especially while driving, helmet use, violence management, weapon safety, and exercise preparedness to prevent injury). Most also recommend annual diet guidance, as well as health guidance regarding sexual behaviors and substance abuse (including anabolic steroids). The key thing to know here is that if adolescents participate in one risky behavior, it is more than likely they are participating in others!

All of the above come from the Guidelines for Adolescent Preventive Services (GAPS).

SUBSTANCE ABUSE

Alcohol and tobacco use remains alarmingly high in adolescents. The mean age for smoking is 12 years, and 12.6 years for alcohol consumption. Girls smoke more often than boys, but boys consume alcohol nearly twice as often as girls. ~ 50% of adolescents use marijuana: the mean age of first use is 14.4 years. Close to 10% of adolescents use cocaine, and ~ 5% use crack.

Table 3-1

RISK FACTORS FOR DEVELOPMENT OF SUBSTANCE ABUSE
Household drug use (especially by parents)
Peer group use
Attention deficit disorder (ADD, ADHD)
Depression
Anxiety disorders
Impulse control problems
Unnecessary, aggressive outbursts

Table 3-2

SUBSTANCE ABUSE TESTING--REASONS TO SCREEN AN ADOLESCENT
Trauma
Unexplained accident
Psychiatric symptoms
School performance deterioration
Unexplained chronic illness
Increased absenteeism
Suicide attempt
Altered mental status

notes

How can you tell if a kid is on drugs?

Signs vary and can be very difficult to interpret (know):
- An increasing degree of emotional and/or physical isolation from family
- Absent or hostile communication
- A decrease in school performance or increased absenteeism
- New disinterest in athletics
- Changes in peer group population
- Involvement in a crime
- Participating in other risky behaviors, including sex

Risk factors for development of substance abuse are listed in Table 3-1.

Now a more controversial question: When is it appropriate to screen an adolescent for substance abuse? The AAP's policy is that drug testing of the older, competent adolescent should be voluntary. However, look for certain signs that make you think about screening (Table 3-2). Almost all drugs can be routinely tested in urine. The one exception is LSD (lysergic acid diethylamide). See Table 3-7 and Table 3-8 at the end of this section for commonly abused substances and their side effects/clinical manifestations.

DEPRESSION

In prepubertal kids, there is no gender difference in rates of depression. However, at post-puberty, girls are 2–3x more likely to experience depression than boys. Co-morbid mental illness is common; and don't forget to look for anxiety disorders, substance abuse, attention-deficit disorder (ADD), and disruptive behaviors.

Look for 9 symptoms, in addition to the major symptoms of depressed mood/irritability and diminished interest (especially on the Board exam!) See Table 3-3. If an adolescent has the major symptoms of depressed mood/irritability, 4 or more of the 9 other findings in Table 3-3, and they occur for > 2 weeks, a "Major Depressive Disorder" is occurring.

Table 3-3

DEPRESSION IN ADOLESCENTS
Weight loss, gain or failure to make expected weight milestones
Decrease or increase in appetite
Insomnia or hypersomnia
Psychomotor agitation or retardation
Fatigue and energy loss
Feelings of worthlessness
Excessive/inappropriate feelings of guilt
Decreased ability to concentrate/think
Recurrent thoughts of death

Note: If these symptoms occur within 3 months of an identifiable stressor, consider this an adjustment disorder with depressed mood. Finally, don't forget that in adolescents, depression can present as sadness or boredom.

Dysthymic disorder presents as a more chronic/depressed state with at least 3 of the 9 symptoms present for at least 1 year, without evidence of specific major depressive episodes.

Bipolar Affective Illness or Cyclothymic Disorder occurs when the adolescent has periods of depression alternating with mania or hypomania.

What else should you look for? Hypothyroidism, nutritional deficiencies, chronic infections (mononucleosis, HIV—if at risk), or a chronic systemic illness (e.g., SLE). Don't forget that substance abuse frequently presents in these ways.

Treatment for depression is complex, and requires a multifaceted approach including medications, such as SSRIs (selective serotonin reuptake inhibitors). Recent literature, however, has called into question the "overuse" of SSRIs in children and adolescents, especially when other therapies have not been attempted prior to using SSRIs. Head-to-head studies demonstrate that tricyclic antidepressants are not as effective as SSRIs for early-onset depression, so avoid them as treatment. Once started, continue SSRIs for a minimum of 6 months. Bipolar disorder requires therapy with lithium, valproic acid, or carbamazepine. If untreated, a major depressive episode can last 7–9 months, and recurrence occurs in 70% of adolescents within 5 years. The earlier the adolescent/child is affected with depression, the more severe and recurrent the depression is likely to be.

When do you hospitalize these adolescents? Hospitalization is appropriate when the patient is suicidal, psychotic, manic, abusing substances, or not responding to outpatient therapy.

EATING DISORDERS

Overview

The incidence of anorexia nervosa and bulimia has increased in recognition and occurrence in the last century. There appears to be a genetic predisposition for eating disorders, and serotonin activity in particular appears to play a role. Neurotransmitters may also play an etiologic role in development of these disorders.

Anorexia Nervosa

Anorexia nervosa occurs in about 1/100 girls, age 16–18 years. The peak incidences usually occur at 2 points in time: ages 14.5 years and 18 years. Some estimates say 25% of these girls may start < age 13! Girls outnumber boys by 10:1. One source says that boys affected generally also may have "gender identity" issues.

Diagnose anorexia nervosa by using the DSM-IV criteria (see Table 3-5). Often, girls appear "normal" before exhibiting this disorder yet, in reality, tend to be overachievers and perfectionists. Other psychiatric disorders are commonly associated, including obsessive-compulsive and affective disorders. Risk periods seem to be during the transition into middle/junior high, high school, and college. Also, these disor-

notes

Quick Quiz

1) What are 7/9 symptoms to look for in depression?
2) Under what conditions should you hospitalize an adolescent with psychological problems?
3) How common is anorexia nervosa? Bulimia?
4) What are the diagnostic criteria for anorexia nervosa?
5) In anorexics, what ECG changes suggest increased risk for ventricular arrhythmias?
6) True or False: Bulimic girls are usually underweight.

ders commonly are preceded by an announced intention to go on a diet. On the Boards, look for the gymnast/ballet dancer!

Early intervention is critical. Conduct a general physical exam, including Body Mass Index, vital signs, and orthostatic measurements. In severe anorexia, heart rates may fall to 20 beats/min, and hypothermia is fairly common. Consider lab tests if the patient has been abusing laxatives and/or diuretics, or inducing vomiting. With laxative and diuretic abuse and excessive vomiting, look for hypokalemia and a hypochloremic metabolic alkalosis. Hematology can also be severely affected, with bone marrow suppression resulting in low WBCs and anemia. In girls, LH, FSH, and serum estradiol levels are low. In boys, testosterone levels are low. In both boys and girls, cortisol and endorphins are elevated. ECG changes: Look for ST-segment depression on exercise stress testing or prolonged QT intervals—these are associated with increased risk of ventricular tachycardias! CHF can occur if the severely debilitated patient is hydrated too rapidly! Daily weight gains should be limited to 0.2–0.4 kg/day!

Treatment is comprehensive and involves psychotherapy (for both the patient and family), behavior modification, and nutritional guidance. Consider pharmacotherapy if depression also is present; SSRIs may be helpful in preventing recurrence.

Table 3-5

DSM-IV CRITERIA FOR DIAGNOSIS OF ANOREXIA NERVOSA
Intense fear of becoming obese, which does not decrease as weight loss occurs
Disturbance in the way the adolescent views her/his own body weight, size or shape (examples: "I feel fat" even though normal or abnormally below weight for height; "My thighs are huge" even though no body fat is visible)
Refusal to maintain body weight over a minimal normal weight for age and height (15% below the norms for weight for height)
In females, absence of 3 consecutive menstrual cycles

Bulimia

Bulimia is even more common than anorexia nervosa—it occurs in 2–5% of girls but < 1% of boys. Adolescents may have anorexia and bulimia concurrently, or may alternate between the two. Generally, these are older girls in the mid-to-late adolescent period. The goal in the bulimic's eye is to lose weight. This is also a DSM-IV diagnosis (see Table 3-4). These adolescents may be of normal weight or slightly overweight. Initial symptoms may include fatigue, bloating, irregular menses, and sore throat (due to excessive vomiting). Physical findings are important, especially on the Board exam!! Look for bilateral parotid gland swelling, calluses on the dorsum of the fingers (from inducing vomiting), and loss of tooth enamel from the acid vomit. Aspiration pneumonia can also occur. If she is using syrup of ipecac, she may induce hypokalemia and resultant cardiac toxicity. Also look for a metabolic alkalosis and elevated amylase levels.

Bulemia often accompanies an obsessive-compulsive or affective disorder. Consider SSRIs in this subset of patients. Interventions must address the binging/purging behavior early on, as well as the underlying psychopathology.

SEXUAL DEVELOPMENT

Female Issues

Breast

Estrogen is the most influential factor in breast development during puberty. It binds to breast tissue and causes growth of the glandular ductal system. Obviously, other hormones, such as progesterone, play important roles. Progesterone affects alveolar growth, as do insulin, growth hormone, etc. Estrogen requires the presence of these hormones for breast growth to occur.

Initial, pubertal breast development occurs as a proliferation of ductal and stromal tissue and fat deposition. This is known as the "breast bud." Puberty results in both lobular-alveolar and ductal growth. Lactation occurs later, and is due to the presence of prolactin and adrenal steroids.

Table 3-4

DSM-IV CRITERIA FOR DIAGNOSIS OF BULIMIA
Recurrent episodes of binge eating (rapid intake of food in a short period of time)
A feeling of "lack of control" over eating behavior during these binges
Regularly has self-induced vomiting, uses laxatives, enemas or diuretics, strict dieting or fasting, or vigorous exercise to prevent weight gain
A minimum average of 2 binge-eating episodes/week for at least 3 months
Persistent concern with body shape/weight

notes

Asymmetrical growth, where one breast will develop more slowly than the other, is fairly common, and this may persist into adulthood. Breast atrophy is a sign of an eating disorder, with associated severe weight loss and loss of breast and fatty tissue. Accessory breast tissue (polymastia) and accessory nipples (polythelia) occur along the mammalian nipple line in 1–2% of girls. Juvenile hypertrophy, a massive enlargement of one or both breasts, may require mammoplasty after completion of breast maturation, particularly in those where the hypertrophy is severe.

Breast masses are fairly common in the adolescent breast, but bloody discharge, skin dimpling, and nipple retraction are not. The most common breast masses are solitary cysts, fibrocystic changes, and fibroadenomas. A solitary cyst is the most common breast mass in the adolescent. > 1/2 of these cysts will resolve in 2–3 months and do not require further study; simply follow up with serial exams. You can use ultrasound if physical examination cannot differentiate cystic from solid masses. Recurrent cysts usually represent fibrocystic change—known as "benign proliferative breast change"—and are due to a physiologic response of breast tissue to cyclic hormones. The most common symptom of fibrocystic changes is bilateral pain in the upper-outer quadrant of the breast. The pain usually begins in the premenstrual cycle and stops soon after menses. Treat with support, using non-steroidal medications for pain. Oral contraceptives also may reduce the frequency and duration of pain.

When do you refer for surgical intervention? Persistence of a mass or enlargement over 3 menstrual cycles warrants referral for an aspiration. This will likely reveal the more common cyst and its fluid. If negative or inconclusive, order an excisional biopsy (wide margins are not usually indicated). Do not use mammography for routine screening or for adolescents with breast masses. Self-breast exam instruction is controversial in this age group, because the risk of breast cancer in this age group is near zero. There is the balance between increasing unnecessary anxiety (almost every mass identified is benign), and fostering a valuable, preventive health routine in adolescents that can strengthen future behavior (self-exams) as an adult. Most breast masses that do not regress or change with hormonal fluctuations turn out to be fibroadenomas—a benign mix of stromal elements, ducts, and acini. The mass is usually painless and rubbery in character. They are usually in the upper, outer quadrant of the breast and range from 1–3 cm. They have no malignant potential. Cystosarcoma phyllodes are rare, and are rapidly growing lesions that have a small risk of becoming malignant. Intraductal papilloma is a benign, slow-growing tumor located under the areola. It may present with a serous, or sometimes bloody, discharge. Primary breast cancer is extremely rare in adolescents. Only 0.2–3% of all breast cancers occur in those < than age 25 years. Breast cancers present in adolescents as a hard, fixed mass with overlaying skin changes, frequently under the nipple. Family history is extremely important, but only ~ 6% will have breast cancer-associated cancer genes. Remember: Ultrasound and biopsy are the procedures of choice.

Mastitis is a localized breast infection that is more commonly seen in newborns and lactating women. You might also see it occasionally in a non-pregnant adolescent. The most common organism identified is *Staphylococcus aureus*; thus, treat with anti-staphylococcal antibiotics, heat, and analgesia.

Amenorrhea

Primary amenorrhea refers to the absence of menses by: 1) age 16 years with normal sexual secondary sexual development (breast development); or 2) age 14 years in the absence of any breast maturation. Others more simply define primary amenorrhea as lack of menses by age 16. Secondary amenorrhea refers to loss of menses for > 3–6 consecutive months with previous regular cycles, or for > 9–12 months in those with previously irregular cycle lengths. Note: pregnancy is the most common reason for secondary amenorrhea, and can also be an etiology of primary amenorrhea for some adolescents. Don't forget, though, that irregular cycles are common in adolescents, so the duration of amenorrhea may or may not be helpful in determining if true secondary amenorrhea is occurring. (Obviously, if an adolescent with irregular cycles presents with amenorrhea for 5 months, you are also going to seriously consider pregnancy as an etiology).

Causes of amenorrhea are central (hypothalamic or pituitary), ovarian, or anatomic (uterus, cervix, vagina).

Central: If the hypothalamus is the culprit, it is usually due to partial or complete inhibition of gonadotropin-releasing hormone (GnRH) release. This can be due to nutritional deficiencies, cystic fibrosis, anorexia nervosa, excessive exercise, stress, or some drug (phenothiazine-like products). Local lesions in the hypothalamus that could disrupt release are comparatively very rare. Don't forget that isolated GnRH deficiency has been associated with Kallmann syndrome and the inability to smell (anosmia). Deficiency of pituitary gonadotropins (isolated gonadotropin deficiency is rare and pituitary gonadotropin deficiency is usually due to panhypopituitarism) may be the result of tumors (most common is craniopharyngioma), infiltrative disease (sarcoidosis, tuberculosis), or infarction. Note: In women who are of reproductive age, the most common pituitary cause of amenorrhea is a prolactin-secreting adenoma (prolactinoma most commonly). Look for galactorrhea too, but it is found in only ~ 60% of young women—but almost always found on the ABP.

Ovarian: Remember that the ovary produces estrogen and progesterone; therefore, if the ovary is malfunctioning, menstrual irregularities are likely. Problems can include gonadal dysgenesis, premature ovarian failure, infection, hemorrhage, and autoimmune oophoritis. Note: 10% of primary amenorrhea is due to gonadal dysgenesis, frequently as a result of Turner (XO) syndrome. Secondary amenorrhea can be associated with gonadal dysgenesis also, particularly mosaic Turner syndrome!

Polycystic ovaries and chronic hyperandrogenic anovulation are common causes of secondary amenorrhea and, occasionally, primary amenorrhea. A clue in 50% of patients with polycystic ovaries is an LH:FSH ratio > 2.5:1. This indicates a chronic hypothalamic dysfunction. Really, anything that in-

notes

Quick Quiz

1) What is the most likely type of breast mass you will find in an adolescent girl?
2) When should you further investigate a breast mass?
3) What is the most common cause of mastitis?
4) What is the most common reason for secondary amenorrhea?
5) Amenorrhea and anosmia should make you consider what syndrome?
6) In a girl with galactorrhea and amenorrhea, what is the most likely etiology?
7) What is significant about the FSH:LH ratio in girls with polycystic ovary disease?
8) Describe signs of androgen excess in amenorrhea.
9) A girl presents with her first menses and hemorrhages to a hematocrit of 20%. It is difficult to stop her bleeding. What is the likely etiology for her excessive blood loss?
10) What is the cancer seen in girls of mothers who took diethylstilbestrol (DES)?

creases circulating androgen hormones will result in amenorrhea, hirsutism, and virilization, as seen in polycystic ovaries. Examples include Cushing syndrome, anabolic steroid abuse, adrenal adenomas, etc.

Anatomic: These are frequently due to a defect in the development of the müllerian duct system, resulting in imperforate hymen, vaginal atresia, or absence/malformation of the cervix or uterus. If any of these is present (with the exception of the absence of a uterus), normal menses occur but is blocked, resulting in painful swelling above the blockage. Rokitansky syndrome is müllerian agenesis with primary amenorrhea and absence/hypoplasia of the vagina, cervix, and/or uterus. Asherman syndrome occurs with uterine synechiae occurring after endometrial disruption/infection, leading to secondary amenorrhea with obstruction/obliteration of the uterine cavity.

How do you assess amenorrhea? Evaluate with the usual complete history and physical but, of course, pay particular attention to where in the hypothalamus-pituitary-gonadal axis there might be a problem. Pubic, axillary, and facial hair development indicate androgen defect/problems. Look at breast and vaginal mucosa for maturation effects of estrogen. Always perform pregnancy testing first! Then ask about things that could cause "central" etiologies, such as weight loss, nutrition, excessive exercise, and/or stress. Look for any physical signs of Turner syndrome and for galactorrhea (prolactinoma).

Signs of androgen excess: hirsutism, acne, voice changes, and clitoromegaly. Pelvic examination is important to identify possible anatomic etiologies.

Lab screens after a negative pregnancy test usually include: LH and FSH to differentiate between a hypothalamic and an ovarian etiology; prolactin level to determine a pituitary microadenoma; and TSH for thyroid difficulties. If you suspect androgen excess during the physical exam, order testosterone and dehydroepiandrosterone levels.

While waiting on these results, perform a progesterone challenge to evaluate if estrogen is present and the anatomy is normal. Give 10 mg of medroxyprogesterone for 7 days, and expect bleeding by days 2–7 after completion of the course. If no bleeding occurs, the anatomy is disrupted or there is not enough estrogen. Next, give 2.5 mg oral conjugated estrogen (Premarin®) for 25 days with 10 mg oral medroxyprogesterone added from day 16–25. If still no bleeding occurs, order pelvic sonogram/CT and hormonal levels, including estradiol levels. Anatomic abnormalities resulting in obstruction usually require surgical correction.

Polycystic ovaries usually require cycling with estrogen and progesterone (usually oral contraceptives). Hirsutism may require electrolysis. If you find a pituitary microadenoma, use bromocriptine. True ovarian failure requires hormone replacement therapy with larger doses of conjugated estrogens and medroxyprogesterone on days 16–25.

Dysfunctional Uterine Bleeding

Dysfunctional uterine bleeding is defined as vaginal bleeding that occurs in cycles < 20 days or > 45 days, lasts > 8 days, results in blood loss > 80 mL, and/or is associated with anemia. Dysfunctional uterine bleeding is further subdivided into primary (most common) and secondary.

Primary dysfunctional uterine bleeding is usually due to an immature hypothalamus-pituitary-gonadal system. Anovulatory cycles are common early in most adolescents and are characterized by large variations in estrogen levels and a lack of progesterone.

Secondary dysfunctional bleeding is usually due to coagulation disorders and underlying disease processes of the vagina, cervix, uterus, and ovary. The most common cause of excessive bleeding that requires hospitalization is the presence of a bleeding disorder. Abnormal bleeding at the time of menarche may be the first sign for some of these diathetic bleeding episodes, especially von Willebrand disease. Others to consider include Factor VIII or IX deficiency, thrombocytopenia, platelet disorders, thalassemia major, and leukemia.

Anatomic causes include lacerations to the vagina, hymenal tears, and foreign bodies. Diethylstilbestrol (DES) used in the 60s and early 70s can cause a rare, DES-related clear cell adenocarcinoma in girls of mothers who took it, which may present as vaginal bleeding. Cervical problems, such as STDs and polyps, also can cause bleeding. Endometritis is an etiology of uterine origin, and usually results from preceding infection. Treatment of secondary dysfunctional bleeding usually involves assistance from a gynecologist, and will not be discussed further here. However, if you discover an underlying cause prior to such referral, obviously you should take care of it.

notes

Dysmenorrhea

This is one of the leading causes of school absenteeism in adolescents, because over 2/3rds of teenage girls have it. We have a pretty good idea what causes this. Most dysmenorrhea is due to prostaglandin production before menses, which causes vasoconstriction and muscular contractions. Remember that the cyclooxygenase pathway of arachidonic acid makes PGE_2, PGD_2, and $PGF_{2\alpha}$, which cause vasoconstriction, followed by vasodilation, and muscle contraction and relaxation. The biggest increase in the prostaglandins occurs just before menses. Alternatively, leukotrienes are involved in some women, because they are produced during the last steps of the lipoxygenase pathway. These agents stimulate smooth muscle to contract. So, based on this information, give cyclooxygenase inhibitors like ibuprofen or naproxen for dysmenorrhea in hopes that it is due to the more common cyclooxygenase pathway, If it commonly occurs and is predictable during the cycle, it may be best to start before the symptoms begin. For women who don't respond, their pain is likely due to the lipoxygenase pathway. Secondary dysmenorrhea is due to other conditions, such as infection, ectopic pregnancy, endometriosis, and other etiologies. Besides agents that inhibit the synthesis of prostaglandins (ibuprofen, naproxen), oral contraceptives are very effective in reducing or eliminating dysmenorrhea.

Male Issues

Breast—Gynecomastia

Gynecomastia occurs in ~ 50% of boys ages 10–16 years, and is most commonly seen around age 14. It is due to a decreased ratio of androgen to estrogen and a change in the sensitivity of breast tissue receptors. The area is usually tender and asymmetric. Most gynecomastia resolves spontaneously within 3 years. Rare causes of gynecomastia to look for (especially on the Boards) are Klinefelter syndrome; anabolic steroid abuse; tumors of the testicles, adrenal, or pituitary; and some illicit drugs, such as marijuana and amphetamines. "Normal" pubertal gynecomastia is usually < 4 cm and does not require specific workup or therapy, because most will resolve spontaneously. If it is "macrogynecomastia," and > 5 cm (similar to a 2–3 Tanner female), it usually will not regress, and may require surgical therapy; recent studies show promise using tamoxifen and testolactone.

Scrotal Masses

3 types of scrotal masses may occur during adolescence: congenital, acquired, and infectious.

Congenital masses include scrotal dermoid, polyorchism, and scrotal rests (abnormal tissue from other organ systems, such as spleen or adrenals). Congenital masses usually require surgery.

Acquired lesions include hydroceles, spermatoceles, varicoceles, torsion of the spermatic cord or the testicular appendage, trauma/hematocele, and neoplasms. Each of these is described in more detail below.

Hydroceles are non-tender and fluid-filled masses, the evaluation of which is helped by ultrasound. Also, they can be transilluminated. Generally, no treatment is required unless they become painful or too large.

Spermatoceles are located in the efferent ductal system, and will present as a nodule above and posterior to the testes. Key things to remember here are: there is no change with Valsalva, and they transilluminate. These do not affect fertility and generally do not require therapy.

Varicoceles are usually idiopathic, but may be secondary to intraabdominal masses, hepatosplenomegaly, etc. In the physical examination section on a Board exam question, you will see the words "bag of worms" as a descriptor. They are usually left-sided and increase with Valsalva. They can decrease spermatogenesis if they last a long time, and you will need to perform surgery if the testicle has become hypotrophic on that side.

Torsion of the spermatic cord is a surgical emergency! Patient presents with acute onset of severe pain and swelling in the testis, inguinal area, and possibly lower abdomen—usually with accompanying nausea/vomiting. The exam will show a diffusely swollen and tender testicle, and the cremasteric reflex is absent. A radionucleotide scan will show decreased uptake in the scrotal images. You might also consider a Doppler ultrasound. A urologist may attempt a manual "detorsion;" if this is not successful, the patient requires emergency surgery for either an orchiopexy or orchiectomy (if necrotic).

Torsion of the testicular appendage affects the appendix testis or appendix epididymis. A common symptom is either sudden or gradual pain at the upper pole of the testis. The examination will show a tender, pea-sized swelling at the upper pole of the testis and the "blue dot" sign (a blue hue visible through the scrotum). Doppler flows and radionuclide scans will show normal-to-increased values (as compared to torsion of the spermatic cord). Treat with analgesics and anti-inflammatories; the torsion will resolve spontaneously in 2–12 days without surgery.

Trauma/hematocele is, as the name implies, due to trauma. It is associated with onset of pain from the trauma, and swelling may or may not be present. Use ultrasound if you are concerned about an enlarging hematocele. Analgesia, ice, and scrotal elevation are helpful. If the hematocele continues to enlarge, surgical drainage is likely necessary.

Neoplasms usually present as painless swelling, unless hemorrhage or necrosis has occurred, which then typically causes pain. The patient may complain of back pain if retroperitoneal lymph nodes are present. 95% are germ cell tumors (most commonly seminoma, embryonal carcinoma, teratoma, and choriocarcinoma), and the other 5% are of stromal tissue origin. Physical exam will usually show an irregularly shaped firm mass. Workup includes hCG (increased in choriocarcinoma, mixed germ cell tumors), α-fetoprotein (yolk-sac tumors and embryonal carcinoma), testicular ultrasound, and CT scan of chest and abdomen. Note: Most seminomas do not produce any markers! Scrotal masses are evaluated with ultrasound or MRI. Treatment includes orchiectomy and peritoneal lymph node dissection, as well as radiation and chemotherapy, depending on the staging. Pre-treatment

notes

Quick Quiz

1) What is the usual etiology for dysmenorrhea?
2) True or False: Gynecomastia in boys is rare.
3) True or False: Gynecomastia in boys is usually tender and asymmetric.
4) Define hydroceles, spermatoceles, and varicoceles.
5) True or False: Torsion of the spermatic cord is a surgical emergency.
6) Which radiologic test is usually best for examining the scrotum and its components?
7) What is the most common cause of epididymitis in an adolescent male?
8) Which form of contraceptive is also effective for preventing sexually transmitted diseases?
9) Name the absolute contraindications for using oral contraceptive pills.

Table 3-6

CONTRAINDICATIONS FOR ORAL CONTRACEPTIVES
ABSOLUTE
Abnormal vaginal bleeding of unknown cause
Estrogen-dependent tumor
Liver disease
Thromboembolic disease
Cerebrovascular events
RELATIVE
Diabetes mellitus
Seizures
Vascular headaches (including migraines)
Severe/moderate hypertension
Tobacco use

sperm banking is recommended. Overall survival is 70%—and > 95% in stages I and II.

Infectious etiologies of scrotal masses include epididymitis and orchitis. In adolescents, epididymitis is usually due to an STD, and in decreasing frequency, to *C. trachomatis, N. gonorrhoeae, E. coli, Pseudomonas,* or Gram-positive cocci. Pain is usually acute at onset, and patients will present with increased urinary frequency, dysuria, urethral discharge, and fever. The examination will show a swollen and tender epididymis. U/A, Gram stain, and culture of discharges and urethra are usually diagnostic. To differentiate epididymitis from torsion, radionucleotide scan and Doppler will show increase uptake and flow, respectively, compared to torsion. Azoospermia can result, even with appropriate therapy. Therapy is discussed later in this chapter, and the key is to treat both *Chlamydia* and gonorrhea.

Orchitis is usually a result of preceding epididymitis. Here, the patient presents with a swollen and tender testicle and fever. If mumps is involved (very rare today due to the vaccine), a preceding or concurrent parotitis is likely. Workup and treatment are the same as with epididymitis—unless mumps is likely, in which case just supportive care is indicated. If atrophy occurs after orchitis, there is a high risk of cancer; bilateral atrophy usually leads to infertility.

CONTRACEPTION

Unfortunately, contraception discussions with adolescents come up on average, 6 + months after initial sexual intercourse. Frequently, with women, these discussions occur during a visit for a missed period. There are numerous forms of contraception available, but the only one that has 100% efficacy is abstinence. However, some other contraceptives get pretty close to that surety level. Oral contraceptives, for example, are 99.9% effective if used correctly. IUDs are 98–99% effective. Male condoms are 97% effective if used "perfectly," but, in real-world situations, are about 87% effective. Female condoms are 95% effective if used as directed by the manufacturer but, in real-world settings, are only 79% effective. A diaphragm with spermicide is 94% effective if used as directed, but in the real world, the rate is ~ 80%. Injectables such as depo-medroxyprogesterone are 99% effective in real-world settings. The L-norgestrel implant had become popular in adolescents, where long-term contraception (5 years) could be achieved, but its manufacturer pulled it from the market. "Periodic abstinence" or "rhythm" methods result in 90–94% effectiveness in "perfect" usage, but in real-world settings, the effectiveness is ~ 80%. The only method, besides abstinence, that prevents against STDs is male condoms; recommend them to adolescents, even if they are using other forms of birth control, to reduce the risk of sexually transmitted diseases.

Absolute and relative contraindications to oral contraceptives (OCPs) are listed in Table 3-6.

Emergency contraception has become a topic of increasing conversation in the United States, with the release of mifepristone (RU-486®). This agent prevents 100% of pregnancies if taken within 72 hours of intercourse. Other methods include combination pill formulations that contain 100 µg ethinyl estradiol + 0.5–1.0 mg norgestrel, with a second pill taken 12 hours later. These agents will work 74% of the time if used in the first 24 hours, but have significant side effects, including nausea/vomiting and menstrual irregularities. Numerous other combinations are reported in the literature.

notes

SEXUALLY TRANSMITTED DISEASES

OVERVIEW

Prevalence of STDs

Well, you knew this would have to be in the Adolescence chapter, right? > 50% of adolescents have had sex by age 16, and 75% by age 19. These groups commonly become infected with sexually transmitted diseases. Prevalence rates vary, but 10–25% of sexually active adolescents have *Chlamydia trachomatis* (many asymptomatic). The reported rates of *Chlamydia* and gonorrhea are highest among females ages 15–19. Of additional concern is that 20–60% of sexually active female adolescents have human papillomavirus DNA, which can predispose to cervical cancer. In this section, we'll go through each of the STDs, hitting on the important things you need to know for each. But first, some closely related topics.

Prevention

Abstinence is the most reliable way to prevent STDs. However, we are dealing with adolescents (see above % who are sexually active), so a male condom is the cheapest and—thinking "real world" here—the most effective means of prevention available. Female condoms appear to be effective as mechanical barriers for viruses, including HIV; however, no studies have really evaluated the effectiveness of these in the prevention of STDs. Vaginal spermicides are not effective in preventing STDs, and rectal spermicides actually may increase risk of transmission because of their role in facilitating damage to rectal cell linings. Vaginal sponges and diaphragms are protective against cervical gonorrhea and *Chlamydia;* however, teens should never rely on either of them to prevent HIV. Don't forget that Hepatitis B is a sexually transmitted disease, and pre-exposure vaccination is very effective in preventing transmission!! Recommend the Hepatitis A vaccine to men who have sex with men (MSM) and/or with illegal drug users (both injection and non-injection).

Reporting and Confidentiality

Syphilis, gonorrhea, chlamydia, and AIDS are reportable diseases in every state. HIV infection and chancroid are reportable in many states. For reporting other STDs, the requirements vary by state. The laboratory or the provider, depending upon the state, can do reporting. STD reports are strictly confidential. In most states, they are, by statute, protected from subpoena.

Pregnant Adolescents

Offer all pregnant women HIV testing. Also do all of the following at the 1st prenatal visit: Syphilis testing, Hepatitis B Surface Antigen (HBsAg), testing *for Chlamydia trachomatis* and *N. gonorrhoeae*, Hepatitis C antibody testing, and Pap smear, if not done in the preceding year.

Do not perform routine serial cultures for Herpes virus (HSV) during pregnancy. You must perform prophylactic cesarean section only if active lesions are present at the time of labor/delivery. The presence of genital warts is not an indication for cesarean section. Do not conduct routine screening of pregnant women for *Trichomonas vaginalis*.

Children

Management of children (i.e., not consenting adolescents) who have STDs are, by definition, victims of sexual abuse; treatment requires incorporating the use of highly skilled individuals, including the pediatrician, laboratory personnel, social workers, psychologists, and child protection authorities. Gonorrhea, syphilis, and *Chlamydia*, if acquired after the neonatal period, are ~ 100% indicative of sexual contact. For other diseases, such as Human Papillomavirus and vaginitis, the association is not as clear.

HIV

Recommend testing for HIV for all who seek evaluation and treatment for STDs, as well as for those exhibiting high-risk behaviors who present with other conditions. Counseling before and after testing is an integral part of the testing procedure. You must obtain informed consent before performing an HIV test. HIV infection is diagnosed by testing for antibodies against HIV-1 and HIV-2. First, you order antibody testing with a sensitive screening test, the EIA, (enzyme immunoassay; formerly ELISA). A Western blot (WB) or an immunofluorescence assay (IFA) confirms repeatedly reactive EIA tests. If the confirmatory test is positive, the patient has HIV infection and is presumed infectious to others. Within 3 months of infection, 95% of those infected will have positive antibodies. More than 99% of infections in the U.S. are due to HIV-1.

Look for the acute retroviral syndrome (especially on the Board exam!!). It is characterized by fever, malaise, lymphadenopathy, and skin rash. (Granted, it looks and sounds like any viral infection, but be suspicious if they present an adolescent with specific risk factors for HIV in the question's history!) It usually occurs in the 1st few weeks of infection, before antibody testing is confirmed positive. The test to order for the acute retroviral syndrome is a HIV PCR-DNA test or, in some centers, HIV plasma RNA (viral load) is used. Current guidelines report possible benefit from early therapy in these patients; quickly refer to an HIV specialist to help make this determination. Further treatment/evaluation of HIV-infected patients is covered in the Infectious Disease Section.

STDs CHARACTERIZED by GENITAL ULCERS

Overview

In the U.S., there are 3 possibilities for STDs characterized by genital ulcers: herpes, syphilis, or chancroid. Granuloma inguinale (Donovanosis) occurs more prominently in other parts of the world.

notes

Quick Quiz

1) How common is sex among adolescents?
2) Who has the highest prevalence rates of gonorrhea, males or females?
3) What are the "reportable" diseases in every state?
4) What screening laboratory tests should be done or offered to a pregnant adolescent?
5) For which viral infection is prophylactic cesarean indicated? Under what conditions?
6) Describe the acute HIV retroviral syndrome.
7) Differentiate the genital lesions of HSV from Syphilis.
8) How do you identify a positive Tzanck prep (multinucleated giant cell)?
9) True or False: Patients on herpes-suppressive therapy who do not have active lesions still may be shedding virus.

Herpes Simplex

Genital herpes is a recurrent, life-long infection. There are 2 types of HSV: HSV-1 and HSV-2. Most genital herpes are HSV-2. > 50 million people in the U.S. have genital herpes infection. Most of these patients have mild or unrecognized infection, but still shed the virus intermittently! Typical lesions are painful, itchy, and with multiple vesicles—a clue that helps to differentiate genital herpes from syphilis and chancroid (see below). See Figure 3-1.

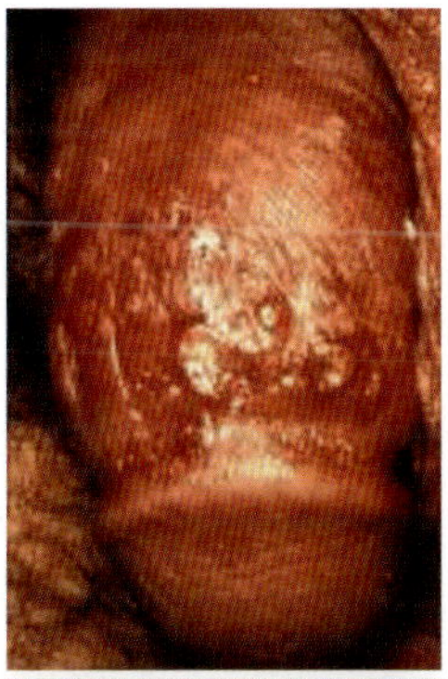

Figure 3-1: HSV -2

Diagnosis: Isolation of HSV in cell culture is the preferred virologic test in patients who present with genital ulcers, especially since the typical, painful, multiple vesicular lesions or ulcerative lesions are absent in many infected individuals.

Reliable, type-specific serologic tests are available. Those that are FDA-approved are IgG-based assays that are type-specific (POCkit HSV2®, HerpeSelect-1 ELISA IgG® or HerpeSelect-2 ELISA IgG®, and HerpeSelect 1 and 2 Immunoblot IgG®).

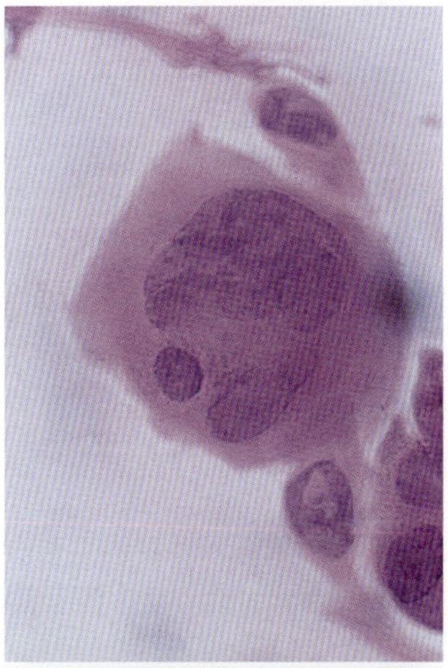

Figure 3-2: Giant Cells

Use these serologic tests in those who have presumed false-negative HSV cultures to diagnose those with unrecognized infection, and to manage sex partners with genital herpes.

PCR technology is helpful for identifying HSV infection of the CNS.

Tzanck preparations are insensitive, nonspecific, and pretty much appear only on Board Exams now! (See Figure 3-2 for the classic multinucleated giant cells).

Treatment of herpes genital herpes: Offer antiviral therapy since it is beneficial to most patients. These drugs will partially control symptoms in initial episodes or recurrences and can be used to suppress future outbreaks. They are most helpful if initiated within 24 hours of symptoms. For episodic, recurrent therapy, many patients experience a prodrome of itching and burning; initiate therapy before physical appearance of lesions. but, these drugs do not eradicate latent virus, nor do they modify recurrences once they are stopped. Three drugs are approved: acyclovir, valacyclovir (the valine ester of acyclovir that provides better oral absorption), and famciclovir (a pro-drug of penciclovir, with better oral absorption than acyclovir). Topical therapy is worthless.

Note: Don't worry about memorizing specific dosages of drugs listed for herpes and other STDs, unless specifically told they are important. Whew!

First clinical episode of Genital Herpes:
- Acyclovir 400 mg t.i.d. x 7–10 days
- Famciclovir 250 mg t.i.d. x 7–10 days
- Valacyclovir 1 g b.i.d. x 7–10 days

Episodic therapy for Recurrent Genital Herpes:
- Acyclovir 400 mg t.i.d. or 800 mg b.i.d. x 5 days
- Famciclovir 125 mg b.i.d. x 5 days
- Valacyclovir 500 mg b.i.d. or 1g/day x 3–5 days

Suppressive therapy for Recurrent Genital Herpes:
- Acyclovir 400 mg b.i.d. daily
- Famciclovir 250 mg b.i.d. daily
- Valacyclovir 500 mg or 1 gm q day

Remember that, even with suppressive and other therapies, subclinical viral shedding still occurs, so encourage adolescents to continue to use condoms.

For those with severe disease or those with disseminated infection, use IV acyclovir 5–10 mg/kg IV q 8 hours.

Herpes and pregnancy: The risk of transmission to the neonate from an infected mother is very high—30–50% if the mother has her 1st episode of genital herpes near delivery. The risk of transmission is < 1% if she acquired the infection in the 1st half of pregnancy, or if she has recurrent herpes at term. Women who have no signs or symptoms (or prodrome) of herpes at delivery may deliver vaginally. Perform cesarean section if lesions are present at the time of delivery. Do not take routine viral cultures at the time of delivery since they do not predict viral shedding.

notes

Syphilis

Overview

Syphilis is a systemic illness due to the spirochete *Treponema pallidum*. There are 3 well-described stages of syphilis, and patients may present at any stage for treatment.

Primary infection is characterized by a painless ulcer or chancre at the site of infection. (See Figure 3-3, chancre).

Secondary infection can vary in appearance and presentation, but frequently will present with a skin rash, mucocutaneous lesions, and lymphadenopathy. Classically, the rash is described as "nickel and dime" lesions on the palms and soles (See Figure 3-4).

Tertiary infection presents later with cardiac, ophthalmic, and auditory abnormalities, and gummatous lesions.

Latent infections, those without clinical manifestations, are detected by serologic testing. Latent syphilis acquired during the preceding year is known as "early latent syphilis," and the patient is generally infectious. "Late-latent syphilis" generally occurs after the 1st year of infection.

Diagnosis

If lesions are present, darkfield examination or direct fluorescent antibody testing of the exudate or tissue is diagnostic. A presumptive diagnosis is possible using 2 serologic tests for syphilis in sequence:

1) nontreponemal tests (Venereal Disease Research Laboratory {VDRL} and Rapid Plasma Reagin {RPR}) and
2) treponemal tests (Fluorescent treponemal antibody absorbed {FTA-ABS} and *T. pallidum* particle agglutination {TP-PA}).

So, first get the nontreponemal test, and then the confirmatory treponemal test. Which one you use doesn't really matter. It mainly depends on the laboratory you are using. The nontreponemal tests correlate fairly well with disease activity. A 4-fold rise or fall in titer is considered a clinically significant difference. Note: You cannot compare a VDRL with an RPR. You must use the same test. Nontreponemal tests usually become nonreactive with time after treatment. However, some patients can persist with low titers; this is known as a "serofast" reaction.

On the other hand, for most patients, treponemal tests (e.g., FTA-ABS) will be positive for life, regardless of treatment. About 15–25% who are treated for primary syphilis will sero-revert after 2–3 years. Because of this, the treponemal tests are not good for looking at therapeutic responses!

Neurosyphilis can be difficult to diagnose in a patient with a positive *serum* test. If the CSF-VDRL is positive, the patient has neurosyphilis. It is a very specific test. In contrast, a negative CSF-VDRL is very insensitive, and will miss many people who really have neurosyphilis. Usually, the diagnosis of neurosyphilis relies on a variety of clinical and laboratory findings: elevated CSF WBC, and elevated CSF protein, with or without clinical manifestations. Recently, some have advocated getting an FTA-ABS test on CSF. It is less specific than a CSF-VDRL, but it is very, very sensitive. Some believe that a negative CSF FTA-ABS excludes neurosyphilis, but this point is still controversial.

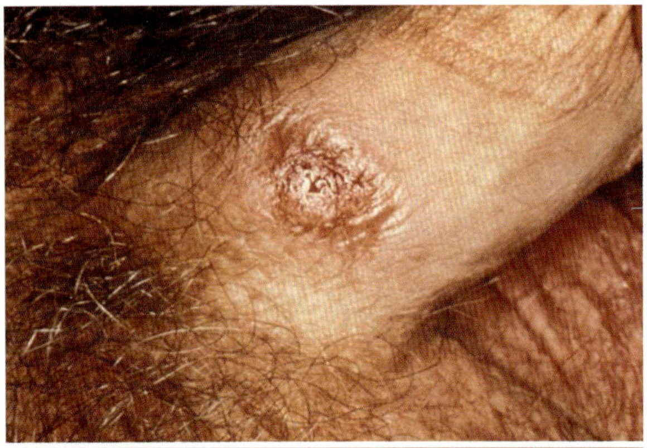

Figure 3-3: Primary Syphilis, Painless Chancre

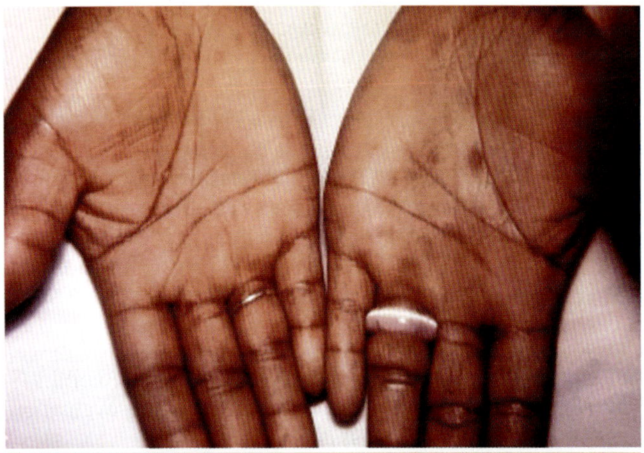

Figure 3-4: Secondary Syphilis, "nickel and dime" rash

Treatment: Drug of Choice for Syphilis

Parenteral penicillin G is the drug of choice for all stages of syphilis. It is the only drug to use in a pregnant woman. If she is penicillin-allergic, desensitize her! The Jarisch-Herxheimer (allergic) reaction is an acute febrile response accompanied by headache, myalgia, and other symptoms within the first 24 hours after beginning treatment for syphilis.

Treatment of Primary, Secondary, and Early Latent Syphilis

Benzathine penicillin G 2.4 million units IM x 1 dose (if the patient is < 48 kg, dose with 50,000 units/kg IM), or

Doxycycline 100 mg b.i.d. x 14 days or tetracycline 500 mg qid x 14 days (use only if non-pregnant and penicillin-allergic!)

Patients should be re-examined clinically and serologically (VDRL or RPR) 6 and 12 months following treatment. Assume patients have failed therapy or been re-infected if they have signs or symptoms that persist, recur, or have a sustained 4-fold increase in titer. Treatment at this point is usually weekly injections of the benzathine penicillin G 2.4 mil-

notes

Quick Quiz

1) Describe the palmar rash of secondary syphilis.
2) How do you diagnose syphilis?
3) What are the specific treatments for primary syphilis, secondary syphilis, and late-latent syphilis?
4) Describe how to diagnose and treat neurosyphilis.
5) A pregnant woman is diagnosed with primary syphilis. She has a history of anaphylaxis to penicillin. What is the best treatment for her?
6) An infant is diagnosed with congenital syphilis. What are possible physical findings to look for? What is the specific treatment necessary?

lion units IM for 3 weeks; also evaluate these patients for HIV, and perform a CSF analysis.

Treatment of Late Latent Syphilis, Tertiary Syphilis, or Syphilis of Unknown Duration

Benzathine penicillin G 2.4 million units IM q week x 3 weeks (If the patient is < 48 kg, use a dose of 50,000 units/kg IM) or

Doxycycline 100 mg b.i.d. x 28 days or tetracycline 500 mg q.i.d. x 28 days (only for non-pregnant, penicillin-allergic)

Evaluate patients with latent syphilis, or syphilis of unknown duration, for evidence of tertiary disease (aortitis, gumma, iritis). If the patient has neurologic or eye signs/symptoms, evidence of active tertiary syphilis (aortitis, gumma, iritis), treatment failure, or HIV infection, also perform a CSF evaluation.

Follow-up includes repeat testing at 6, 12, and 24 months.

Treatment of Neurosyphilis

Know that CNS disease can occur at any stage of syphilis, from primary to tertiary. Clinical clues of neurologic involvement include: cognitive dysfunction, motor or sensory deficits, ophthalmic or auditory symptoms, cranial nerve palsies, or classic meningitis symptoms. Note: A great presentation is a young person with hearing loss!! In this scenario, always think neurosyphilis! CSF is indicated in all of these cases. Also, don't forget about uveitis!

Preferred: Aqueous crystalline penicillin G 3–4 million units IV q 4 hours, or 18–24 million units/day as continuous infusion for 10–14 days.

Alternate: Procaine penicillin 2.4 million units IM q day + probenecid 500 mg q.i.d. x 10–14 days.

(Some experts will also give benzathine penicillin G 2.4 million units IM q week x 3 weeks at the end of neurosyphilis therapy.)

If penicillin-allergic, you can use ceftriaxone 2 grams/day IM/IV x 10–14 days (but some get cross-reactivity); most desensitize the patient.

Follow-up: If you initially find increased CSF WBCs, repeat CSF every 6 months until CSF WBCs are normal. CSF-VDRL and CSF protein decreases much more slowly than CSF WBCs, and may not be normal until ~ 2 years out. If the CSF is not normal after 2 years, re-treatment is probably indicated.

Congenital Syphilis

Diagnosis of congenital syphilis is complicated, because we have no definitive test for the infant. Transplacental transfer of IgG antibodies occurs, as does transfer of maternal non-treponemal and treponemal antibodies.

If an infant is born to a mother with a +VDRL or +RPR, examine the infant for clinical findings of congenital syphilis:

- nonimmune hydrops
- jaundice
- rhinitis
- hepatosplenomegaly
- skin rash
- pseudoparalysis of an extremity.

Because of these complexities, the CDC has come up with different scenarios to help us sort this out:

1. Infants with proven or highly likely disease have:
- An abnormal exam
- 4-fold or greater serum VDRL or RPR than the mother's
- Positive darkfield or fluorescent antibody test of body fluid

For these infants the following are recommended:
- CSF for VDRL, cell count and protein
- CBC
- Other tests, if clinically indicated: long-bone x-rays, CXR, liver functions, cranial ultrasound, eye and hearing screens.

Treat infants in this category of proven or highly likely congenital syphilis:

Aqueous crystalline penicillin G 50,000 units/kg/dose IV q 12 hours during the first 7 days of life, then q 8 hours thereafter to complete 10 days, or procaine penicillin 50,000 units/kg/dose IM q day x 10 days.

If you miss > 1 day of therapy, you have to restart at day 1.

2. Infants with normal physical examination and a serum-quantitative, nontreponemal-serologic titer the same or < 4x the mother's titer, and one of the following findings:
- Mother was not treated, or treatment status is unknown
- Mother was not treated with penicillin
- Mother was treated < 4 weeks before delivery
- Mother's syphilis is staged early, and her nontreponemal test has not changed 4-fold

For these infants the following are recommended:
- CSF for VDRL, cell count and protein
- CBC
- Long-bone x-rays

Treatment of this set of patients is varied and slightly controversial:

Most recommend treating with the same as "proven" above, although some say a single dose of benzathine penicillin G 50,000 units/kg/dose IM is acceptable, if the evaluation (CSF, CBC, long-bone films) is normal.

notes

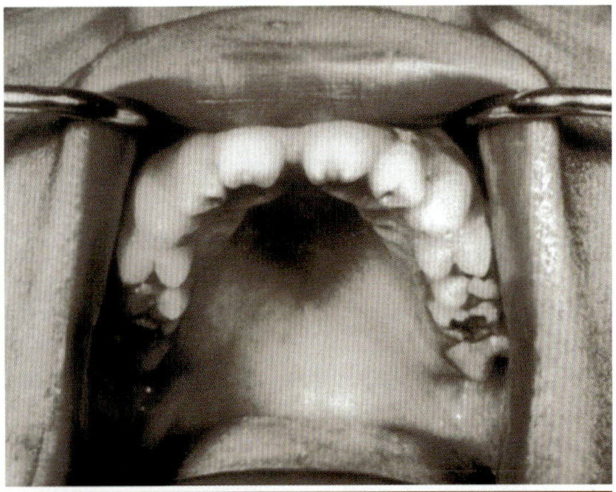

Figure 3-5: Hutchinson Teeth

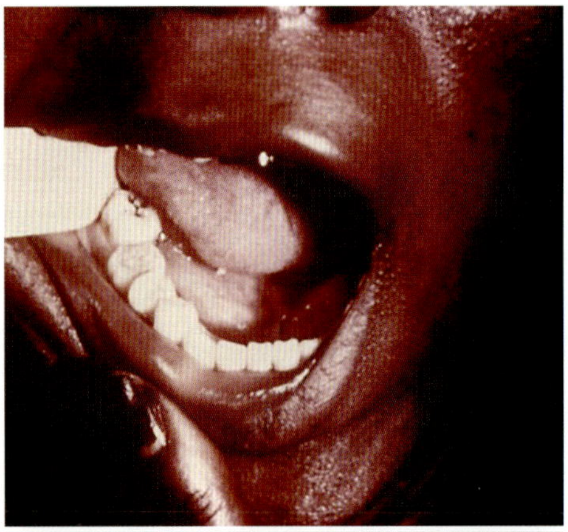

Figure 3-6: Mulberry Molar

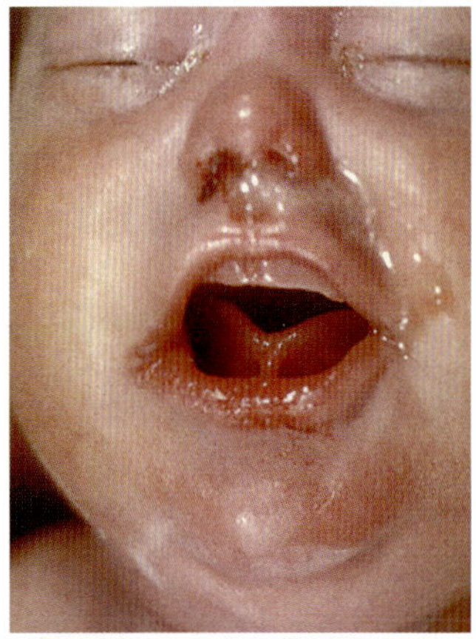

Figure 3-7: "Snuffles"

3. Infants who have a normal physical examination and a serum-quantitative, nontreponemal-serologic titer the same or < 4-fold the maternal titer and all of the following are true:

- Mother was treated during pregnancy, and treatment was appropriate > 4 weeks before delivery
- Mother's nontreponemal titers decreased 4x for early syphilis, or remained stable and low for late syphilis
- Mother has no evidence of relapse or reinfection

For these infants, no further evaluation is necessary.

Give these infants benzathine penicillin G 50,000 units/kg/dose IM x 1.

4. Infants with a normal physical examination and a serum–quantitative-nontreponemal serologic titer the same or < 4x the maternal titer and:

- Mother's treatment was adequate before pregnancy
- Mother's nontreponemal serologic titer remained low and stable before and during pregnancy, and at delivery (VDRL ≤ 1:2; RPR ≤ 1:4)

These infants require no further evaluation.

Treatment: No treatment is recommended; however, some specialists would treat with a single IM injection, as in #3 above.

Here are some congenital syphilis pictures that could show up on the Board Exam:

- Hutchinson Teeth Figure 3-5; note the notching.
- Mulberry molar: The first lower molar is now "dome-shaped" due to congenital syphilis. Figure 3-6 .
- Syphilitic rhinitis ("Snuffles"), highly infectious. Figure 3-7.

Conclusion for neonatal syphilis: On the Board Exam, if you are ever in doubt about whether to treat, just do it! It is likely the right answer 95% of the time ☺.

Chancroid

Chancroid is much rarer than either herpes or syphilis but can occur in the U.S., especially in discrete outbreaks. The infection is due to *Haemophilus ducreyi*, which must be cultured on special culture media. See Figure 3-8. There is no FDA-approved PCR test available for this organism. Patients present with painful ulcers (unlike syphilis) and inguinal adenopathy. See Figure 3-9.

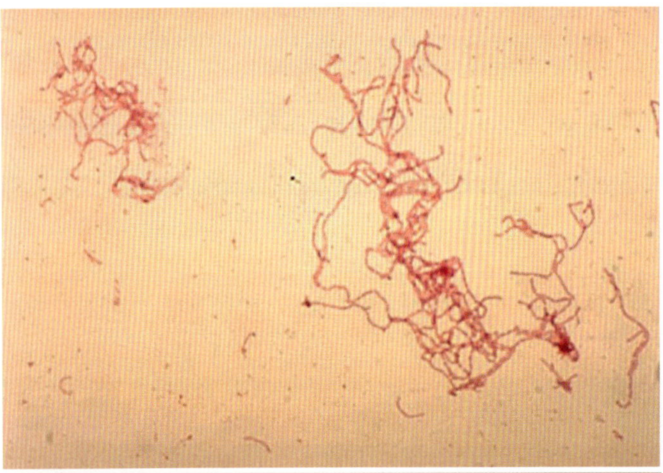

Figure 3-8: Chancroid

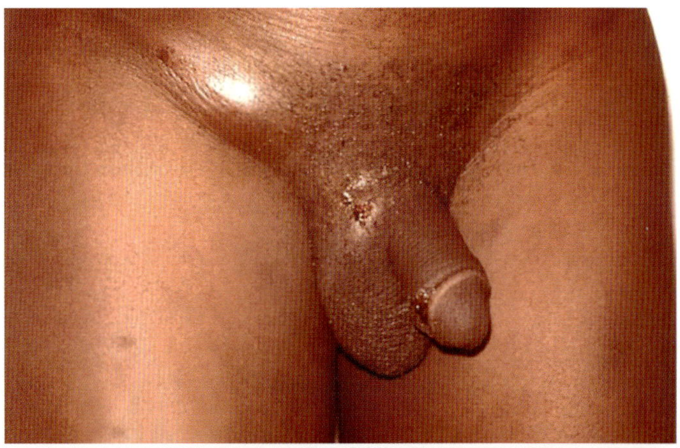

Figure 3-9: Chancroid with Inguinal Lymphadenopathy

notes

Quick Quiz

1) What organism is responsible for chancroid?
2) How does chancroid present, compared to syphilis?
3) How does Granuloma inguinale present?
4) What is the organism responsible for Granuloma inguinale? Can you spell it correctly? Can you pronounce it?
5) What organism is responsible for Lymphogranuloma venereum?

Diagnosis of chancroid can be made on a clinical basis:

1. One or more painful genital lesions are present
2. No evidence of syphilis by darkfield examination of ulcer exudate, or a serologic test for syphilis done at least 7 days after the onset of the ulcers
3. The clinical presentation is consistent and regional lymphadenopathy, if present, is consistent
4. HSV testing was performed on the ulcer and is negative

painful ulcers and suppurative inguinal adenopathy is pathognomonic for chancroid.

Treatment of chancroid:

- Azithromycin 1 gram x 1, or
- Ceftriaxone 250 mg IM x 1, or
- Ciprofloxacin 500 mg b.i.d. x 3 days, or
- Erythromycin 500 mg t.i.d. x 7 days

Granuloma Inguinale (Donovanosis)

Granuloma inguinale is caused by *Calymmatobacterium granulomatis*. It is rare in the U.S. It presents as a painless, progressive ulcerative lesion without regional lymphadenopathy (See Figure 3-10). These lesions are extremely vascular and can easily bleed on contact. Diagnose by visualizing dark-staining Donovan bodies on tissue-crush preparation or biopsy.

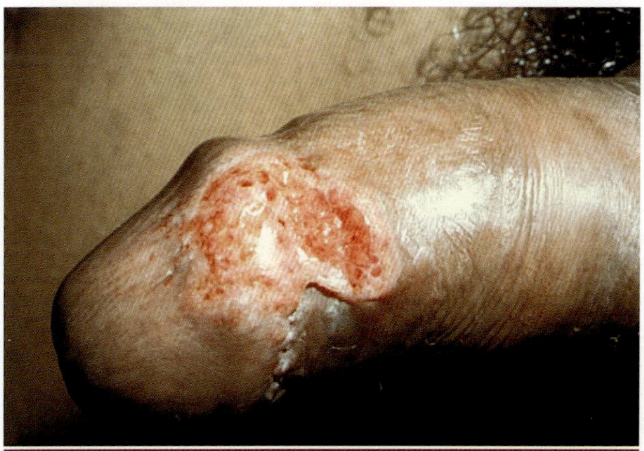

Figure 3-10: Granuloma Inguinale

Treatment:

- Doxycycline 100 mg b.i.d. x 3 weeks, or
- Trimethoprim-sulfamethoxazole DS b.i.d. x 3 weeks

Use either for a minimum of 3 weeks, or until all lesions heal. Alternatives can include:

- Ciprofloxacin 750 mg b.i.d. x 3 weeks, or
- Erythromycin 500 mg q.i.d. x 3 weeks, or
- Azithromycin 1 gm q week x 3 weeks

Lymphogranuloma Venereum

Lymphogranuloma Venereum (LGV) is due to *Chlamydia trachomatis serovars* L1, L2, or L3 (the L's go with Lymphogranuloma). Patients present with a genital ulcer at the site of inoculation, followed by unilateral tender inguinal and/or femoral lymphadenopathy. The ulcer has usually disappeared before the patient seeks treatment. Use serology for diagnosis, and a complement fixation titer ≥ 1:64 is consistent with LGV.

Treatment: Doxycycline 100 mg b.i.d. x 21 days
Alternative: Erythromycin 500 mg q.i.d. x 21 days

STDs with URETHRITIS and CERVICITIS

Chlamydial Infections

Men: Urethritis is due to an infection that classically presents as a urethral discharge or mucopurulent/purulent material with occasional dysuria. Asymptomatic infections are common. The main 2 organisms to worry about in men are *Neisseria gonorrhoeae* and *Chlamydia trachomatis*. It is called "Nongonococcal" urethritis (NGU) if Gram-negative intracellular diplococci are not seen on urethral smears. *C. trachomatis* is the most common cause of NGU, but other organisms such as *Ureaplasma urealyticum*, *Mycoplasma genitalium*, *Trichomonas vaginalis*, and Herpes simplex have been described. Make diagnosis by Gram stain. If Gram stain shows ≥ 5 WBCs/oil field, this is highly sensitive and specific for urethritis. Also, you can do a leukocyte esterase test on first-void urine or microscopic examination of first-void urine for ≥ 10 WBCs/high power field. If these are not found, do specific tests for *N. gonorrhoeae* and *C. trachomatis*.

Treatment of chlamydial infections in men:

- Azithromycin 1 g x 1 dose, or
- Doxycycline 100 mg b.i.d. x 7 days

Alternative:

- Erythromycin 500 mg q.i.d. x 7 days, or
- Erythromycin ethylsuccinate 800 mg q.i.d. x 7 days, or
- Ofloxacin 300 mg b.i.d. x 7 days, or
- Levofloxacin 500 mg q day x 7 days

notes

Some patients will have recurrent or persistent urethritis. Evaluate for *T. vaginalis*, and also ensure that any partners are treated. If you are assured of compliance and the partners have been treated, use the following for treatment:

- Metronidazole 2 g x 1 dose

plus

- Erythromycin 500 mg q.i.d. x 7 days, or erythromycin ethylsuccinate 800 mg q.i.d. x 7 days

Women: Mucopurulent cervicitis (MPC) is often asymptomatic, but some women have discharge or vaginal bleeding, especially after sexual intercourse. MPC can be due to *C. trachomatis*, *N. gonorrhoeae*, or neither. Test with culture or nucleic acid amplification procedures to identify the organism responsible. Also consider empiric therapy for a woman who has suspected gonorrhea or *Chlamydia* if the patient's risk factors suggest a high prevalence and there is a good likelihood that she will not return for therapy.

Chlamydial infections in sexually active adolescents are quite common, and most are asymptomatic. Annually screen sexually active adolescent women, even those without symptoms. The concern is pelvic inflammatory disease (PID), increased risk of ectopic pregnancy, and infertility. Treat both *Chlamydia* and gonococcal infections.

Treatment for MPC:

- Azithromycin 1 g x 1 dose, or
- Doxycycline 100 mg b.i.d. x 7 days

Alternative treatment for MPC:

- Erythromycin 500 mg q.i.d. x 7 days, or
- Erythromycin ethylsuccinate 800 mg q.i.d. x 7 days, or
- Ofloxacin 300 mg b.i.d. x 7 days, or
- Levofloxacin 500 mg q day x 7 days

Many believe that adolescents should be retested in 3–4 months to look for recurrence.

Treatment of MPC in pregnant women:

- Erythromycin 500 mg q.i.d. x 7 days, or
- Amoxicillin 500 mg t.i.d. x 7 days

Alternative:

- Erythromycin 250 mg q.i.d. x 14 days, or
- Erythromycin ethylsuccinate 800 mg q.i.d. x 7 days, or
- Erythromycin ethylsuccinate 400 mg q.i.d. x 14 days, or
- Azithromycin 1 g x 1 dose

Note: Erythromycin estolate is contraindicated in pregnancy due to increased risk of hepatotoxicity. Also, always have the pregnant women return for followup testing to assess for cure.

Gonorrheal Infections

Most men are symptomatic, while most women are not. Gonorrheal infections in women can cause the same complications as *Chlamydia* infections, including PID, increased risk of ectopic pregnancy, and infertility. Usually, treatment for gonorrhea also includes therapy for chlamydia. Of recent concern in the U.S. has been the emergence of quinolone-resistant *N. gonorrhoeae* (QRNG), especially in the State of Hawaii (~ 15 %!!).

The following are for uncomplicated gonococcal infections of the cervix, urethra, and rectum:

- Cefixime 400 mg x 1, or
- Ceftriaxone 125 mg x 1, or
- Ciprofloxacin 500 mg x 1, or
- Ofloxacin 400 mg x 1, or
- Levofloxacin 250 mg x 1

plus—If *Chlamydia* has not been ruled out:

- Azithromycin 1 g x 1, or
- Doxycycline 100 mg b.i.d. x 7 days

Alternative treatments for gonorrhea:

- Spectinomycin 2 g IM x 1 (use only if quinolone or cephalosporin can't be used)

Note: The FDA has not approved quinolones in children < age 18. However, the CDC okays the use of quinolones in those children weighing > 45 kg (99 lbs).

For treatment of uncomplicated gonococcal infections of the pharynx:

- Ceftriaxone 125 mg IM x 1, or
- Ciprofloxacin 500 mg x 1

plus, if *Chlamydia* has not been ruled out:

- Azithromycin 1 g x 1, or
- Doxycycline 100 mg b.i.d. x 7 days

Pregnant women: Do not use a quinolone or tetracycline. Use a cephalosporin for gonorrhea, and either erythromycin or amoxicillin for *C. trachomatis*. If she is allergic to cephalosporins, the only option (on the Board examination) is spectinomycin 2g IM for the treatment of gonorrhea.

DISSEMINATED GONOCOCCAL INFECTION

This is a classic Board topic. [know!] Disseminated gonococcal infection (DGI) accompanies bacteremia. It can present as petechial or pustular skin lesions, asymmetrical arthralgia, tenosynovitis, or frank septic arthritis. See Figure 3-11, with left knee showing arthritis with a skin lesion over the knee. It can also present as perihepatitis (Fitz-Hugh-Curtis syndrome—look out for the adolescent female with right-upper quadrant abdominal pain!). More about this in the Infectious Disease section.

Treatment of disseminated gonococcal infection:

- Ceftriaxone 1 gm IM/IV q 24 hours

Alternatives:

- Cefotaxime 1 g IV q 8 hours, or
- Ceftizoxime 1 g IV q 8 hours, or
- Ciprofloxacin 400 mg IV q 12 hours, or
- Ofloxacin 400 mg IV q 12 hours, or
- Levofloxacin 250 mg IV q day, or
- Spectinomycin 2 g IM q 12 hours.

notes

Quick Quiz

1) Know the main treatments for all of the STDs.
2) How often should you screen an asymptomatic adolescent who is sexually active for STDs?
3) For every STD, also be sure to know the treatment regimen for pregnant women!
4) What are the characteristics of bacterial vaginosis infection?
5) Should you treat male partners of a woman with bacterial vaginosis?

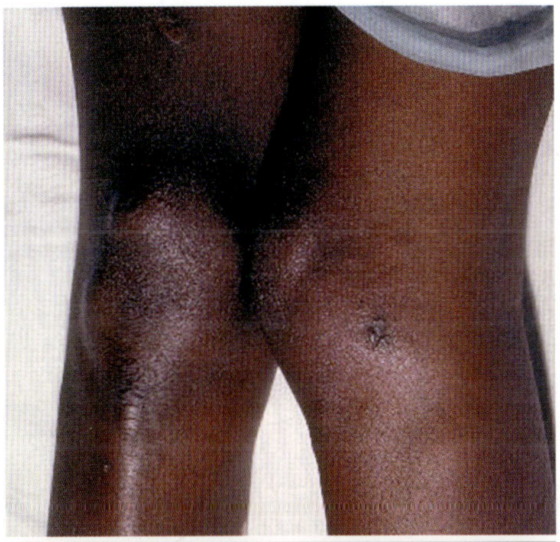

Figure 3-11: GC Septic Arthritis

Continue the above for 24–48 hours, until you see improvement; then you might change treatment to 1 of the following to complete at least 1 week of therapy:
- Cefixime 400 mg b.i.d., or
- Ciprofloxacin 500 b.i.d., or
- Ofloxacin 400 mg b.i.d., or
- Levofloxacin 500 mg q day.

If meningitis occurs, use ceftriaxone 1–2 g IV q 12 x 10–14 days. For endocarditis, prescribe 4 weeks of therapy at the same dosages.

INFECTIONS with VAGINAL DISCHARGE

Overview

3 diseases most commonly cause vaginal discharge:
1) Trichomoniasis (due to *Trichomonas vaginalis*)
2) Bacterial vaginosis (due to replacement of normal flora by other organisms, including *Gardnerella vaginalis*)
3) Candidiasis (usually due to *Candida albicans*)

Do pH testing to determine the etiology of the infection. Bacterial vaginosis and trichomoniasis usually elevate the pH to > 4.5. Presence of an amine odor after adding KOH to the discharged material indicates bacterial vaginosis. You will see *T. vaginalis* as motile organisms on a wet mount, and clue cells for bacterial vaginosis. Yeasts are visible on KOH for candidal infection.

Bacterial Vaginosis

Bacterial vaginosis (BV) is a clinical syndrome due to the replacement of the normal flora, particularly *Lactobacillus sp.*, in the vagina. The *Lactobacillus* is frequently replaced by anaerobes (*Prevotella* and *Mobiluncus*), *Gardnerella vaginalis*, and *Mycoplasma hominis*. BV is the most common cause of vaginal discharge. Treatment of male sexual partners is not beneficial.

Clinical diagnosis requires 3 out 4 of the following findings:
1) Homogenous, white, noninflammatory discharge that smoothly coats the vaginal walls
2) Clue cells on microscopic examination
3) pH of vaginal fluid is > 4.5
4) Fishy odor of vaginal discharge before or after the addition of 10% KOH

Treatment of bacterial vaginosis:
- Metronidazole 500 mg b.i.d. x 7 days, or
- Metronidazole gel 0.75%, one full applicator intravaginally, q day x 5 days, or
- Clindamycin cream 2%, one full applicator intravaginally at bedtime x 7 days

Alternatives:
- Metronidazole 2 grams x 1 oral dose, or
- Clindamycin 300 mg b.i.d. x 7 days, or
- Clindamycin ovules 100 g intravaginally q bedtime x 3 days

Pregnant women:
- Metronidazole 250 mg t.i.d. x 7 days, or
- Clindamycin 300 mg b.i.d. x 7 days

We know that BV is associated with abnormal pregnancy outcomes (premature rupture of membranes, chorioamnionitis, preterm labor, preterm birth, post-cesarean wound infection); so far, topical therapy is not effective in pregnancy. Risk of teratogenicity with the use of metronidazole in pregnancy has been recently disputed.

Trichomoniasis

Trichomoniasis is due to the protozoa *Trichomonas vaginalis*. Most men are asymptomatic, while most women have symptoms, such as malodorous yellow-green discharge with vulvar irritation. Asymptomatic infection also can occur in women. You usually can see the organisms on wet mounts, or they can be cultured. (See Figure 3-12).

notes

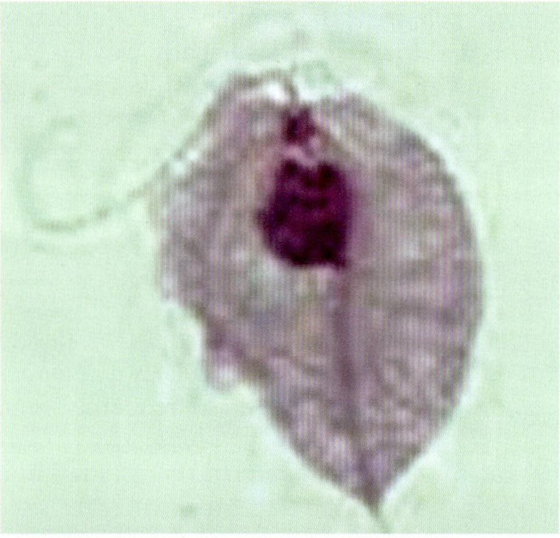

Figure 3-12: Trichomonad

Treatment of trichomoniasis:

- Metronidazole 2 grams x 1 dose, or
- Metronidazole 500 mg b.i.d. x 7 days

Recently, treatment failure has become more common, and most recommend retreating with metronidazole 500 mg b.i.d. x 7 days. If retreatment fails, use 2 grams q day x 3–5 days. Give pregnant women the standard 2-gram dose x 1.

Vulvovaginal Candidiasis

Vulvovaginal candidiasis is usually due to *Candida albicans*, but other candidal species can be involved. Typical symptoms include itching and vaginal discharge. Most women will have at least 1 episode of vulvovaginal candidiasis during their lifetime, and most of these will be uncomplicated. Complicated vulvovaginal candidiasis is defined as recurrent, severe non-albicans, or in women with uncontrolled diabetes, debilitation, immunosuppression, or pregnancy. Another common risk factor is recent antibiotic use.

Diagnose uncomplicated vulvovaginal candidiasis by doing a wet prep or Gram stain or culture for the organism. Candida vaginitis is usually associated with a pH < 4.5. KOH is very helpful.

Treatment of uncomplicated vulvovaginal candidiasis:

Intravaginal agents:

- Butoconazole 2% cream 5 g intravaginally x 3 days, or
- Butoconazole 2% cream 5 g sustained release x 1 dose, or
- Clotrimazole 1% cream 5 g intravaginally for 7-14 days, or
- Clotrimazole 100 mg vaginal tablet x 7 days, or
- Clotrimazole 100 mg vaginal tablet, 2 tablets x 3 days, or
- Clotrimazole 500 mg vaginal tablet x 1 dose, or
- Miconazole 2% cream 5 g intravaginally x 7 days, or
- Miconazole 100 mg vaginal suppository x 7 days, or
- Miconazole 200 mg vaginal suppository x 3 days, or
- Nystatin 100,000 unit vaginal tablet x 14 days, or
- Tioconazole 6.5% ointment 5 g intravaginally x 1, or
- Terconazole 0.4% cream 5 g intravaginally x 7 days, or
- Terconazole 0.8% cream 5 g intravaginally x 3 days, or
- Terconazole 80 mg vaginal suppository, x 3 days, or

Oral Agent:

- Fluconazole 150 mg oral tablet x 1

OK…please do not memorize all of these for the Board exam!! They won't ask you to differentiate between these, or to know that if you use the terconazole 0.8% cream, you need to do it for only 3 days. Just know that the topicals work, and 1 oral agent works!! Male partners may need to be treated topically if there is recurrence in the female partner, or if the male has evidence of balanitis.

Complicated Vulvovaginal Candidiasis

Recurrent vulvovaginal candidiasis is usually defined as having 4 or more recurrences/year; please be sure to consider HIV in these patients on the Board examination, especially if you can't seem to get rid of the candidal infection. Do vaginal cultures to try and identify an unusual species such as C. glabrata. Usually, these patients require longer initial therapy of 7–14 days for topicals, or a repeat dose of fluconazole 3 days later for oral treatments. Some of these women may require maintenance antifungals, which they can take once weekly as vaginal suppositories or oral agents (fluconazole, itraconazole, etc.). Generally, continue these for 6 months.

Severe vulvovaginitis is characterized by extensive vulvular erythema, edema, excoriation, and fissure formation. Here again, longer treatment duration is usually necessary, and is the same as outlined above for recurrent vulvovaginal candidiasis.

Non-albicans vulvovaginal candidiasis can be difficult to treat. Longer duration of therapy with a non-fluconazole azole drug is recommended. If there is recurrence, use 600 mg boric acid in a gelatin capsule—vaginally, daily x 2 weeks.

Compromised hosts do not respond well to therapy. In these situations, encourage the patient to modify conditions as much as possible.

Pregnant patients frequently get vulvovaginal candidiasis, and only topical azole therapy x 7 days is recommended.

PELVIC INFLAMMATORY DISEASE

Pelvic inflammatory disease (PID) is a catchall phrase for inflammatory disorders of the upper female tract, including any combination of endometritis, salpingitis, tubo-ovarian abscess, and pelvic peritonitis. Most of the time, organisms obtained through sexual intercourse are the culprits, including *N. gonorrhoeae* and *C. trachomatis*. But other normal vaginal flora have also been found to be responsible, including anaerobes, *Gardnerella vaginalis*, *Haemophilus influenzae*, enteric Gram-negative rods, and Group B Streptococcus (*Streptococcus agalactiae*). CMV, *Mycoplasma hominis*, and *Ureaplasma urealyticum* also have been implicated.

Symptoms for PID vary, and it is sometimes a difficult diagnosis to make. Many women with PID have subtle or mild symptoms. Laparoscopy can be very helpful if you suspect salpingitis, but this diagnostic tool is usually not immediately accessible. Unfortunately, no single item in the history, physical, or laboratory is very sensitive or specific in making

notes

Quick Quiz

1) How is trichomonas treated? How about in a pregnant woman?
2) Name ALL the treatments for vulvovaginal candidiasis. (Just kidding). Name the only oral therapy approved.
3) Name several PID treatments.
4) Describe when to hospitalize a patient with PID.

the diagnosis, and using a combination of tests reduces either the sensitivity or specificity, making it less likely to be helpful. Many cases of PID are undiagnosed because of failure to recognize the mild/subtle symptoms of the disease in many women.

Because it is such a difficult diagnosis to make, the CDC has defined minimum criteria for making the diagnosis. This will be very sensitive but, unfortunately, not very specific. The important thing is not to miss a diagnosis of PID because of the potentially adverse, long-term outcomes (sterility, abscess, etc.). Generally, you start empiric therapy for PID if a sexually active woman presents with uterine/adnexal tenderness or cervical motion tenderness, and you can't find another explanation.

Other things can be helpful in making, or supporting, the diagnosis:

- Temperature > 101° F
- Abnormal cervical or vaginal mucopurulent discharge
- Presence of WBCs on saline microscopy of vaginal secretions
- Elevated ESR
- Elevated C-reactive protein
- Documentation of cervical infection with *N. gonorrhoeae* or *C. trachomatis*

(Laboratory tests (ESR, CRP) may be helpful, but not commonly done.)

Note: If the cervical discharge is normal, and you find no WBCs on wet prep, the diagnosis of PID is unlikely.

The most specific criteria for diagnosing PID (but these are rarely done!) include:

- Endometrial biopsy for histopathologic evidence of endometritis
- Transvaginal sonogram or MRI to show thickened, fluid-filled tubes, with or without free pelvic fluid or tubo-ovarian complex
- Laparoscopic evidence of PID

Sometimes, some of the above are done if the diagnosis is in doubt, or if certain aspects of the case warrant further evaluation. Sorry this is vague, but at least for the Pediatric Boards, you won't need to know the indications for these procedures. For the Boards, if there is any question that this might be PID, treat!

When do you hospitalize women with PID? This is also difficult, but know these general guidelines:

1. Surgical emergencies cannot be excluded (appendicitis)
2. Pregnancy
3. Clinical response to oral antimicrobial therapy is inadequate
4. The patient is unable to follow or tolerate an outpatient oral regimen (some would say most adolescents fall into this category, but actually no data are available that suggests that adolescents benefit from hospitalization for treatment of PID)
5. Severe illness, nausea, and vomiting, or high fever are present
6. You suspect or find a tubo-ovarian abscess

Treatment of PID: OK, here is the nightmare: there are many acceptable therapies for PID. Generally, the Boards will give you standard regimens, which will be the first ones listed here. For completeness, we give them all to you.

Parenteral treatments for PID (first line):

- Cefotetan 2 g IV q 12 hours, or
- Cefoxitin 2 g IV q 6 hours

  plus
- Doxycycline 100 mg orally or IV q 12 hours

You can stop parenteral therapy after she has shown improvement for 24 hours, then complete 14 days of doxycycline.

Another parenteral protocol for PID:

- Clindamycin 900 mg IV q 8 hours

  plus
- Gentamicin-loading dose of 2 mg/kg IV/IM, followed by maintenance dose of 1.5 mg/kg q 8 hours. (You can also use single, daily dosing.)

Still more alternative therapies for PID (least used):

- Ofloxacin 400 mg IV q 12, or
- Levofloxacin 500 mg IV q day

  with or without
- Metronidazole 500 mg IV q 8 hours, or
- Ampicillin/sulbactam 3 g IV q 6 hours

  plus
- Doxycycline 100 mg orally or IV q 12 hours

Quinolones would not be used when other agents are available.

After improvement has occurred, stop the parenteral therapy and use doxycycline 100 mg b.i.d., or clindamycin 450 mg q.i.d. to complete 14 days of therapy. You will sometimes be asked to use this regimen if the patient is cephalosporin-allergic.

What about outpatient therapy?

notes

Outpatient treatments for PID:

- Ceftriaxone 250 mg IM x 1, or
- Cefoxitin 2 g IM x1, and Probenecid 1 g x 1 orally, or
- Other 3rd generation cephalosporins
  plus
- Doxycycline 100 mg b.i.d. x 14 days
  with or without
- Metronidazole 500 mg b.i.d. x 14 days

Other outpatient treatments for PID:

- Ofloxacin 400 mg bid, or
- Levofloxacin 500 mg q day x 14 days
  with or without
- Metronidazole 500 mg b.i.d. x 14 days

Note: This is what you are more likely to see on the Peds Boards because of desire not to use quinolones in children < age 18. The CDC has quinolones as recommendations for those under 18, but the FDA has not approved them for this indication. For the Boards, if they have them listed, it is probably OK to use, unless an alternative is listed—but be very careful that they aren't trying to trick you into using a quinolone on a pregnant young adult!

For outpatient therapy, if no clinical improvement occurs within 72 hours, hospitalize the patient and place on a parenteral regimen.

EPIDIDYMITIS

For adolescent males, the most common causes of epididymitis are *C. trachomatis* and *N. gonorrhoeae*. You occasionally may see Gram-negatives, such as *Escherichia coli* in males who engage in anal intercourse. Treat most as outpatients unless there is severe pain or complication, or you are uncertain of the diagnosis (testicular torsion, infarction). Most adolescents present with unilateral testicular pain and tenderness, with findings of hydrocele and palpable swelling. Adolescents, in particular, are prone to testicular torsion, and you should always consider it in the differential diagnosis. Immediately refer patient to a urologist if you suspect testicular torsion.

For diagnostic purposes, do the following:

- Gram-stained smear of urethral exudate, or intraurethral swab to look for ≥ 5 PMNs/oil immersion field and N. gonorrhoeae
- Intraurethral exudate culture, or a nucleic acid amplification test (either swab or first-void urine) for *N. gonorrhoeae* and *C. trachomatis*
- First-void uncentrifuged urine exam for WBCs if the urethral Gram stain is negative. Also, culture and Gram stain of urine.
- Syphilis and HIV testing

Treatment for epididymitis: Always start empiric antibiotics pending laboratory results. Also, recommend bed rest, scrotal elevation, and treat for pain relief.

If the epididymitis is most likely due to gonococcal or chlamydial infection (as it will be in a majority of adolescents):

- Ceftriaxone 250 mg IM
  plus
- Doxycycline 100 mg b.i.d. x 10 days.

If, for some reason, you suspect an enteric Gram-negative organism is responsible, or the patient is allergic to cephalosporins and/or tetracyclines:

- Ofloxacin 300 mg b.i.d. x 10 days. or
- Levofloxacin 500 mg q day x 10 days

HUMAN PAPILLOMAVIRUS INFECTION (HPV)

There are > 30 different types of Human Papillomavirus (HPV) that can infect the genital tract. Most infections are asymptomatic and subclinical. HPV types 6 or 11 usually cause visible warts. Besides the genital area, HPV types 6 and 11 can produce warts in the conjunctival, nasal, oral, and laryngeal areas.

The HPV types we're most concerned about are those that are strongly associated with cervical neoplasia, and those that also can be found with squamous intraepithelial neoplasia of the penis, anus, and vulva, as well as squamous cell carcinoma. These are HPV types 16, 18, 31, 33, and 35. You probably should memorize these. (One way I remember is to think—well, at 16 and 18, most teenagers are "bad" and 31, 33, and 35 are "bad" because they are odd years early in your 30s.)

The warts due to HPV can occur on the penis, vulva, scrotum, perineum, perianal skin, vagina, urethra, anus, and/or mouth. Intra-anal warts occur in those who have had receptive anal intercourse. Perianal warts, on the other hand, can occur in both men and women without a history of anal sex.

Aim treatment at removing symptomatic warts. Unfortunately, treatment does not eliminate infectivity of the virus. No particular one of the available treatments is superior to the others. In general, warts on moist surfaces, and/or in intertriginous areas, respond better to topical treatment, as opposed to warts on drier surfaces, which don't usually respond very well to topicals. Change treatments if there is not great improvement after 3 provider-given treatments, or if the warts have not completely cleared by 6 treatments.

Recommended regimens for external genital warts:

Patient-applied:

- Podofilox 0.5% solution or gel, or
- Imiquimod 5% cream

Provider-applied:

- Cryotherapy with liquid nitrogen or cryoprobe, or
- Podophyllin resin 10%–25%, or
- Trichloroacetic acid (TCA) or bichloracetic acid (BCA) 80–90%, or
- Surgical removal

notes

Quick Quiz

1) What causes epididymitis in adolescent men?
2) Which HPV can predispose to cancer?
3) List therapy for HPV.
4) List therapy for HPV in a pregnant woman.
5) Which adolescents should get Hepatitis A vaccine?
6) How do you protect someone who is exposed to active Hepatitis A? Hepatitis B?
7) True or False: There is effective prophylaxis for hepatitis C exposure.

Alternatives include: intralesional interferon or laser surgery.

Recommended regimens for vaginal warts:
- Cryotherapy with liquid nitrogen, or
- TCA or BCA 80–90%

Recommended regimens for urethral meatus warts:
- Cryotherapy with liquid nitrogen, or
- Podophyllin 10–25%

Recommended regimens for anal warts:
- Cryotherapy with liquid nitrogen or
- TCA or BCA 80–90%, or
- Surgical removal

Recommended regimens for oral warts:
- Cryotherapy with liquid nitrogen, or
- Surgical removal

Pregnancy Issues: Do not use imiquimod, podophyllin, or podofilox during pregnancy. HPV can cause respiratory papillomatosis in infants and children and, therefore, most recommend removal of genital warts if they occur during pregnancy. Do not perform a cesarean delivery solely to prevent HPV infection in the newborn. However, cesarean delivery may be indicated if genital warts are obstructing the pelvic outlet, or if vaginal delivery would result in excessive bleeding.

Subclinical Genital HPV Infection: Note: DNA or RNA tests for screening subclinical genital HPV infection is not recommended. Also, do not treat if you diagnose this infection by colposcopy, biopsy, acetic acid application, or the detection of HPV by laboratory tests. If coexistent squamous intraepithelial lesions are present, treatment management depends on histopathologic findings.

CERVICAL CANCER SCREENING

Adult and adolescent women with a history of STDs are at increased risk for cervical carcinoma. Therefore, most recommend that, when a patient presents for a possible STD, a Pap smear also be performed. If the Pap smear shows high-grade squamous intraepithelial lesions (high grade-SIL: includes moderate dysplasia/cervical intraepithelial neoplasia (CIN) 2, severe dysplasia/CIN3, and carcinoma *in situ*), refer her for colposcopy and biopsy. For those with low-grade SIL (cellular changes associated with HPV and mild dysplasia/CIN 1), follow up with Pap, and if repeat tests are positive, refer for colposcopy.

Pap tidbits:

Pap should be done annually in *all sexually active adolescent females*. (Adult guidelines have recommendations for spacing out routine Pap smears to every 3 years after 3 negative smears). Remember:
- Pap is not a screening test for STDs.
- Do Pap only when the woman is non-menstruating.
- Mucopurulent discharge is not a contraindication for Pap.
- Pap testing is usually performed last, because it is not affected by prior testing collections/procedures.
- Perform Pap test on pregnant women as routine, prenatal care.

VACCINE-PREVENTABLE STDs

Overview

Vaccines are currently available to prevent hepatitis A and hepatitis B, which are both potential sexually transmitted diseases. Trials are underway to investigate vaccines for HIV, HPV, and herpes. Don't forget, when you see an adolescent (especially on the Board exam), offer him/her hepatitis B vaccination if she/he is unvaccinated. Give hepatitis A vaccine to adolescent men who have sex with men, and adolescents who abuse IV drugs.

Hepatitis A

If an unvaccinated person is exposed through household, sexual contact, or by sharing IV drugs with a person with hepatitis A, give a single IM dose of Immune Globulin (0.02 ml/kg) as soon as possible, but not > 2 weeks after exposure. Hepatitis A vaccine alone is not recommended for post-exposure prophylaxis.

Hepatitis B

If an unvaccinated person is exposed through sexual contact, or by sharing IV drugs with a person with hepatitis B, give hepatitis B Immune Globulin (HBIG) and hepatitis B Vaccine, at separate sites at the same time, within 14 days of the most recent exposure. For children and adolescents with household exposure, vaccinate with hepatitis B vaccine. HBIG is not necessary. For victims of sexual abuse where the offender is not known to have acute hepatitis B, HBIG is not required, but give the vaccination.

Hepatitis C

No vaccine is available for hepatitis C, and prophylaxis with immune globulin is not effective in preventing HCV infection.

notes

PROCTITIS, PROCTOCOLITIS, and ENTERITIS

These can be sexually transmitted entities, depending upon an individual's sexual practices.

Proctitis is inflammation limited to the rectum (the distal 12 cm) and is usually associated with anorectal pain, tenesmus, or rectal discharge. The most common pathogens are usually *N. gonorrhoeae*, *C. trachomatis*, *T. pallidum*, and HSV. It is mainly seen in those who participate in receptive anal intercourse. The recommended treatment regimen for these patients is ceftriaxone 125 mg IM plus doxycycline 100 mg b.i.d. x 7 days.

Proctocolitis has similar symptoms to proctitis, but patients also have diarrhea, abdominal cramps, and inflammation of the colonic mucosa. Organisms causing this are likely to be *Campylobacter*, *Shigella*, and *Entamoeba histolytica*. Proctocolitis can be acquired by the oral or fecal-oral route. Aim treatment at the offending agent.

Enteritis presents as diarrhea and abdominal cramping without signs of proctitis or proctocolitis. It can be seen in those with sexual practices that include oral-fecal contact. *Giardia lamblia* is the most common pathogen identified. Treat with metronidazole.

ECTOPARASITIC INFECTIONS

Note

Lice and scabies can be sexually transmitted, and must be included in the differential for an adolescent presenting with persistent pruritus or nits.

Pediculosis Pubis

Patients will usually present with itching because of the presence of nits or lice in their pubic hair. See Figure 3-13 for a photo of *Phthirus pubis* (crab louse).

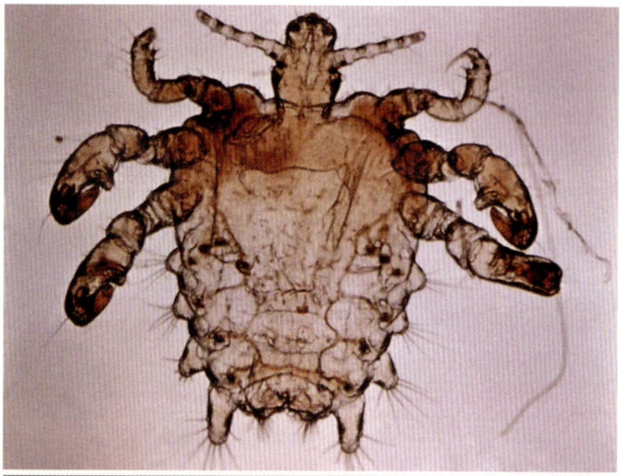

Figure 3-13: *Phthirus pubis*, "Crab Louse"

Treatment of pediculosis pubis includes applying:

- Permethrin 1% cream to affected areas for 10 minutes,
  or
- Lindane 1% shampoo for 4 minutes (do not use in pregnant or lactating women),
  or
- Pyrethrins with piperonyl butoxide for 10 minutes

Do not apply these to the eyes. Treat eyelash involvement with occlusive ophthalmic ointment to the eyelid margins b.i.d. x 10 days. All bedding and clothing must be decontaminated (machine washed and machine dried using heat; or dry cleaned). Retreatment may be necessary if you observe lice or eggs at the hair/skin junction.

Scabies

Scabies requires sensitization to the organism, *Sarcoptes scabiei.* (See Figure 3-14). The first time a person is infested with *S. scabiei*, it may take weeks before pruritus develops;

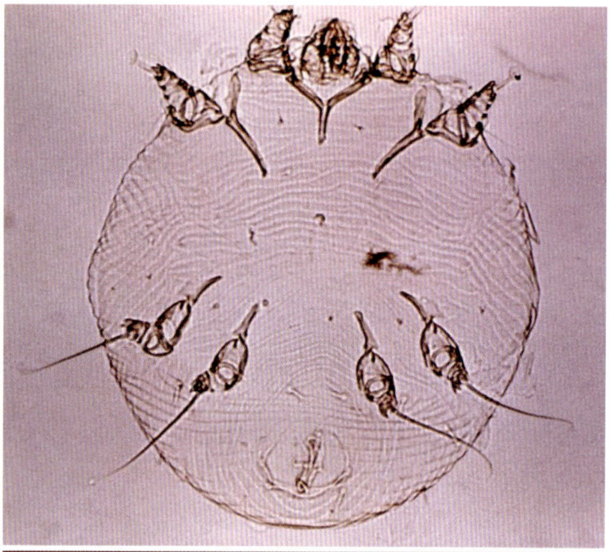

Figure 3-14: *Sarcoptes scabiei*

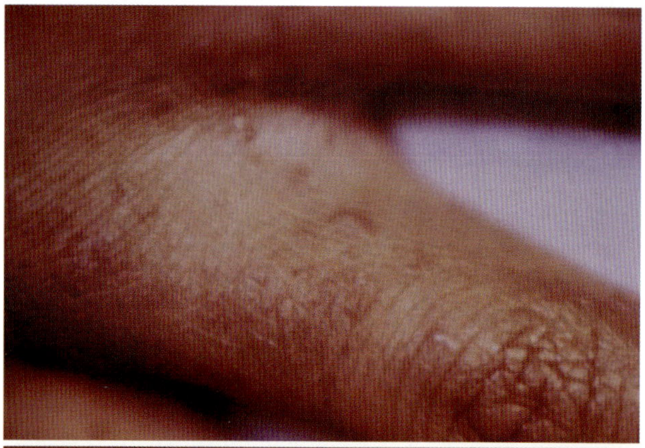

Figure 3-15: Scabies

notes

Quick Quiz

1) What is the therapy for lice in a pregnant woman?
2) Name an effective therapy for scabies.
3) What are the organisms responsible for scabies and lice?

however, on the next exposure, itching will occur within 24 hours. Burrows in the webs of the fingers and toes are common; the pruritus is intense. (See Figure 3-15).

Treatment for scabies:

Apply permethrin 5% cream all areas of the body from the neck down, and wash off after 8–14 hours.

Alternative treatments are:

- Lindane 1% (but many avoid lindane because of neurotoxicity): apply 1oz. of lotion or 30 grams of cream in a thin layer to all areas of the body from the neck down and thoroughly wash off after 8 hours, or
- Ivermectin 200 µg/kg orally, repeated in 2 weeks.

Do not apply lindane after a bath, or to someone with extensive atopic dermatitis, because seizures have been reported. Aplastic anemia has also been reported after use of lindane.

Decontaminate bedding and clothing, as with lice above.

The rash and itching of scabies may persist for up to 2 weeks after treatment.

Table 3-7

SUBSTANCE ABUSE AND THEIR KEY CLINICAL FINDINGS/EFFECTS - 1 of 2		
Drug	Symptoms/Signs	Lab/Other Effects
Marijuana	Impairment of short-term memory, decreased performance in driving, loss of critical judgment, time perception distortion	Plasma testosterone levels decreased as well as spermatogenesis, decreased glucose tolerance, antiemetic effect, significant fall in intraocular pressures (good for glaucoma)
Tobacco	Chronic cough, phlegm and wheezing	Increased hemoglobin/hematocrit, increased platelet aggregation
Toluene (airplane glue)	Relaxation and "pleasant" hallucinations for 2 hours	Toluene is excreted rapidly in the urine and may be detected by looking for hippuric acid
Gasoline	Euphoria followed by violent excitement and then coma	Pulmonary hypertension, restrictive lung defects, peripheral neuropathy, acute rhabdomyolysis, hematuria
Amyl nitrite, butyl nitrite (room deodorizers)	Euphoria, enhanced musical appreciation and aphrodisiacs; headaches, syncope	Hypotension, transiently inverted T waves and depressed ST segments; methemoglobinemia, increased intraocular pressures
LSD (Lysergic acid diethylamide)	Very potent hallucinogen 3 stages: 1) Somatic (physical effects--dizziness, dilated pupils, flushing, increased temp, tachycardia) 2) Perceptual (changes in vision and hearing- "seeing smells" or "hearing" colors) 3) Psychic effects (changes in sensorium- delusional ideation, body distortion, psychosis)	Not associated with a withdrawal syndrome. "Flash-backs" common years after use.

notes

Table 3-8

SUBSTANCE ABUSE AND THEIR KEY CLINICAL FINDINGS/EFFECTS - 2 of 2		
Drug	Symptoms/Signs	Lab/Other Effects
MDMA (Ecstasy, methylenedioxymetha-mphetamine)	Euphoria, heightened sensual awareness, increased "emotional" energy. Nausea, jaw-clinching, teeth grinding and blurred vision are common. Anxiety, psychotic episodes can occur.	
PCP (Phencyclidine, angel dust)	Cramps, diarrhea and hematemesis. Euphoria, nystagmus, ataxia and hallucination. Higher doses--psychosis with use of verbal abusive language. Higher levels still result in cardiac arrhythmias and seizures. Coma (unique for PCP) has absence of respiratory depression, presence of muscle rigidity, hyperreflexia and nystagmus.	Urine drug screen is helpful in diagnosis.
Cocaine	Euphoria, decreased fatigability, paranoid ideation. Seizures can occur.	Pupillary dilatation, tachycardia, hypertension. Think in young person with MI--look for cocaine.
Amphetamines	Hypertension, hyperpyrexia and seizures occur.	Cardiac conduction abnormalities. Cerebrovascular damage. Withdrawal syndrome: Early--depression, agitation, anergia; Intermediate--loss of energy, limited interest in surroundings, anhedonia; Final--drug craving returns. Do NOT use phenothiazines for treatment of withdrawl! (hypotension and seizures)
Opiates	Euphoria, decrease in pain, pinpoint pupils.	Severe vasodilation. Respiratory depression. Pulmonary edema. Loss of libido. Constipation. Withdrawal occurs 8 hours without heroin over a period of 24-36 hours--first finding seen is yawning, then lacrimation, mydriasis, insomnia, "goose flesh," diarrhea, and systolic hypertension. Diazepam helpful.
Anabolic Steroids	Acne, keloids, stria, hirsutism, gynecomastia, testicular atrophy and azoospermia. Rage, depression, mania, and libido alterations.	Hepatitis, increased risk of hepatocellular carcinoma. Fluid retention is common. Growth retardation because of early epiphyseal closure.

notes

Infectious Disease

MedStudy

2nd Edition
Pediatrics Board Review
Core Curriculum

Infectious Disease

Authored by J. Thomas Cross, Jr., MD, MPH, FAAP
and Robert A. Hannaman, MD

Many thanks to

M. Suzanne Whitworth, MD
Pediatric Infectious Disease
Cook Children's Hospital
Fort Worth, TX

Table of Contents

Infectious Disease

BACTERIA

GRAM-POSITIVE BACTERIA

Staphylococcus aureus

Staphylococcus aureus is a common inhabitant of skin and mucous membranes. It can cause self-limited disease such as impetigo or serious, life-threatening infections. Bacteremia is especially common among IV drug users and hemodialysis patients. It is also a cause of toxic shock syndrome (TSS), staphylococcal epidermal necrolysis, and staphylococcal scalded skin syndrome. Pathogenicity (which is not the same as resistance to antibiotics!) is associated with production of entero- and exotoxin, coagulase, and leukocidin. In chronic carriers, *S. aureus* is found in nasal mucosa, skin, or rectal cultures, but not in the blood.

The percentage of methicillin-resistant *S. aureus* (MRSA) infections has grown substantially due to the previous indiscriminate use of methicillin and similar antibiotics. In most hospitals, 15–20% of *S. aureus* isolates are MRSA. In some tertiary care centers, the percentage is > 50%! Unfortunately, MRSA is now frequently seen in community-acquired infections as well!

In carriers, it is difficult to eradicate. You can try topical mupirocin ointment (Bactroban®) and oral rifampin or clindamycin, but even with these, it still recurs. In all cases of bacteremia and serious infection with MRSA, vancomycin is the only drug of choice (although there are newer agents, such as linezolid; for the Boards, vancomycin will be your choice). (Linezolid {Zyvox®} is a newer antibiotic, but is quite expensive and generally should be reserved for patients intolerant of vancomycin). Although other drugs may be used for their synergistic effect (gentamicin and rifampin), vancomycin is always required. In some skin and soft tissue infections, other antibiotics may be effective, including TMP/SMX or clindamycin, each +/– rifampin. Note: Resistance to quinolones is rapidly developing.

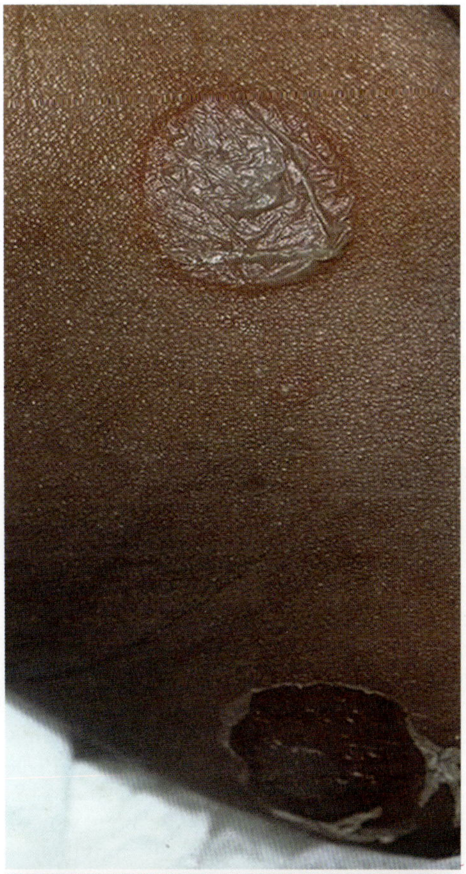

Figure 4-1: Bullous Impetigo

Skin infections are common with *Staphylococcus aureus*, especially impetigo, which also is due to *Streptococcus pyogenes*. This presents as red-crusted papules and pustules, often at the site of a prior insect bite. "Bullous impetigo" is usually staphylococcal in origin; it presents as flaccid, coalescent pustules with bullae on previously normal skin (see Figure 4-1). *Staphylococcus* is the usual cause of furuncles (boils) and carbuncles.

If, on the ABP examination, they tell you a child has *Staphylococcus aureus* bacteremia, be very suspicious of endocarditis or osteomyelitis (*S. aureus* is the most common cause of osteomyelitis, except in sickle cell patients)! Also, *S. aureus* bacteremia will frequently "seed" many sites in the body. If a catheter is involved, usually you must remove it and, in addition, treat with antibiotics.

Children with cyanotic congenital heart disease have an increased risk of staphylococcal brain abscess. Also, children who undergo neurosurgical procedures, especially shunt revisions, are at increased risk for staphylococcal infection.

Toxic Shock Syndrome (TSS)

TSS often presents with red skin, hypotension, fever, diarrhea, and hypocalcemia. With young women, TSS is usually associated with menstruation and tampon use. A young woman with the focus in the uterus may have a bloody discharge or be menstruating. Do not treat the hypocalcemia unless either symptoms or ECG signs develop. Any time there is a post-surgical toxic shock, any device implanted during the surgery must be immediately removed (prosthetic device, implant, etc.). See Table 4-1—Toxic Shock Syndrome.

Another cause of TSS is *Streptococcus pyogenes*. This usually results from a progressive skin infection—especially post-op and with chickenpox! Note: In staphylococcal TSS, blood cultures are usually negative, whereas in streptococcal TSS, blood cultures are usually positive!

Table 4-1

CRITERIA FOR DIAGNOSIS OF TOXIC SHOCK SYNDROME
- Temp > 38.9°C
- Systolic blood pressure < 90 mmHg (or < 5% for age < 16 years)
- Rash with subsequent desquamation (palms/soles especially)
- Involvement of > 3 organ systems: GI, muscular, mucous membranes, renal, liver, blood, CNS
- Negative serology for RMSF, leptospirosis, measles

notes

Staphylococcal Scalded Skin Syndrome (SSSS)

S. aureus can cause an exfoliating dermatitis mediated by exfoliating toxin. In young infants, it is known as Ritter syndrome. Bacteremia may or may not be present. Fever is common, and minimal friction applied to the skin results in removal of the superficial layers of epidermis; this is known as Nikolsky sign. (see Figure 4-2). Older children can have a similar syndrome without the skin sloughing; it presents with red, tender skin that looks like Group A Streptococcus scarlet fever.

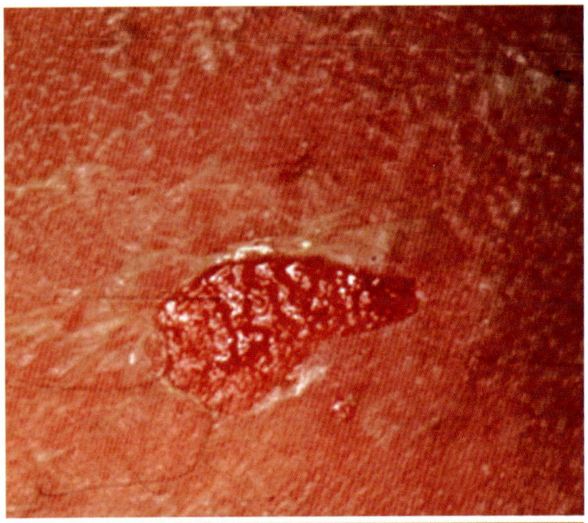

Figure 4-2: Staphylococcal Scalded Skin Synd.

Staphylococcus aureus Food Poisoning

S. aureus is the most common cause of food poisoning in the United States. Eating preformed enterotoxin from food that is contaminated is what causes it. Incubation period is < 4–6 hours, and the patient presents with nausea, vomiting, and abdominal cramps. Fever may be present. Most have a self-limited disease, but some children can have severe dehydration. This is typically associated with meats and cream-filled baked goods.

Staphylococcus epidermidis, S. saprophyticus, other Coagulase-negative Staphylococci

S. epidermidis and *S. saprophyticus* are examples of coagulase-negative Staphylococci. *Staphylococcus epidermidis* is almost always methicillin-resistant. It is the most common cause of both catheter-related bacteremia (catheter gets contaminated as it passes through the skin) and bacteremia occurring post-op when anything foreign was left in the body (prosthetics, including heart valves and joints, pacemakers, CNS shunts, etc.) Be especially on the look-out for VP-shunt infections with this organism. Treat with vancomycin +/- rifampin +/- gentamicin. *S. saprophyticus* causes UTIs in adolescent females.

S. epidermidis is responsible for ~ 1/3 of the bacteremias in children receiving chemotherapy for childhood malignancies; it also accounts for the majority of bacteremias in neonates in NICUs. The key factor for both is the presence of an intravascular catheter.

Additionally, *S. epidermidis* is a common "contaminant" in blood cultures and other cultures. A single blood culture that is positive for *S. epidermidis*, without an underlying prosthetic device or risk factors, is usually a contaminant. However, this is more difficult to discern in NICUs where, generally, a positive culture must be initially treated if there is suspicion of infection.

Streptococcus pneumoniae

Remember: You need functioning spleen and antibodies to defend against the encapsulated *S. pneumoniae* and *H. influenzae*—so both infections are seen more often in:

- Asplenic patients (anatomically or functionally asplenic, including those with sickle cell disease)
- Very young and old patients
- Patients with hypogammaglobulinemia (i.e., any antibody dysfunction or decrease)

S. pneumoniae is the most common cause of otitis media. Amoxicillin remains the drug of choice even in the era of increasing resistance. However, increase dosages to 80–100 mg/kg/day for children at increased risk of resistant pneumococcal infection—children in daycare settings, on recent antibiotics, with recurrent OM, or < 2 years of age.

Pneumococcus is also the most common bacterial cause for bacteremia, meningitis, and pneumonia. Risk factors for invasive pneumococcal disease include the following heritages: Native Americans, Alaskan natives, or African-Americans. For children 2–11 months of age, any underlying CNS, cardiac, or renal abnormality increases the risk.

In children, "occult bacteremia without a focus" accounts for ~ 60% of all pneumococcal invasive disease. This "syndrome" occurs in febrile children 3–36 months of age. It occurs in 3% of all children in these ages with a temperature > 39°C (102.2°F). The use of conjugated pneumococcal vaccine (Prevnar®) has resulted in a decrease in this disorder.

S. pneumoniae is the most common cause of bacterial pneumonia in children older than 1 month of age (*viruses*, however, cause more pneumonia than any other etiology!). In children with documented pneumonia, 1–3% will have a positive blood culture. Most do well without complications.

In infants > 2–3 months of age, pneumococcus is the most common cause of bacterial meningitis and has the highest rate of complications. The mortality rate is 7%; ~ 1/3 have severe morbidity with neurologic sequelae. Meningitis is discussed later in this section.

Depending on the geographic location, 10–60% of those with *S. pneumoniae* develop some degree of resistance to penicillin (PCN), usually by alterations in PCN-binding proteins (this is not the same as β-lactamase resistance). For bacteremia without evidence of meningitis, use ceftriaxone until PCN sensitivity is known. Empiric treatment of presumed *S. pneumoniae* meningitis should always include both vancomycin and cefotaxime or ceftriaxone until susceptibility is known.

notes

Quick Quiz

1) If a child presents on the Board exam with bacteremia due to MRSA, what is the only effective therapy?
2) What organisms commonly cause impetigo?
3) List the criteria for the diagnosis of toxic shock syndrome.
4) What is Nikolsky sign?
5) What is the most common cause of food poisoning in the U.S.?
6) What is the most common organism found in catheter-related and VP-shunt infections?
7) Which types of patients are at highest risk for pneumococcal sepsis?
8) How do you treat otitis media?
9) What is the empiric therapy for pneumococcal meningitis?
10) How may an infant with *S. pyogenes* infection present?
11) Describe the rash of scarlet fever.

For outpatients with otitis media or pneumonia and allergic to PCN, give a cephalosporin, clindamycin, doxycycline (for adolescents), or quinolone.

Remember: Postsplenectomy pneumococcal sepsis can be rapidly fatal, and can present with flu-like symptoms, purpura, and DIC (test question will have Howell-Jolly bodies on peripheral smear).

Streptococcus pyogenes (Group A Streptococcus)

S. pyogenes is the only species in Group A, beta-hemolytic streptococcus. It may cause one or more of the following:

- Pharyngitis
- Impetigo
- Streptococcal TSS
- Rheumatic fever
- Acute glomerulonephritis
- Scarlet fever

The major protein on its cell surface is the "M protein." The M protein occurs in > 80 antigenically distinct types, and defines which strains are rheumatogenic, which cause glomerulonephritis, which are toxigenic for toxic shock syndrome, etc.

Pharyngitis

Streptococcal pharyngitis (usually *S. pyogenes*) is more likely with each of these 3 findings:

1) Temp > 100°
2) Tender cervical lymphadenopathy
3) Exudative tonsils

If you don't find any of these, the chance of *Streptococcus* is < 3%; 1 finding = 20%; 3 findings = 50%. In children > 2 years of age who have cough, rhinorrhea, or other symptoms of URI with "sore throat," it is not streptococcus! Infants will not present with pharyngitis, but rather, with thick, purulent, nasal discharge (known as streptococcosis), low-grade fever, and decreased feeding. Some children will have abdominal pain or vomiting. Streptococcal disease is most commonly seen in the winter and spring, and in children > 3 years of age.

Conduct a throat culture or rapid diagnostic test in children you suspect have streptococcal pharyngitis. Just because the throat is red, has exudates, and "looks like strep" does not mean it is. Culture is the gold standard and takes 1–2 days for results. It is perfectly appropriate to wait on culture results before giving antibiotic therapy. The risk of rheumatic fever is alleviated as long as you start antibiotics within 9 days of infection, so waiting 1–2 days is not going to be a problem. Others prefer the rapid tests, using latex agglutination or enzyme immunoassay. These have a sensitivity of ~ 90%, and a specificity approaching 100%. Recent optical immunoassay has shown to be even more sensitive. If using a less-sensitive rapid test, and the test is negative, get a throat culture so you will not miss treating a true-positive infection.

Scarlet Fever

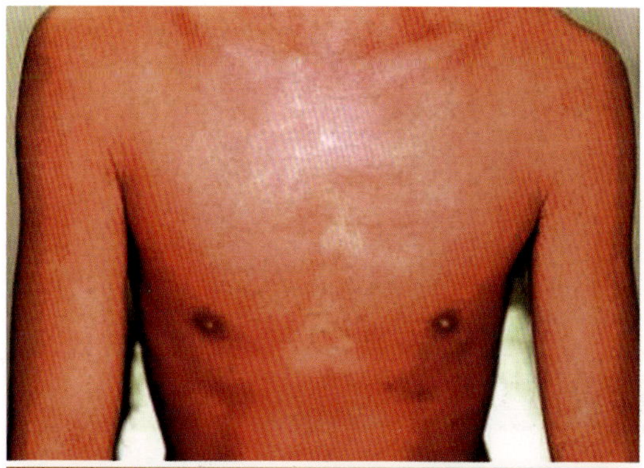

Figure 4-3: Scarlet Fever

Scarlet fever occurs when a child presents with a fine, diffuse red rash with acute streptococcal pharyngitis. The rash is due to pyrogenic exotoxins, and SPE A, B, C, and F.

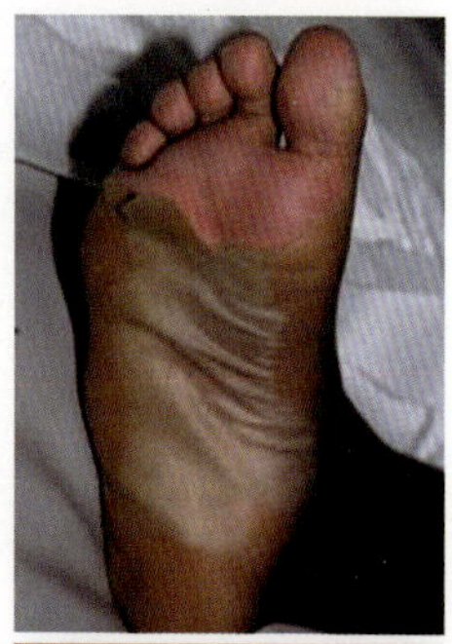

Figure 4-4

The rash usually appears 24–48 hours into the illness but can appear as the first sign. The rash has a "sandpaper" quality, begins on the neck and upper chest, and spreads. (see Figure 4-3).

The rash is especially prominent in the flexor skin creases of the antecubital fossa and produces what are known as Pastia lines; these lines are pathognomonic for scarlet fever. Also, the mouth area is pale and de-

notes

scribed as "circumoral pallor." The rash lasts ~ 1 week, then fades with desquamation of the trunk, hands, and feet (see Figure 4-4).

Impetigo, Superficial Pyoderma, Erysipelas

Impetigo or superficial pyoderma is the most common form of skin infection caused by *S. pyogenes*. It is common after minute injuries to the skin, such as insect bites, scabies, or minor trauma. The child is usually afebrile and does not have pain. It is most common in children ages 2–5 years. It also is common for other family members to become infected.

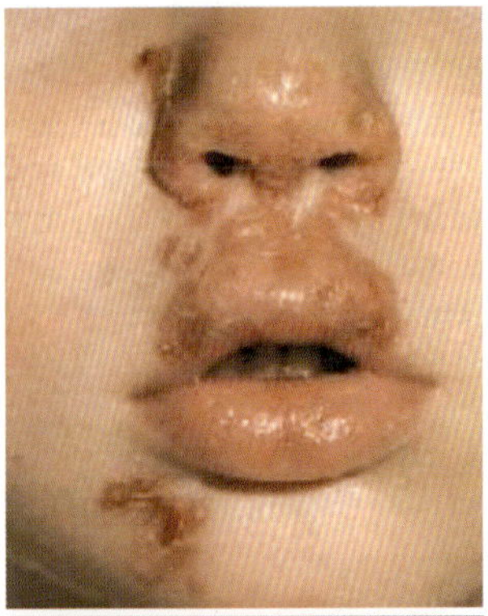

Figure 4-5: Impetigo

The lesions of impetigo are "honey-crusted" and may be oozing purulent material. (See Figure 4-5). The lesions most commonly occur around the mouth, nose, and extremities. One strain, M49, is highly associated with the development of poststreptococcal glomerulonephritis.

Erysipelas (see Figure 4-6) is an acute streptococcal infection of the deeper layers of skin and underlying connective tissues. It is rare in children. In contrast to impetigo, the skin is tender. It is common to see and feel a well-demarcated line between infected and uninfected skin. Lymphangitis can also occur. "Leading edge" cultures may be useful for detecting the organism.

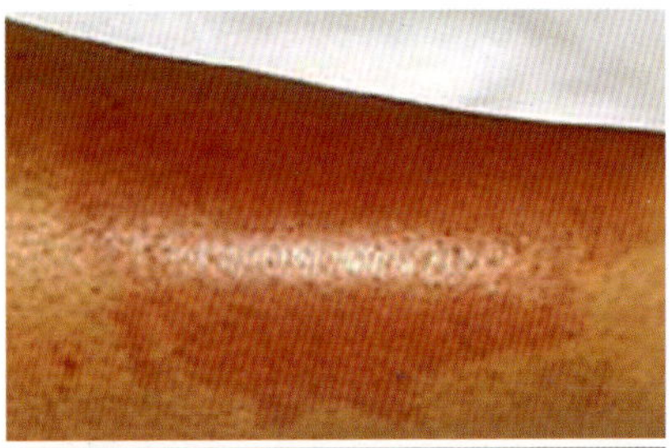

Figure 4-6: Erysipelas

Cellulitis from Group A streptococcus can be very serious; in some cases, it can become deep-seated and lead to necrotizing fasciitis, which is infection that causes destruction down to the subcutaneous tissue level. There is severe pain and swelling, and the skin becomes bluish and dusky in appearance. After 4–6 days, frank gangrene can occur. Surgical debridement is the treatment of choice, along with IV PCN and clindamycin. Recent/concurrent varicella infection is an identified risk factor. Note that cellulitis due to *S. pyogenes* can also be responsible for poststreptococcal glomerulonephritis, but not rheumatic fever.

As noted above, *S. pyogenes* can cause toxic shock syndrome. Remember: With Streptococcal toxic shock, blood cultures are more likely to be positive!

Rheumatic fever and acute poststreptococcal glomerulonephritis are discussed in Rheumatology and Nephrology sections, respectively.

Treatment

Penicillin is the drug of choice for *S. pyogenes* infection. For streptococcal pharyngitis, use PCN V at a dose of 40 mg/kg/day. Generally, most use 250 mg 2–3 times a day. The most common reason for PCN failure is non-adherence. If compliance is an issue, administer a single IM dose of benzathine PCN G 600,000 U for children weighing < 27 kg (60 lb.) or 1.2 million U for children weighing > 27 kg.

Even in compliant patients, eradication of *Streptococcus* does not occur in 15%. Most believe that many of these failures occur in *S. pyogenes* "carriers."

If the child is PCN-allergic, use cephalexin, cefadroxil, or other cephalosporins. Oral erythromycin or azithromycin is acceptable for those allergic to both PCNs and cephalosporins. However, it recently has been reported that ~ 5–10% of *S. pyogenes* are resistant to erythromycin or azithromycin. Most do not recommend using azithromycin if the child can tolerate PCN.

Recurrent *S. pyogenes* can be a difficult management issue. Many are colonized, or there is "ping-ponging" going on in the household: Spread from one family member to another, back and forth. Clindamycin (20 mg/kg/day x 10 days) is effective in eradicating the carrier state. Very few may require tonsillectomy.

Treatment of impetigo usually involves treating for both *S. pyogenes* and *S. aureus* infection, commonly with cephalexin. Skin *S. pyogenes* may cause acute glomerulonephritis even with treatment, but skin *S. pyogenes* ***cannot*** cause rheumatic fever. [Pharyngeal strains of *S. pyogenes* can cause both rheumatic fever (prevented with therapy) and glomerulonephritis (not prevented with therapy)].

In children with a history of acute rheumatic fever or rheumatic cardiac disease, use 1.2 million U of benzathine PCN G IM every 3–4 weeks, or oral PCN or sulfadiazine daily (for those PCN-allergic). Additionally, some recommend treating all household contacts of a case of rheumatic fever or poststreptococcal glomerulonephritis to rid the household of the potentially offending strain—but a majority of experts recommend only targeted chemoprophylaxis in household contacts ≥ 65 years of age, or those who have other risk factors for potentially invasive *S. pyogenes* disease (HIV, varicella, DM, chemotherapy, etc.).

Group B Streptococcal Infection (Streptococcus agalactiae)

S. agalactiae (Group B) is a common cause of infection in the newborn and young infant. It is a major cause of newborn pneumonia, bacteremia, and meningitis (this is why ampicillin is included in the empiric treatment for meningitis; ampicillin is also used for *Listeria* and *Enterococci* in this age group). It is associated with UTIs in pregnant women, and is also a cause of postpartum endometritis and bacteremia. It can originate from a GU reservoir.

notes

Quick Quiz

1) What areas of the body are commonly affected by impetigo?
2) How does erysipelas differ from impetigo?
3) What is a risk factor for necrotizing fasciitis due to *S. pyogenes* infection?
4) What is the drug of choice for *S. pyogenes* infection? If a child has anaphylaxis to penicillin and you are uneasy about using cephalosporins, what is an acceptable alternative therapy?
5) Differentiate "early-onset" and "late-onset" Group B Streptococcal disease.
6) What type of streptococci are common organisms in endocarditis?
7) What organism is responsible for pharyngitis in college outbreaks?

There are "early" and "late-onset" Group B streptococcal infections in the newborn/early infancy period.

Things to know about *early* onset:

- Median time of onset is 1 hour! (max is 7 days)
- Obstetric complications are common
- Prematurity is common
- Septicemia is the most common presentation (45%)
- Pneumonia is next most common (40%)
- Meningitis occurs in < 10%
- The most common serotypes are Ia, Ib, II, III, and V
- Case fatality rates are 5–15%

Things to know about *late* onset:

- Median onset is 27 days (range: 7 days–3 months)
- Bacteremia without a focus is the most common presentation (50%)
- Meningitis is next most common (40%)
- Osteomyelitis (especially proximal humerus), septic arthritis (hip, knee, ankle), cellulites, or adenitis (unilateral, facial, genital or inguinal areas) occur in < 10%
- Serotype III is responsible for 90%
- Case fatality rates are 2–6%

There is a "late-late onset," which occurs > 3 months out. This usually occurs in premature infants as a bacteremia without a focus, but this is usually considered to be associated with IV lines. The case fatality rate is < 1%.

Do not use antigen detection in urine. Blood cultures are the gold standard, but if the infant has been/is on antibiotic therapy, antigen detection in serum and CSF may be helpful.

Initial treatment is with PCN G + an aminoglycoside. On confirmation of group B streptococcus as the etiology, continue PCN G for 10 days for pneumonia and sepsis, and 14 days minimum for meningitis. Septic arthritis requires 2–3 weeks, while osteomyelitis requires 3–4 weeks. Treat non-meningitis cases with 200,000 U/kg/day, and meningitis with 400,000–500,000 U/kg/day.

For bacteremia, repeat blood cultures 24–48 hours into therapy. For those with meningitis, repeat lumbar puncture 24–48 hours into therapy (some recommend repeat lumbar puncture at the end of therapy to document resolution of inflammatory response). If there are still significant numbers of WBCs, or an elevated protein, many continue treatment for another week, then repeat the lumbar puncture. With meningitis, many also recommend a CT/MRI before completion of therapy.

Prevention of group B strep infection with maternal prophylaxis is reviewed in the Newborn section.

β-hemolytic Group C, G, Non-hemolytic Group D (Streptococcus bovis), and Viridans Streptococci

These organisms are normal flora of the mouth, GI tract, and female genital tract. Viridans (Latin for "green") streptococci refer to a group of 18+ species, which now are subdivided into *Streptococcus anginosis* (previously *milleri*), *mitis, salivarius*, and *mutans*. Viridans streptococci are not particularly pathogenic but, because they are frequently present in transient bacteremia episodes after dental procedures or mucous membrane injury, they can cause disease. Toothbrushing causes bacteremia ~ 40% of the time! In particular, *S. mutans*, *S. sanguis*, and *S. mitis* adhere more easily to damaged heart valves.

Viridans streptococci are common organisms in endocarditis. They make up ~ 1/3 of cases. The majority of children who have endocarditis also have some underlying congenital heart defect—or have had rheumatic fever.

Group C streptococci cause pharyngitis, particularly in college student outbreaks. Numerous case reports show that Group C and G streptococci may occasionally cause bacteremia, pneumonia, epiglottitis, osteomyelitis, endocarditis, UTIs, and other systemic infections.

Group D streptococcus (*S. bovis*) rarely causes disease in children, although some cases of endocarditis have occurred in neonates. It is more common (although still rare) in adults. If found in adults, search for colon cancer.

Groups C, non-hemolytic D, and G are susceptible to PCN. Viridans streptococci have increased rates of resistance, and you must guide therapy for endocarditis by susceptibility testing. Vancomycin is the drug of choice if patient is PCN-resistant.

For endocarditis, viridans streptococci or *S. bovis* (MIC ≤ 0.1 µg/ml) that is highly susceptible to PCN, treat with 4 weeks of IV PCN or ceftriaxone. Many add gentamicin for 5 days to kill synergistically. For MICs between 0.1– 0.5 µg/ml, use PCN and gentamicin for 2 weeks, followed by PCN alone for 2 more weeks. For resistant viridans streptococci (MIC ≥ 0.5 µg/ml), use 4–6 weeks of PCN or ampicillin plus gentamicin, or use vancomycin alone.

notes

Enterococcus

Two species of *Enterococcus* are responsible for the majority of infections in humans—*E. faecalis* and *E. faecium*. *E. faecalis* is responsible for ~ 90%. The source of these organisms is usually either the GI or urinary tract. ~ 1/2 of newborns become colonized with enterococci by the first week of life. The organism is easily spread by fomites, especially in the hospital setting.

There are 3 main types of infection in children/infants:

1) UTI
2) Polymicrobial abdominal infections
3) Bacteremia/sepsis

Few enterococci infections occur in "normal" infants. Most with UTIs have an indwelling urinary catheter.

Most neonatal enterococcal infections are nosocomial and occur after the second week of life, usually with bacteremia due to line infection or necrotizing enterocolitis. Common symptoms include bradycardia, fever, apnea, and abdominal distention.

Almost all enterococci are resistant to all cephalosporins and penicillinase-resistant PCNs, and moderately resistant to the aminoglycosides. *E. faecium* is one of the few organisms resistant to imipenem, and is causing great problems with rapidly emerging, strong resistance to vancomycin ("VRE").

If sensitive, vancomycin, PCN, and ampicillin are only inhibitory, but (!)... an aminoglycoside + any of these is effective treatment. So you must treat sensitive enterococcal sepsis or endocarditis with vancomycin, PCN, or ampicillin, in addition to gentamicin. Resistance to these antibiotics is increasing, so it is imperative that you do sensitivity testing.

Listeria monocytogenes

Listeria monocytogenes infections are associated with decreased cellular immunity syndromes like AIDS, lymphoma, and leukemia, but you may also see them in neonates and pregnant women. For some reason, it is not actually seen as much as expected in patients with AIDS. The highest incidence occurs in infants < 1 month of age. The case fatality rate of listerial meningitis is 15% overall, which ranks it behind only *S. pneumoniae*, at 21%. (Case fatality rates for the other common meningitis organisms: *H. influenzae* is 6%, *N. meningitidis* is 3%, and group B streptococcus is 7%).

Neonates generally get the infection from their colonized mothers postnatally, transplacentally, via premature rupture of membranes, or via fecal contamination from the mother at the time of birth. Environmental sources of the organism include sheep, goats, other livestock, and poultry. Infection can occur with direct contact with contaminated milk products (especially goat cheese!!), meats, or vegetables soiled with manure.

On the Board examination, be careful of a neonate for whom you are told the laboratory has preliminarily identified an organism from blood or CSF as "diphtheroids." Remember: *Listeria* is a Gram-positive rod and can mimic the appearance of contaminant "diphtheroids."

Like enterococcus, *Listeria* is resistant to cephalosporins (again, this is why ampicillin is included in the empiric treatment for meningitis in the elderly or neonates). Also as with enterococci, PCN and ampicillin are only inhibitory but (!)...an aminoglycoside in combination with either of these is very effective treatment, usually given for 2–3 weeks.

Even so, most mild-to-moderate cases of listeriosis do not require an aminoglycoside. But, treat resistant or serious cases with PCN or ampicillin in combination with an aminoglycoside; vancomycin or TMP/SMX if patient is allergic to PCN. Because aminoglycosides do not penetrate the CSF well, use very high-dose PCN or ampicillin to treat listerial meningitis. Again:

- Mild-to-moderate listeriosis: Amp
- Serious/resistant: Amp + aminoglycoside
- Listerial meningitis: high-dose Amp +/- aminoglycoside

Corynebacterium diphtheriae

Corynebacterium diphtheriae causes diphtheria. Tonsillopharyngeal diphtheria is an upper respiratory infection with a gray-white pharyngeal membrane (Figure 4-7), hoarseness, sore throat, and a low fever (< 101°)! Low fever! See Figure 4-9, showing the conjunctivitis and classic "bull neck" seen with diphtheria infection. The incubation period is 2–4 days. Laryngotracheobronchial diphtheria occurs in ~ 10% and results in hoarseness, strider, and respiratory compromise. Nasal diphtheria is more common in infants and younger children. These children have a profuse, mucoid, grayish discharge. It is the mildest type and rarely causes toxic manifestations.

Toxic effects include myocarditis with possible cardiac failure, renal effects, and polyneuritis. 10% develop myocarditis, which typically occurs in the 1st week of infection. Arrhythmias are common. Renal failure is rare, but proteinuria, cylindruria, or microscopic hematuria is common. Usually, the neural involvement includes isolated peripheral nerve palsies or a Guillain-Barré-like syndrome.

Treatment is erythromycin, mainly to render the patient noncontagious, as opposed to being therapeutic. Second choice is PCN. Always give diphtheria antitoxin with the antibiotic. Also, after recovery, immunize patients with diphtheria toxoid.

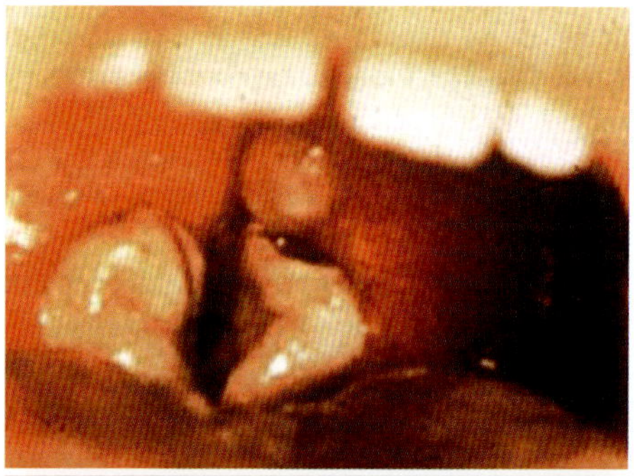

Figure 4-7: Pharyngeal Membrane

notes

Quick Quiz

1) What is the best antibiotic(s) for treatment of bacteremia due to Enterococcus faecium?
2) Which age group has the highest incidence of *Listeria* infection?
3) True or False: A blood culture grows an organism preliminarily identified as "diphtheroids" with final identification available tomorrow. In a neonate, it is probably safe to assume that this organism is a contaminant.
4) What food products have a risk of carrying *Listeria*?
5) Describe the clinical syndrome produced by *Corynebacterium diphtheriae*.
6) How do you treat diphtheria?
7) Fried rice left out un-refrigerated may grow this bacteria which can cause a self-limited gastroenteritis. What is the bug?

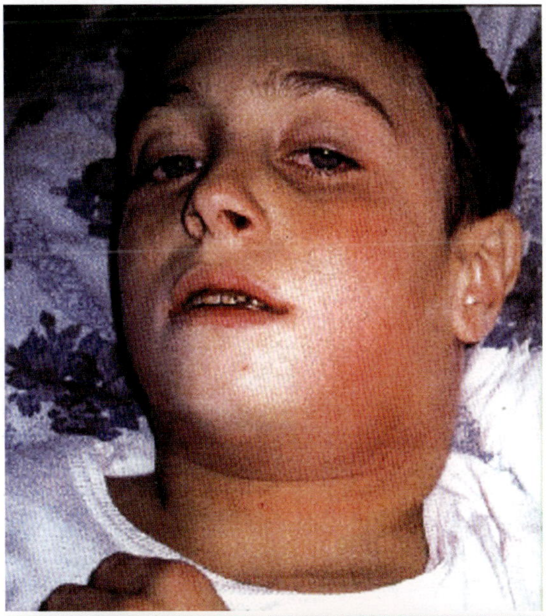

Figure 4-9: Diphtheria, Bull Neck Conjunctivitis

Corynebacterium jeikeium (JK) is especially a problem in neutropenic patients and bone marrow transplant units, where it is a cause of IV catheter-related infections. JK is resistant to most drugs. Vancomycin is the only effective agent.

Arcanobacterium haemolyticum (previously *Corynebacterium haemolyticum*) causes a pharyngitis similar to that of *S. pyogenes*, with a desquamative scarlatiniform rash and lymphadenitis. Most commonly, the infection occurs in the adolescent age group. It is effectively treated with PCN, erythromycin, or tetracycline.

Bacillus anthracis

Bacillus anthracis are large, Gram-positive rods (bacilli) that cause anthrax. There are 3 types of anthrax: cutaneous (95%, See Figure 4-8), gastrointestinal, and pulmonic ("woolsorters disease"). Because of recent bioterrorist attacks, this organism will appear on the Boards! [Know it!] Inoculation occurs from handling contaminated hides/wool or—less naturally—via malicious contamination, such as in the mail. The cutaneous form of anthrax starts as a painless papule that vesiculates and forms a painless ulcer, then a painless black eschar, often with a lot of non-pitting, painless induration and swelling. *B. anthracis* produces a tripartite exotoxin, consisting of edema factor, protective antigen, and lethal factor. Both edema factor and lethal factor require protective antigen to be active. Treatment of choice for anthrax is penicillin G (if sensitive) or a quinolone. Second choice may be tetracycline. Prophylaxis for exposures is ciprofloxacin for 30–60 days, unless the MICs of the organism indicate PCN susceptibility.

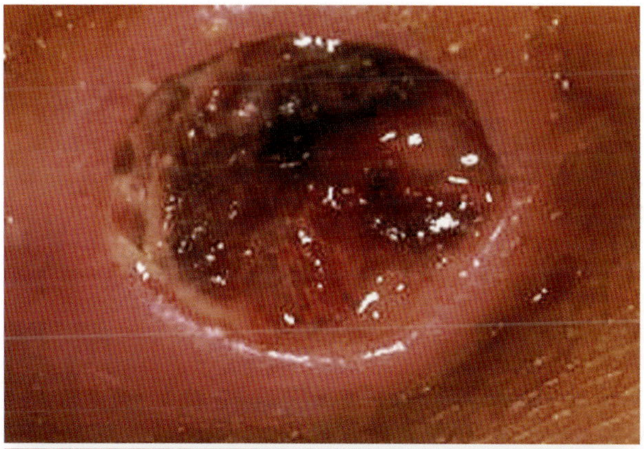

Figure 4-8: Anthrax Ulcer (painless)

Bacillus cereus

Bacillus cereus is a close relative of *Bacillus anthracis*. It can cause 2 forms of gastroenteritis: 1) A short incubation (1–6 hr) emetic type, due to preformed heat stable toxin, and 2) A longer incubation (8–16 hr) diarrheal type, due to enterotoxin production *in vivo* in the GI tract. The emetic form is associated with fried rice left at room temperature. This gastroenteritis is self-limited and necessitates only symptomatic treatment.

Diagnosis is usually clinical, but you can look for *B. cereus* spores from stool or emesis, or by isolating the toxin from the suspected food item.

B. cereus is an occasional cause of infection in contact lens wearers, after a traumatic eye injury, and is a possible cause of IV catheter-related infections. Treat serious disease with vancomycin.

notes

Clostridium species

Clostridium is a strict, anaerobic, Gram-positive rod.

- *Clostridium difficile* causes antibiotic-associated colitis.
- *Clostridium botulinum* causes botulism—the most potent toxin known! It blocks presynaptic acetylcholine release. This is discussed further in the Neurology section.
- *Clostridium perfringens* is one of the most common causes of food poisoning in the U.S. It presents as a 24-hour (or less) diarrheal illness, and is associated with contaminated meat.
- *Clostridium septicum*: The majority of patients with *C. septicum* sepsis have an associated GI malignancy—this is seen mostly in adults.
- *Clostridium tetani* is the cause of tetanus.

As mentioned above, antibiotic-associated colitis is caused by *Clostridium difficile* (antibiotic-associated diarrhea is usually just a side effect of the medicine). Symptoms can occur up to 3 weeks after the antibiotics are stopped. To diagnose, do a stool assay for the *Clostridium difficile* cytotoxin. A toxin assay is required because 5% of healthy persons have *C. difficile* in their stool, and not all of the *C. difficile* organisms produce the cytot oxin. Treatment: Stop the antibiotics and give 7–14 days of metronidazole. You could use oral vancomycin, but it is more expensive ($300+)! Concerns about developing resistance make metronidazole the drug of choice. Other treatments are bacitracin, rifampin, or bile-binding resins (cholestyramine, etc), which bind the toxin. Relapse rates are ~ 30%. This is usually due to the spores becoming active; just repeat the same treatment!

So a common Board scenario/question: A child has *C. difficile*-associated diarrhea. You treat her with metronidazole. She gets better. She returns 2 weeks after resolution of her diarrhea with a relapse. What do you use to treat her again? Metronidazole.

Use bacitracin, rifampin, and cholestyramine as adjuncts in complicated cases.

Cellulitis and gas gangrene can be caused by *C. septicum, perfringens, tetani*, or *novyi*. Most gas gangrene is due to *C. perfringens*. The main toxin in all *Clostridia* is the "alpha toxin." For acute antibiotic treatment of *C. perfringens*, use PCN (tetracycline or clindamycin if patient is PCN-allergic).

Tetanus is an acute illness due to the exotoxin produced by *C. tetani*. This clostridium is commonly found in soil and in normal human fecal flora 2–30% of the time. The highest incidence occurs in people who live on farms. Tetanus in children is rare in the U.S. However, in developing countries, it kills 400,000 neonates yearly.

Two forms of tetanus are observed: 1) Generalized, with widespread distribution of toxin; and 2) Local, with toxin only near the portal of entry. In children, the generalized form is more common. The incubation period is 5–12 days. The portal of entry, typically a wound, appears to be inconsequential. The infection begins with increasing stiffness of muscles of the neck, jaw, and large muscles of the back and lower extremities. Usually, by 24 hours into the illness, there is marked stiffness of the jaw and neck. The spasms of tetanus

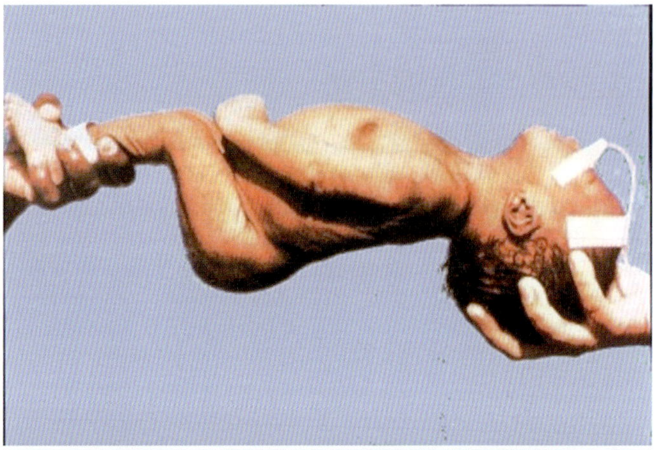

Figure 4-10: Tetanus in Newborn

are characteristic: Stimuli such as a loud noise, a touch, or a flashing light can each cause paroxysmal contraction of the whole body and lasts for 5–10 seconds. The body is rigid like a board, the head is pulled back, the back is arched, the fists are clenched, and the thumbs abducted. (See Figure 4-10). The child's jaw is completely immobile, and the face has a tonic expression, known as "risus sardonicus:" Raising of the eyebrows, narrowing of the palpebral fissures, downward/outward moving of the angles of the mouth, and pressing of the upper lip to the teeth. The affected person does not lose consciousness. Death results from eventual respiratory failure.

Neonatal tetanus, or "tetanus neonatorum," results from the cultural habit of placing manure or soil on/in the umbilical stump. The illness starts on day 3–10 of life, and presents with the child crying excessively and unable to suck. Quickly ensuing are trismus (persistent contraction of the masseter muscles), tonic contractions, spasms, and seizures. Death occurs from hypoxia, exhaustion, and lack of calories. Mortality rates approach 75%.

Diagnosis is clinical. Aim treatment at providing a quiet, stimulus-free environment. Manage with continuously administered neurologic blocking agents and mechanical ventilation. It is vital to use parenteral fluids and careful nutritional support.

Tetanus antitoxin is required. Metronidazole is now the preferred antibiotic, although PCN G is also acceptable.

What about tetanus prophylaxis for routine wound management? Let's consider some cases involving a sweet girl named Marla:

- Marla has a staple injury (a clean, minor wound). She has had either an unknown number of tetanus immunizations, or a known number < 3. Give her Td (or DTaP if < 7 years of age).
- Marla has a staple injury (a clean, minor wound). She has had ≥ 3 prior tetanus immunizations, with the last immunization < 10 years ago. She requires no further immunization at this point.

notes

Quick Quiz

1) What is the treatment for a recurrence of *C. difficile* diarrhea?
2) How do you treat tetanus?
3) Know the tetanus scenarios listed for Marla in the text.
4) What age groups have the highest incidence of meningococcal infection?
5) What laboratory test is recommended in children with meningococcemia to screen for an immunologic deficiency?
6) What is the treatment for meningococcemia?

- Marla has a staple injury (a clean, minor wound). She has had ≥ 3 prior tetanus immunizations, and her last immunization was > 10 years ago. She requires a booster Td today.
- Marla steps on a dirty nail with cow feces on it. Her dog licks the foot after the injury. She has an unknown number of immunizations or a known number < 3. Give her Td (or DTaP if she's < 7 years of age) and human tetanus immune globulin (TIG).
- Marla steps on a dirty nail with cow feces on it. Her dog licks the foot after the injury. She has had ≥ 3 tetanus immunizations in the past, with the most recent < 5 years ago. She requires no vaccine.
- Marla steps on a dirty nail with cow feces on it. Her dog licks the foot after the injury. She has had ≥ 3 tetanus immunizations in the past, and her last immunization was 5.5 years ago. She requires Td (or DTaP if she is < 7 years old).

Here, then, are the protocols:

- Wound is dirty and either the child has had < 3 tetanus immunizations or the immunization history is unknown—use TIG + immunize.
- Wound is clean and immunizations are up-to-date (most recent < 10 years)—no treatment.
- Wound is dirty and immunizations are up-to-date, with most recent immunization < 5 years—no treatment.

GRAM-NEGATIVE BACTERIA

Neisseria meningitidis

Neisseria meningitidis (meningococcus) is a *Gram-negative diplococcus* that is an occasional, ordinary inhabitant of the upper respiratory tract. Carrier rates normally are 2–30% in normal populations. In an epidemic, the carrier rate approaches 100%! Meningococcus usually does not cause disease, because specific antibodies (humoral defense) and complement lyse the organisms as they enter the bloodstream. There are 5 clinically significant serogroups based on the antigenic differences between their capsular polysaccharides. These groups are A, B, C, W-135, and Y. In the U.S., serogroups B, C, and Y each account for 30% of the cases reported.

Meningococcus is now the 2nd leading cause of meningitis (after pneumococcus). The highest incidence of infection is seen in children < 2 years of age, the period of waning maternal IgG antibodies. A 2nd increase in incidence occurs in adolescents ages 15– 19. Highest rates occur in the winter and early spring. Most adults have developed natural immunity against the meningococcus.

Patients with terminal complement deficiency (C5–C9), or those deficient of properdin, are especially prone to meningococcemia. Ensure that all patients with bacteremia or meningitis have a CH50 or CH100 assay. ~ 20% of children with systemic meningococcal disease will end up having a complement deficiency.

Meningococcemia presents with fever, hypotension, diffuse purpuric lesions, and DIC. > 60% will have a petechial rash. (See Figure 4-11).

Penicillin G is the treatment of choice; for the PCN-allergic, give fluoroquinolones (to adults) or 3rd generation cephalosporins—if rash only—to children. If the child is allergic to PCN and cephalosporin, chloramphenicol is the drug of choice. With prompt treatment, the mortality rate from men-

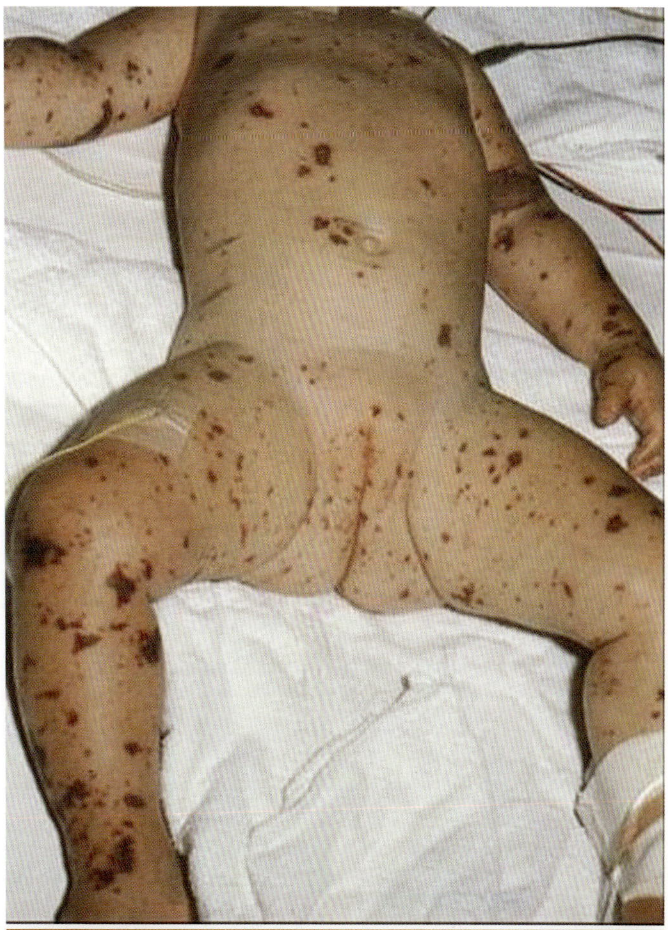

Figure 4-11: Meningococcemia

notes

ingococcemia is 10%. Hearing loss is a common complication of meningococcal meningitis.

Who should receive prophylaxis? Household, daycare, and close intimate contacts. Give rifampin 10 mg/kg (max dose 600 mg) q 12 hours x 2 days; or ceftriaxone 125 mg IM for children < 12 years, or 250 mg IM for children > 12 as an alternative. Ceftriaxone is the drug of choice for an exposed pregnant woman! You can give a one-time dose of ciprofloxacin (1 time, 500 mg) in adults > 18. These drugs are better than PCN for eradicating the carrier state, because they concentrate in the throat mucosa. Give a patient with meningococcus prophylaxis before leaving the hospital (obviously, if they received ceftriaxone or cefotaxime for treatment, they are covered).

What about the nurse who took the blood pressure when the patient came in? Or you're the physician who spent 30 minutes in the room with the patient before making your astute diagnosis? No, you don't take prophylaxis unless you have close intimate contact, such as with intubation or mouth-to-mouth resuscitation. I know this is different from what most people do in the "real world," where ciprofloxacin is given out like candy on Halloween. But for the Board examination, as the provider, you take prophylaxis only under these circumstances involving contact with oral secretions!

Vaccine is available for serogroups A, C, Y, and W-135. Remember: 30% of infections are due to serogroup B, so you are still missing a good chunk of infections. But vaccinate children who are splenectomized, or have functional asplenia (kids with sickle cell), and those with complement or properdin deficiencies. It is a polysaccharide vaccine, so it works only in kids > 2 years of age. All military recruits receive it, and most recommend that all college freshmen who will be living in campus dormitories be vaccinated as well. In January 2005, a new conjugated meningococcal vaccine was released (Menactra™); more info in the Health Supervision chapter.

Neisseria gonorrhoeae

Sexually Transmitted Disease

Neisseria gonorrhoeae is a common cause of sexually transmitted disease. It is a Gram-negative organism that is usually found as diplococci. The penicillinase-producing strains of *N. gonorrhoeae* now account for 50% of cases in many areas of Asia and Africa, and are also common in the U.S. The sexually transmitted disease aspects (cervicitis, PID, urethritis, etc.) are discussed in the Adolescent section, as is disseminated gonococcal infection in adolescents—which is very important to know for the Boards!

Gonococcal Ophthalmia

Gonococcal ophthalmia can occur at any age (presumably from self-inoculation; I really don't want to think about that). Most cases occur in the newborn as the infant passes through an infected birth canal. The use of 1% silver nitrate, 0.5% erythromycin, or 1% tetracycline ointment significantly reduces incidence.

Infants will present 2–7 days after delivery with bloody, green, or serosanguineous discharge from the eyes. If this occurs, the first thing to do is get a Gram-stained smear and culture for *N. gonorrhea*! If the discharge occurs < 48 hours, it is almost always due to a chemical reaction to the prophylaxis. If it occurs 7–14 days post-birth, it is almost always due to *Chlamydia trachomatis*. Also, do a blood culture and lumbar puncture in infants with presumed gonococcal conjunctivitis.

Complications of gonococcal ophthalmia can include iridocyclitis and corneal ulcerations.

Ceftriaxone 50 mg/kg IM or IV x 1 is sufficient for treating ophthalmia neonatorum, although many receive antibiotics for 2–3 days, until blood and CSF cultures are confirmed negative.

Moraxella catarrhalis

Moraxella catarrhalis (formerly *Branhamella catarrhalis* [formerly *Neisseria catarrhalis*!]) is a Gram-negative diplococcus that causes respiratory infections. It is the 3rd most common cause of otitis media and sinusitis in children (behind *S. pneumoniae* and non-typeable *H. influenzae*). Rarely, it can cause bacteremia, particularly in immunocompromised children.

Almost all *Moraxella* strains produce β-lactamase. Amoxicillin/clavulanic acid, cefuroxime, cefprozil, cefpodoxime, erythromycin, tetracycline, and TMP/SMX are all generally effective agents.

Pseudomonas aeruginosa

Pseudomonas aeruginosa is a small Gram-negative rod with a single flagellum. *Pseudomonas* is commonly found in cystic fibrosis (see Pulmonology section). Consider *Pseudomonas aeruginosa* if there is a history of nail-puncture wounds (especially if through a tennis shoe), osteomyelitis and endocarditis in IV drug abusers, bacteremia in burn patients, and chronic otitis externa (can be especially severe in diabetics). You might see ecthyma gangrenosum (round, indurated, black lesion with central ulceration) with pseudomonal bacteremia. *Pseudomonas* is the cause of "hot tub rash," which people get from improperly chlorinated hot tubs (this is usually self-limited).

Treatment is with broad-spectrum PCNs, such as piperacillin/tazobactam and ticarcillin/clavulanic acid; or cephalosporins, such as ceftazidime and cefepime, or aminoglycosides. Quinolones are also effective, as are imipenem and meropenem. [Know: Never use ceftriaxone for *Pseudomonas* infection.]

Burkholderia cepacia and B. pseudomallei

Until recently, *Burkholderia cepacia* and *B. pseudomallei* used to be known as *Pseudomonas species*. *B. cepacia* is common in cystic fibrosis, is very difficult to treat, and has a poor prognosis. *B. pseudomallei* is a common infection in children in Southeast Asia (known as melioidosis), and can result in localized infection or septicemia. Treatment is even more difficult than for *Pseudomonas aeruginosa*; both are resistant to

notes

Quick Quiz

1) After exposure to a child with meningococcemia, who should receive prophylaxis in the community?
2) After exposure to a child with meningococcemia, which health care workers should receive prophylaxis?
3) Who should receive the meningococcal vaccine?
4) What age group is most commonly affected by gonococcal ophthalmia?
5) For eye discharges after delivery, what is responsible for the discharge if it occurs within 48 hours after delivery? 2–7 days after delivery? 7–14 days after delivery?
6) What is the treatment for uncomplicated gonococcal ophthalmia?
7) True or False: Most *Moraxella* produce β-lactamase.
8) A child steps on a nail through his tennis shoe. What organisms would you be concerned about if he developed an osteomyelitis in the foot?
9) Iguana = What organism?
10) What location do many *Shigella* infections occur?
11) Which requires many fewer organisms for transmission? *Shigella* or *Salmonella*?
12) What laboratory finding is common in *Shigella* infections?

aminoglycosides! Quinolones, doxycycline, chloramphenicol, and trimethoprim may be helpful.

Salmonella

Salmonella are Gram-negative bacilli that are usually motile. Non-typhoidal salmonella are a fairly common cause of diarrhea. Because the bacteria are not host-adapted, like *S.* serotype Typhi (formerly known as *S. typhi*), they can be found in many different non-human host animals. Frozen foods (especially chicken), milk, and eggs can spread it. Baby chicks, iguanas, turtles, and other exotic pets may also be sources of infections. Treatment increases the risk of developing a carrier state; so for uncomplicated gastroenteritis, do not give antibiotics! However, give antibiotic therapy for *Salmonella* diarrhea in children < 6 months of age and older children with immunocompromising diseases (HIV, agammaglobulinemia, etc.).

Salmonella serotype Typhi is, unlike most *Salmonella,* non-motile and encapsulated. It causes *typhoid fever*, usually from contaminated food, milk, or water. Adults are more likely to be carriers, because *S.* serotype Typhi tends to seed in gallstones. (Did "typhoid Mary" have gallstones?) The infection tends to cause *leukopenia.* The classic "rose spots" form on the trunk about a *week* after the fever starts; these look like little, 2–3 mm angiomas. Perform 3 sets of blood cultures; bone marrow culture is the most sensitive test for diagnosis of *S.* serotype Typhi.

Typhoid *vaccine* is recommended for travelers (> 2 years old) who go outside of the usual tourist areas of Latin America, Asia, and Africa.

Treatment of typhoid fever: options include 3rd generation cephalosporins, ampicillin, TMP/SMX, quinolones, and chloramphenicol, depending on sensitivities. Carriers without gallbladder disease or stones can usually be cleared with 6 weeks of ampicillin + probenecid. (The probenecid decreases clearance and causes a higher blood level of the ampicillin.)

Shigella

Shigella sonnei is the most common serotype in the U.S., with *S. flexneri* 2nd in frequency. Highest incidences occur in daycare centers, residences for the mentally ill, and persons living on Native American reservations. Children ages 1–4 years have the highest incidence, with a peak between July and October. Outbreaks also occur due to contaminated pools and lakes. Food-borne outbreaks, especially from fresh fruits and vegetables, also occur.

Person-to-person transmission of *Shigella* plays a key role (unlike *Salmonella* infection). *Shigella* can infect with only 10–100 organisms vs. the thousands to millions for *Salmonella.*

Incubation is most often 24–48 hours. Most children's infection begins with fever, malaise, poor appetite, vomiting, and/or headache. Diarrhea is usually watery and can progress within hours or days to dysentery: frequent small stools with mucous or blood accompanied by lower abdominal cramps and tenesmus.

Rectal prolapse occurs in 5–8%. Peripheral WBCs are usually elevated; bandemia is very common. Seizures occur with increased frequency with *Shigella* infection.

Treat with ceftriaxone, cefixime, and azithromycin. Nalidixic acid is cheap and also effective. TMP-SMX and ampicillin used to be the drugs of choice, but resistance has made them all but useless for *Shigella* infection.

E. coli

E. coli is a Gram-negative, lactose-fermenting, motile rod belonging to the Enterobacteriaceae family. *E. coli* is a common cause of UTI. It also is a cause of meningitis in the neonate.

There are > 200 different serotypes, with 5 phenotypes causing diarrhea:

1) Enteropathogenic (EPEC): Causes acute and chronic diarrhea in infants. Treat with TMP-SMX or oral gentamicin.
2) Enterotoxigenic (ETEC): Causes watery diarrhea in infants and "traveler's diarrhea." TMP-SMX is the drug of choice.
3) Enteroinvasive (EIEC): Causes diarrhea and fever.
4) Enterohemorrhagic (EHEC) and also now known as STEC (Shiga-toxin producing *E. coli*): Responsible for hemolytic uremic syndrome. No antibiotics (see below).
5) Enteroaggregative (EaggEC): Persistent diarrhea in children in developing countries and in travelers.

notes

In general, do not give antimotility agents! Bismuth subsalicylate (Pepto-Bismol®) is useful for ETEC infections.

Enterohemorrhagic (EHEC, STEC) outbreaks of ***E. coli* *O157:H7***: food-borne infections are becoming more frequent—especially in the U.S. The incidence of *E. coli* O157:H7 infection is > *Shigella*! Dairy cattle appear to be a major reservoir, and the disease is linked to eating undercooked beef and unpasteurized milk or apple juice. This *E. coli* produces a Shiga toxin (STX), which may cause bloody diarrhea, hemorrhagic colitis, *hemolytic uremic syndrome* (HUS), and can simulate TTP. Culture requires sorbitol-enhanced agar. HUS classically has the triad of kidney failure, thrombocytopenia with purpura, and hemolytic anemia. Treatment with antibiotics is contraindicated! It appears that treating these patients infected with O157:H7 strains increases the risk of HUS.

Haemophilus influenzae

Overview

Haemophilus influenzae is a small, "pleomorphic," Gram-negative coccobacillus. *H. influenzae* type b (Hib) used to be the most common cause of meningitis and serious bacteremia in children. However, the introduction of the *H. influenzae* vaccine quickly reduced the incidence of encapsulated *H. influenzae* type b (the etiology of severe invasive disease), to the point where it has become almost nonexistent in some centers. Today, non-typeable strains are still responsible for a large number of mucosal infections, including conjunctivitis, otitis media, sinusitis, and bronchitis.

In newborns, incidence of non-typeable *H. influenzae* has increased for bacteremia and meningitis. Most of the organisms are picked up traversing the birth canal from the mother. ~ 80% of cases occur in the 1st day of life. *In utero*, infection also occurs. Because of this increased incidence, many have stopped using ampicillin and gentamicin in the newborn, which will not cover β-lactamase-producing *H. influenzae*.

Vaccine use has also resulted in "herd immunity," whereby those not vaccinated have some protection because of the reduced incidence of nasopharyngeal carriage for pathogenic strains. Many of these infections are more historical, but you still need to know them for the Boards!

Meningitis

Symptoms are nonspecific for *H. influenzae* meningitis. Peak age is < 1 year. ~ 1/3 of children have seizures with *H. influenzae* meningitis. Petechial rash also occurs, as in meningococcal infection. Other sites of infection are common, including septic arthritis or buccal cellulitis. Common complications include subdural empyema, brain infarcts, cerebritis, ventriculitis, brain abscess, and hydrocephalus. Mortality is ~ 5%. Long-term sequelae occur in 15–30% of survivors, with sensorineural hearing loss the most common. Other sequelae include language disorder, mental retardation, and developmental disorders.

Prior to, or concurrent with, antibiotics (ceftriaxone or cefotaxime), use dexamethasone 0.6 mg/kg/day divided q 6 hours x 2 days to prevent hearing loss and neurologic sequelae.

Epiglottitis

Epiglottitis occurs primarily in children ages 2–7 years with an abrupt onset of high fever, dysphagia, and drooling. The epiglottis is described as "cherry red." These kids have the "I'm going to die" look. Most would not try and examine the oropharynx of an **uncooperative** child with possible epiglottitis without the presence of an adequate airway or anesthesia/ENT in the operating room. For children in whom the diagnosis is certain—based on presentation and clinical examination—intraoral examination is likely unnecessary. In those in whom the diagnosis is unclear, many experts advocate the use of a tongue depressor in a **cooperative** child. You must view individual factors for each case. (Further therapy issues are in the Pulmonology section).

Septic Arthritis/Osteomyelitis

Before the Hib vaccine was available, *H. influenzae* was the most common cause of septic arthritis in children < age 2 years. Septic arthritis of the hip and shoulder require surgical drainage.

Buccal Cellulitis

Buccal cellulitis previously was virtually always caused by *H. influenzae* infection, but now the vaccine has all but prevented this infection from occurring. If present, the child was almost always bacteremic with *H. influenzae*. Buccal cellulitis is palpable on both sides of the cheek, purplish in color, and these children are very toxic in appearance.

Periorbital or preseptal cellulitis was commonly due to *H. influenzae* also. Today, pneumococcus is the most common etiology for bacteremic periorbital cellulitis. A significant portion of cases of preseptal cellulitis is related to minor trauma of the eyelids or insect bites, and is due to *S. aureus* or a Group A Streptococcus.

Occult Bacteremia

Occult bacteremia with *H. influenzae* is very different from occult bacteremia with pneumococcus. Pneumococcal "occult" bacteremia will usually spontaneously resolve without therapy, while bacteremia with *H. influenzae* will result in 30–50% developing meningitis or other deep, focal infection from occult bacteremia!

Pneumonia

Pneumonia from *H. influenzae* used to cause ~ 1/3 of bacterial pneumonia in the pre-Hib vaccine era. Today, it is rare. Most cases have pleural effusion; blood cultures are positive in 90%.

Treat invasive *H. influenzae* with a 3rd generation cephalosporin—either ceftriaxone or cefotaxime. You can use ce-

notes

Quick Quiz

1) Name the diseases with which *E. coli* O157:H7 is associated.
2) What food products are associated with *E. coli* O157:H7?
3) What age are newborns at greatest risk for serious disseminated disease from nontypeable *H. influenzae*?
4) What is the most common long-term sequela of *H. influenzae* meningitis?
5) Know the treatment for *H. influenzae* meningitis.
6) How is the epiglottis described in acute epiglottitis?
7) What is buccal cellulitis associated with?
8) What is the most common cause of bacteremic periorbital cellulitis?
9) What is a common cause of periorbital cellulitis if a bug bite or scratch was the inciting injury?
10) True or False: You should treat all occult bacteremias due to *H. influenzae* with parenteral antibiotics.
11) What is the drug of choice for otitis media? What if you suspect or find a β-lactamase producing *H. influenzae*?
12) A daycare center in a commune (that does not allow immunizations) has 2 cases of *H. influenzae* meningitis. What should the other children in the daycare center receive?
13) How is *Yersinia pestis* transmitted?
14) How is plague diagnosed? Treated?
15) What organism is associated with "pseudoappendicitis syndrome" in older children and adolescents?

furoxime (2nd generation) for non-meningitis infection, but with caution because it does not cross the blood-brain barrier well. Treat uncomplicated Hib meningitis with IV therapy for 7–10 days; septic arthritis requires 14–21 days. Those with osteomyelitis, pericarditis, or empyema are generally treated for 4–6 weeks IV, followed by oral therapy. Occult Hib infection requires therapy to prevent focal infection from developing.

For noninvasive disease, such as otitis media and sinusitis, amoxicillin is the drug of choice. If amoxicillin fails, use agents active against β-lactamase-producing strains, including amoxicillin/clavulanic acid, TMP-SMX, azithromycin/clarithromycin, cefuroxime axetil, cefixime, cefpodoxime, etc.

Chemoprophylaxis is important for those exposed to invasive strains of *H. influenzae*. The rules for who gets prophylaxis are quite complicated, and I have to re-read the guidelines several times to make sense of it. In general, for the exam, you'll give prophylaxis. Give rifampin 20 mg/kg (max 600 mg) q day x 4 days to household contacts and daycare attendees (although, hopefully, most of them are immunized).

Yersinia

Yersinia pestis

Yersinia pestis is a Gram-negative coccobacillus that causes plague. Reservoir is wild rodents. It is transmitted by fleas or direct contact, such as skinning animals, and has high mortality. The bubonic type causes large, localized lymphadenopathy ("buboes") that suppurate. (see Figure 4-12). If not treated, it can lead to sepsis and death. The bubonic type also may lead to a pneumonic form that is rapidly transmitted to bystanders by coughing. (Again, bioterrorism has brought this organism back to the Board exam!)

Note: Plague and tularemia present similarly (adenopathy after hunting, etc.), except that the geographic locations are different—desert SW for plague vs. Arkansas, Missouri, and Oklahoma for tularemia.

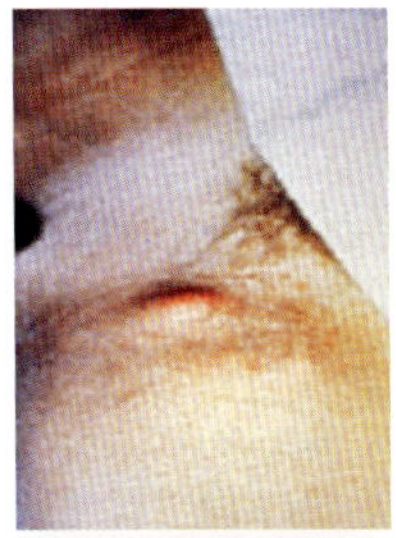

Figure 4-12

Diagnose plague by aspirating the lymph nodes or by serology.

Treat plague with streptomycin. 2nd line choices: Tetracycline or quinolones.

Yersinia enterocolitica

Yersinia enterocolitica is a small, Gram-negative coccobacillus. It produces entero- and endotoxin. Most humans become infected from ingesting contaminated food, milk, or water. Pigs are commonly infected, so those who handle pork products, especially chitterlings, are at increased risk. A fairly common scenario is for a grandmother (or grandfather) to prepare chitterlings, or handle raw pork, and then feed or handle the baby without washing her hands well—resulting in the infant becoming colonized, and then infected. Contaminated blood transfusions have also been implicated in some cases. *Yersinia* is found in ~ 1% of diarrheal illnesses.

Older children and adolescents present with the "pseudoappendicitis syndrome," which can be due to *Yersinia pseudotuberculosis* or *Y. enterocolitica*. This appears just like appendicitis.

Adults are more likely to get the reactive arthritis and erythema nodosum associated with *Yersinia* infection.

Bacteremia occurs in the very young and in those with iron overload (especially children who are transfusion-dependent with sickle cell disease, aplastic anemia, etc.).

Treat with TMP-SMX, aminoglycosides, tetracycline, 3rd generation cephalosporins, and quinolones.

Legionella pneumophila

The Legionellae family comprises many species—of which *Legionella pneumophila* causes 80–90% of human Legionellae infections. Legionella infections are rare in children. Legionellae are aerobic, Gram-negative bacilli that require a particular media (enriched, buffered, charcoal yeast extract) to grow.

Legionella is contained in water, and modes of transmission are multiple—with aspiration the most likely.

notes

Legionella pneumophila infection (legionellosis) causes legions of problems. Multisystem disease is the clue! Patients often have diarrhea and CNS symptoms (H/A, delirium, and *confusion)*, in addition to the pneumonia. Presentation is similar to, and often confused with, *Mycoplasma pneumoniae.* Like *M. pneumoniae,* the CXR looks much worse than the exam indicates. It can also cause "Pontiac fever," which is a multisystem flu-like illness without pneumonia.

Treat moderate infections with azithromycin—or quinolones. Erythromycin is also effective. If severely ill, add rifampin.

Klebsiella

Klebsiella is a rare cause of pneumonia, bacteremia, and meningitis in children. It also can cause UTIs, but is much less common than *E. coli*. Most *Klebsiella* are uniformly resistant to ampicillin.

Brucella

Brucellosis is a zoonosis caused by an aerobic Gram-negative bacillus that, worldwide, is usually caused by *B. melitensis* (goats, sheep, and camels). Other strains: *Brucella abortus* (cattle), *B. suis* (pigs), and *B. canis* (dogs). It is often transmitted to humans via unpasteurized milk or cheese, by inhalation (work-related), or by handling carcasses. It affects the heart (especially suspect in culture-negative endocarditis), lungs, GI tract, GU (orchitis, abortion), and endocrine glands (thyroiditis, adrenal insufficiency, SIADH). Granulomatous hepatitis can also occur. Check for brucellosis in an FUO workup! Confirming the diagnosis is difficult. Cultures may take up to 6 weeks to grow. In some types, you can do serotyping (looking for increasing specific IgM titers).

Treatment requires combination therapy:

Doxycycline x 4–6 weeks + aminoglycoside (streptomycin, gentamicin, or netilmicin) x 2 wks, or

Doxycycline + rifampin x 4–8 wks.

Quinolones are effective for acute disease but may have a higher relapse rate.

For children < 8 years, it is very difficult to treat. Most recommend TMP-SMX for 4–6 weeks. Add gentamicin with rifampin for serious or complicated infections.

Francisella tularensis

Francisella tularensis is a small, Gram-negative pleomorphic bacillus that causes tularemia ("rabbit fever"). It is found in many animals, and is especially prevalent in Arkansas, Missouri, and Oklahoma. It is transmitted by ticks and blood-sucking flies; the organism may also be ingested or inhaled. Typically, patients with tularemia present with a sudden onset of fever, chills, myalgias, and arthralgias, followed by an irregular ulcer at the site of inoculation. Known as the "Ulceroglandular form," it may persist for months. Regional lymphadenopathy develops, and these nodes may necrose and suppurate. Other forms include: glandular (without the ulcer), oculoglandular (conjunctival and lymph node), oropharyngeal (sore throat), pneumonic (pneumonia), and typhoidal (septicemic form).

Base diagnosis of tularemia on the typical clinical syndrome, and confirm with serologic testing for *Francisella tularensis*. Differentials include plague, which occurs mostly in the desert SW.

Treat with streptomycin, gentamicin, or tetracycline if not severely ill.

Bartonella

Bartonella henselae causes cat-scratch disease or, in the immunocompromised patient, bacillary angiomatosis. (Who sang "Cat-Scratch Fever"?) Cat-scratch disease is characterized by > 3 weeks of chronic, tender, regional cervical/axillary lymphadenopathy, a history of cat contact or scratch, and a primary skin lesion, which appears as a small, nondescript, pink papule (~ 60% have the skin lesion). See Figure 4-14. Dog contact may be responsible in some cases. The enlarged node (See Figure 4-13) can persist for months, but usually resolves. 10% will have systemic symptoms, which can include encephalopathy (2.4%), seizures, blindness due to neuroretinitis (1.4%), hepatosplenomegaly, oculoglandular fever, and FUO. The oculoglandular syndrome of Parinaud is one of the more common atypical presentations.

Diagnosis is usually clinical; however, use of PCR and serum antibodies is available.

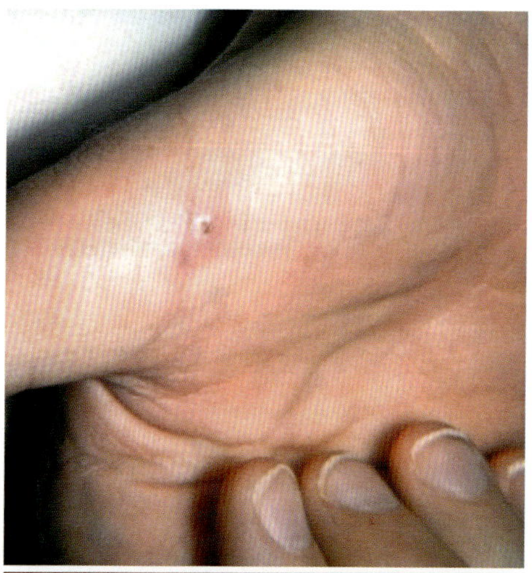

Figure 4-14: Cat-Scratch D., 1° Lesion

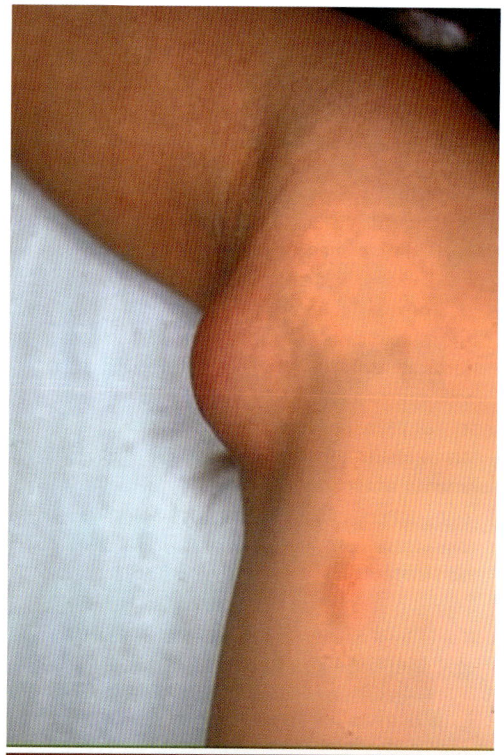

Figure 4-13: Cat-Scratch D., Adenopathy

notes

Quick Quiz

1) For which type of atypical pneumonia is multisystem disease a diagnostic clue?
2) What antibiotics may be useful in cat-scratch disease?
3) What do you suspect in a neonate with *Citrobacter* growing in the CSF?
4) Where does the rash occur with RMSF (to the right of this question is not the correct answer)?

Do not incise and drain because a persistent sinus tract infection will likely develop. Node biopsy may be required in atypical cases to confirm the diagnosis, and Warthin-Starry silver stain would identify granulomas and bacteria.

Treatment is supportive, although recently, azithromycin and rifampin have been shown to reduce the time for lymph node swelling to resolve.

Bacillary angiomatosis occurs mainly in HIV-infected adults. The skin lesions of bacillary angiomatosis are identical to "verruga peruana." Treatment: Erythromycin +/- rifampin, depending on severity. (Ted Nugent is the answer to the question from above.)

Helicobacter pylori

Helicobacter pylori is a Gram-negative, spiral, flagellated bacillus. It causes gastritis and PUD, and is a risk factor for adenocarcinoma of the stomach. Infection is frequently acquired in childhood, and remains asymptomatic for life in most individuals. More in the GI section.

Citrobacter

Citrobacter is rare. However, if the Board Exam mentions a neonate with *Citrobacter* growing in a blood or CSF culture, immediately get a CT/MRI of the head to look for brain abscess!

RICKETTSIAE

Rickettsia

Rickettsia rickettsii, a Gram-negative coccobacillus, causes Rocky Mountain spotted fever (RMSF)—[know!] This disease has a 3% mortality. Classic signs and symptoms include a rash, fever, headache, arthralgias (but *not* overt arthritis), and a history of recent exposure to ticks. The peak incidence is in children ages 5–9 years. It is common in the Carolinas, Georgia, Virginia, Missouri, Oklahoma, and Texas. The rash occurs on the distal extremities. (See Figure 4-15). It progresses from maculopapular to petechial. Most infected persons get the rash, but few get all of the classic signs/symptoms. Patients may also present with diarrhea and abdominal pain.

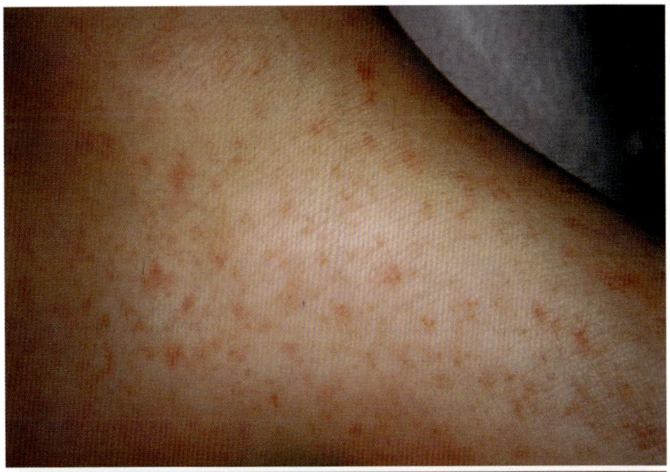

Figure 4-15: Rocky Mountain Spotted Fever (RMSF)

Other rickettsial infections include *R. typhi* (endemic typhus), *R. prowazekii* (epidemic typhus), *R. conorii* (Mediterranean spotted fever), and *Coxiella burnetii* (Q fever).

Know: Q fever is a zoonosis that is transmitted to humans mainly by inhalation of the aerosol released from the infected animal. Q fever is seen in abattoir (slaughterhouse) workers, and in people exposed to an infected animal's products of conception during birthing. Buzzwords: Cattle or Cats + Cilled (☹!) or Conception = Coxiella (Q fever).

Diagnose by serology (IFA usually), or by staining tissue specimens (biopsy) obtained from the site of the rash—the staining method is very specific, but not very sensitive—and do this before you give antibiotics.

Treat **all** *Rickettsia* infections with tetracycline/doxycycline or chloramphenicol. Vaccines have no effect.

Ehrlichiosis

Ehrlichia infection (ehrlichiosis) has been called "spotless Rocky Mountain Fever." There are two forms of the disease: 1) "Human Monocytic Ehrlichiosis" (HME), and 2) Human Granulocytic Ehrlichiosis (HGE). The organism is small, Gram-negative, and obligately intracellular. HME is due to *E. chaffeensis,* and is mainly prevalent in Texas, Oklahoma, Missouri, and Arkansas; HGE is likely due to either *Anaplasma phagocytophilia* (formerly *E. phagocytophilia)* or *E. equi,* and predominates in the Northeast and Midwest. There is frequently a rash in children. The organism affects the monocytes or neutrophils, and patients typically present with the viral picture of fever, headache, and leukopenia. They may also have thrombocytopenia. Think of this in a Board exam presentation of pancytopenia and tick bite! Diagnosis is usually by serologic testing, but the organism can be isolated in culture from blood/CSF, by PCR, or by detection of an intraleukocytoplasmic cluster of bacteria (morulae). (See Figure 4-16).

Treat ehrlichiosis with doxycycline/tetracycline.

notes

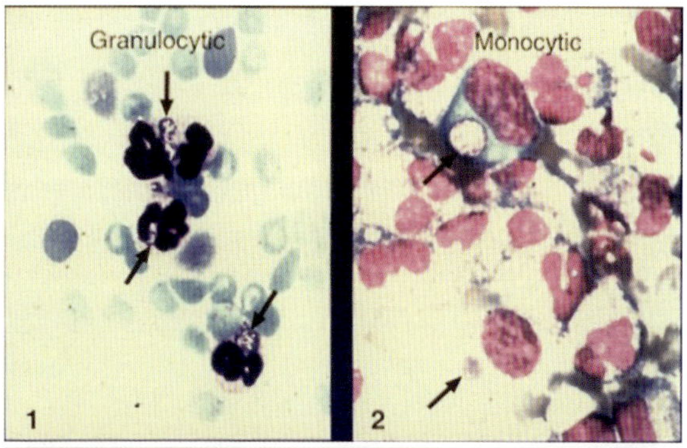

Figure 4-16: Morulae seen in Ehrlichiosis

Note: there are reports of dual infection with *Ehrlichia* + *Babesia microti* (an intra-RBC protozoan parasite) and *Ehrlichia* + *Borrelia burgdorferi* (Lyme) in the endemic northeast areas.

GRAM-VARIABLE

Gardnerella vaginalis (previously called *Haemophilus vaginalis*) is Gram-variable. Treat with metronidazole. It is associated with a vaginosis.

ACID-FAST

Overview

All *Mycobacteria* are acid-fast (RED on a green background).

- *M. scrofulaceum* and *M. avium-intracellulare* cause lymphadenitis in children (See Figure 4-17); treat by ***excising*** the nodes! Do **not** ***incise*** the node—it will cause a chronic draining lesion!
- *M. leprae* causes leprosy. Transmission is probably via person-to-person respiratory droplets. Diagnose with Fite stains of skin or nerve.
- *M. marinum is* the "fish tank bacillus." It causes nonhealing skin ulceration in people working around fish tanks. It often causes strings of lesions along the lymphatic channels. Treat *M. marinum* with ethambutol + rifampin or clarithromycin + rifampin
- *M. tuberculosis*, which will be covered now.

Mycobacterium tuberculosis

Overview

TB is a favorite Board exam topic. For good reason—the incidence of TB has been increasing since 1988. This is mainly due to TB associated with HIV infections.

Tuberculosis infection occurs when aerosolized, contaminated droplets (coughed up by a person with the disease) are inhaled by another, and the droplet or droplet nucleus reaches an alveolus. This is almost always a latent infection, called latent tuberculosis infection (LTBI). It may be an active infection in HIV patients. [Know: We no longer do "prophylaxis" after a positive PPD, but rather "treat" the LTBI.] Note: Children commonly don't spread the organism by the respiratory route, and most children get their tuberculosis infection from an adult. So if they ask you about the likelihood of spread from a 4-year-old to another 4-year-old in daycare, the answer is No. It is likely an adult is responsible for spread if an outbreak occurs in a daycare facility.

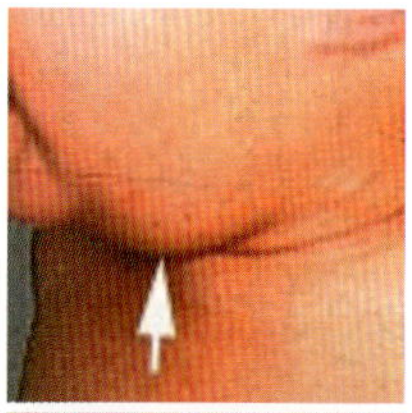

Figure 4-17

TB disease may occur days to years after initial infection, if at all. 90% remain disease-free. The risk of conversion is 5% within 2 years and another 5% thereafter. HIV patients are an exception, and have 40% risk of conversion within several months.

Non-latent primary TB infection (in other words, occurring with the initial tuberculosis exposure, followed immediately by pulmonary disease)—commonly seen in adolescent and adult HIV patients—is primarily a lower-lobe disease (reflecting normally increased airflow to the lower lobes), while latent TB disease (again, pulmonary disease occurring months to years after the initial exposure) is primarily an upper-lobe/apical disease.

Report all persons with current TB disease or suspected current TB disease to the state or local health department.

Presentations in Children/Adolescents/Adults

Most children with tuberculosis infection have no signs or symptoms at any time! Infants and adolescents are more likely to have symptoms. Infants are most likely to have nonproductive cough, mild dyspnea, and wheezing, especially at night. CXR will show hilar lymphadenopathy—this is your clue on the Board examination! Frequently, the lymph node swelling will compress bronchial structures and result in air trapping, hyperinflation, and lobar emphysema.

Children with pulmonary tuberculosis will frequently have a local, asymptomatic pleural effusion. However, pleural effusions are infrequent in children < 6 years. Pleural effusions associated with *M. tuberculosis* have a lymphocyte count of 1,000–6,000/mm^3, a low-glucose, elevated protein, and elevated LDH. Pleural fluid is usually AFB smear-negative, but a pleural biopsy increases the yield.

Tuberculous pericarditis occurs in 4/1000 children infected with tuberculosis, and may present as a rub or distant heart sounds. Fluid is usually negative for the organism.

Meningitis is the most serious complication in children, and occurs in 3/1000 untreated children with tuberculosis. It most commonly occurs in children ages 6 months–4 years. (It can occur in children < 3 months if the infant's mother had disseminated tuberculosis with placental involvement). A caseous lesion usually forms in the cerebral cortex or meninges during the occult lymphohematogenous dissemination of the initial infection. This caseous lesion enlarges and forms what is known as a "Rich focus," and seeds the subarachnoid space. It also can cause a communicating hydrocephalus. SIADH is common.

A tuberculoma is another serious complication in children, and presents clinically as a brain tumor. Tuberculomas are rare in the U.S., but make up 40% of brain tumors in developing areas of the world. In children, the lesions are infratentorial, near the cere-

notes

Quick Quiz

1) What signs/symptoms do most children with tuberculosis present with?
2) How may tuberculous pericarditis present?
3) How common is tuberculous meningitis and what age group is most commonly affected?
4) What will the serum sodium likely be (high, low, or normal) in a patient with symptomatic tuberculous meningitis?
5) How will an older adolescent with pulmonary tuberculosis present?
6) Who should be screened for tuberculosis?

bellum. Headache, seizures, and fever are the most common symptoms. Tuberculomas are rare but if they occur, they frequently—and paradoxically—do so after the patient has started anti-tuberculosis medications!

The most common extrapulmonary manifestation in children is lymph node involvement. The most common sites are the tonsillar, anterior cervical, and submandibular nodes.

Common presenting signs of TB disease in adolescents and adults include fever, weakness, night sweats, and weight loss. Look out for these teens and adults on the board examination! They'll be coughing all over the kids who are asymptomatic, and you'll have to know to check them for tuberculosis! Symptoms of pulmonary disease in adolescents and adults are cough, pleuritic chest pain, and hemoptysis. The chest x-ray may show an upper-lobe infiltrate and hilar lymphadenopathy. The hilar adenopathy is usually out of proportion to the size of the infiltrate. Acid-fast stains of the sputum may show "red snappers," and you can also send sputum for PCR and culture. In older adolescents and adults, most TB disease is pulmonary; 15% is extrapulmonary. Figure 4-18 shows a cavitary apical lesion.

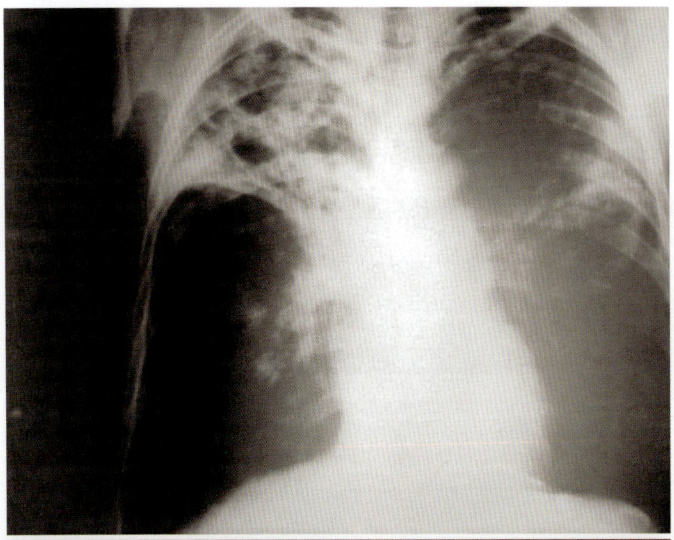

Figure 4-18: TB with Cavitary Apical Lesion

Screening for Latent TB Infection (LTBI)

Who gets screened? High-risk groups including:
- HIV or high risk for HIV
- Close contacts of those with TB disease
- IV drug abusers
- Low-income, medically underserved populations
- The homeless
- Migrant workers
- Residents of long-term care facilities (nursing homes and jails)

How are they screened? Two methods:

The tuberculin skin test is the best and most widely used, but for people easily lost to follow-up, such as in some jails and homeless shelters, screen for actual disease (chest x-ray and sputum for AFB).

Note: Tuberculin skin tests are positive in most infected people, but 10% of children will be initially anergic, then eventually react, suggesting that tuberculosis itself may contribute to the anergy. The tuberculin skin test is contraindicated only if there has been a necrotic skin reaction to previous tests. However, you can give the skin test if the child has had the BCG vaccine (used in some non-U.S. countries as a TB vaccine). Because most of these people were vaccinated as infants, the PPD will probably be valid; thus, interpret and respond accordingly.

The standard Mantoux skin test is an intradermal injection of 0.1 ml (5 tuberculin units) of purified, protein derivative (PPD) tuberculin in the forearm. Evaluate the injection site after 48–72 hours. The reading is based on the diameter of the indurated/swollen area—not the red area—measured perpendicularly to the long axis of the forearm.

The current recommendations as to what constitutes a positive reading from the CDC (listed below) take into account the degree of clinical suspicion of LTBI. The following list shows how a particular diameter of induration may be a positive test in one group, but negative in another. All the following are considered positive skin tests:

5 mm is positive for those in the high-risk group, including persons with:
- HIV or major, cell-mediated dysfunction
- Fibrotic changes on CXR, consistent with prior TB
- Close contact with a documented case
- Patients with organ transplants and other immunosuppressed patients (who are receiving the equivalent of ≥ 15 mg/day of prednisone for ≥ 1 month)

10 mm is positive for those in the moderate-risk group:
- Homeless persons
- Recent immigrants (≤ 5 years) from high-prevalence countries
- IV drug abusers who are HIV-negative

notes

- Prisoners
- Health care workers!
- Nursing home patients and staff
- Diabetics
- Persons undergoing immunosuppressive therapy (equivalent of < 15 mg/day prednisone)
- Children < 4 years old

15 mm is positive for the low-risk group. This includes most people in the community.

Remember this by: HIV+, abnormal chest X-ray, close contacts, severely immunocompromised = 5 mm; no risk factors and ≥ 4 years of age = 15 mm; all the rest = 10 mm.

False-negative skin tests. Think: A) too recent an exposure, or B) anergy.

A) It takes up to 10 weeks to turn positive after exposure, so if a recently exposed patient has a negative skin test, recheck 10–12 weeks after exposure.

B) It used to be that the CDC recommended all HIV patients and other patients suspected of being anergic have 2 other skin tests simultaneously, in addition to the PPD. This is no longer recommended!!

Treatment of LTBI

This section is summarized in Table 4-2.

Who Gets Treated for LTBI?

What do you do if the patient has a positive skin test? [Know!] A positive skin test indicates that the patient has, or has had, LTBI, but not necessarily active disease. If the patient has had no previous TB workup, do a workup for active disease: a chest x-ray and a sputum (if old enough), or morning gastric aspirate for acid-fast bacteria (AFB) smear, PCR, and culture.

If disease is present, treat for tuberculosis, as discussed in the next section.

If no disease is present, treat all previously untreated persons with positive PPDs. This includes the 80-year-old and the 1-year-old HIV-positive, and HIV-negative. Recent or old seroconverters. (Simple, huh?)

What about neg PPDs? Treat all with negative PPD who are close contacts to patients with active TB disease for 10–12 weeks, then recheck with another PPD. If the repeat PPD is positive, continue for 9 months. If the repeat PPD is negative, stop. That's it!

Table 4-2

TREATMENT OF LATENT TUBERCULOSIS INFECTION	
Positive PPD Determination based on Pre-existing Conditions In Infants, Children, and Adolescents	
Certain groups are at high risk of developing TB ***disease*** once ***infected***. These people are candidates for treatment ***regardless*** of their age -- after ensuring active infection is ***not*** present. The current optimum treatment regimen for ***all*** patients is 9 months of daily INH. See text for teatment of drug-resistant organisms. Treat ALL the following (ALL ages!):	
PPD Result (induration)	**In Children with the Following Conditions**
≥ 5mm is positive in this high-risk group	In close contact with known or suspected contagious cases of tuberculosis disease Suspected to have tuberculosis disease: - Findings on chest radiograph consistent with active or previously active tuberculosis - Clinical evidence of tuberculosis disease Receiving immunosuppressive therapy or with immunosuppressive conditions, including HIV infection
≥ 10 mm is positive in these moderate-risk groups	At increased risk of disseminated disease: - Those younger than 4 years of age - Those with other medical conditions, including Hodgkin disease, lymphoma, diabetes mellitus, chronic renal failure, or malnutrition With increased exposure to tuberculosis disease: - Those born, or whose parents were born, in high-prevalence regions of the world - Those frequently exposed to adults who are HIV infected, homeless, users of illicit drugs, residents of nursing homes, incarcerated or institutionalized, or migrant farm workers - Those who travel to high-prevalence regions of the world
≥ 15 mm is positive in this low-risk group	4 years of age or older without any risk factors
PPD negative but HIGH RISK	High risk contacts of ACTIVE cases

notes

Quick Quiz

1) What are considered high-risk, moderate-risk and low-risk groups for tuberculosis?
2) What are the "cut-offs" for a positive PPD in the groups listed in the previous question?
3) A child has a positive PPD. What is the workup if they are asymptomatic?
4) If a child with a positive PPD has no disease present after their workup, what is the necessary treatment? What is the treatment if they have active disease identified?
5) Which children should receive pyridoxine with INH therapy?
6) True or False: You should routinely monitor laboratory in patients on anti-tuberculosis medications.
7) What is the concern of ethambutol use?

How do you treat LTBI?

Treatment of LTBI: Give isoniazid (INH) (10–15 mg/kg/day, max 300 mg/day) to eradicate the TB infection before it can develop into the disease. Again, the risk of conversion is 5% within 2 years for "normal" persons, and ~ 40% within several months for those with HIV. Optimal duration of treatment of LTBI is 9 months.

Treat everyone with INH, except those with known exposure to INH-resistant organisms, or history of INH intolerance. In these cases, give rifampin for 4 months instead. In the CDC's Core Curriculum on TB (2000), the recommendation was PZA + rifampin combination therapy. This has proven too toxic, and is no longer recommended (2002).

Treatment of Tuberculosis

Treatment: The emergence of multidrug-resistant strains has changed the treatment of TB disease. We will first define the 4-drug and 3-drug regimens (know!).

The 4-drug regimen consists of

1) Isoniazid (INH)
2) Rifampin
3) Pyrazinamide (PZA)
4) Either ethambutol (oral preferred) or streptomycin (injection)

The 3-drug regimen consists of the first 3 drugs (**R**ifampin, **I**NH, and **P**ZA.

To remember: **R**est **I**n **P**eace for the TB patient who doesn't get **R**ifampin, **I**NH, and **P**ZA).

In the U.S., initially treat all patients with TB disease for 2 months with 4-drug therapy **unless** criteria for 3-drug therapy are met (see below). Give the first 3 drugs for the full 2 months—drop the 4th drug if susceptibility testing shows sensitivity to the first 3 drugs. After the first 2 months, give INH and rifampin for an additional 4 months. Give HIV-infected patients on protease inhibitors rifabutin instead of rifampin. Duration of therapy (6 months total) for HIV-infected patients is the same for those on a Rifabutin regimen.

Give drugs daily for the first 2 months, then 2 x per week thereafter, although this is fairly flexible.

All patients must be observed taking the medication unless you can absolutely assure compliance. Treatment is the same for extrapulmonary TB.

When can 3 drugs be used? Only if there is a slight chance of drug-resistant infection. All of the following criteria must be met:

- New TB patient and < 4% primary resistance to INH in the community
- No known exposure to a patient with a drug-resistant infection
- Is not from a high-prevalence country

Younger children frequently are given 3 drugs instead of 4 because of the inability to monitor ethambutol toxicity (visual acuity) in the younger-age groups.

Vitamin B6 (pyridoxine) is also given to some with INH-containing regimens to prevent peripheral neuropathy and mild, central nervous system effects. Give to children on milk- or meat-deficient diets, those with nutritional deficiencies, and symptomatic HIV-infected children and pregnant adolescents.

Some other scenarios, but likely not on the ABP:

- If the patient cannot take PZA, give INH and rifampin for a total of 9 months
- If the TB is resistant to INH only, stop INH and give the other 3 drugs for 6 months (total), or rifampin and ethambutol for 12 months
- Multidrug-resistant TB (i.e., to at least INH and rifampin) is difficult, and treatment is based on sensitivities

Side effects: **INH**, **rifampin**, and **PZA** are all hepatotoxic.

INH: In all patients on INH regardless of age, monitor monthly only for signs/symptoms of liver toxicity. Laboratory testing is indicated only if signs or symptoms develop!

Ethambutol is not hepatotoxic, but it can cause a decrease in visual acuity. Often, decreased color perception is the first sign of this deterioration. It is usually reversible if you discontinue the drug quickly. Patients should have an ophthalmologic exam before treatment, and periodic checks thereafter (Snellen chart, gross confrontation eye exam, and question the patient). Any inflammatory disease of the eyes is at least a relative contraindication for ethambutol.

Streptomycin is an older aminoglycoside. It tends to cause vertigo and ataxia in children. Ototoxicity and nephrotoxicity are less common in children than adults.

Nocardia

Nocardia asteroides is only weakly acid-fast (easily missed). Its shape is beaded, branching, and filamentous. It usually

notes

starts as a lung infection—occasionally causing a thin-walled cavitary lesion. It can cause focal brain abscesses and a neutrophilic chronic meningitis (most chronic meningitides are lymphocytic). Nodular skin lesions are common. It is hard to isolate.

Usual treatment is with high-dose sulfonamides or TMP/SMX. In severely ill patients, add combinations of drugs, including Amikacin + imipenem. Minocycline is another alternate choice for those sulfa-allergic.

Cryptosporidium/Isospora belli

Cryptosporidium and *Isospora belli* are both acid-fast and common causes of chronic diarrhea in adolescent and adult patients with AIDS. The *Isospora* are large and oval shaped; treat infection with TMP/SMX. Infection with *Cryptosporidia* (small and round) is usually self-limited in immunocompetent patients and requires no treatment. In immunocompromised patients, many have tried paromomycin and albendazole with varying success.

OTHER ORGANISMS

Actinomyces is an anaerobic organism that causes an infection, in which there are growing, characteristically yellow, "sulfur" granules that are actually clusters of organisms. The usual presentation of actinomycosis is cervicofacial involvement caused by a dental infection. (See Figure 4-19). Actinomyces is a cause of PID when there is an IUD in place. The organism can also be associated with appendicitis. It occasionally causes a chronic neutrophilic meningitis (as do *Nocardia* and fungi).

Treat with PCN or ampicillin. Second choice is tetracycline.

Chlamydia are obligate intracellular parasites. *Chlamydophila psittaci* (formerly *Chlamydia psittaci), Chlamydia trachomatis*, and *Chlamydophila pneumoniae* (formerly *Chlamydia pneumoniae* and TWAR) are pathogenic in humans.

- *C. psittaci*: Found in psittacine and other birds, and causes psittacosis (pneumonia and *splenomegaly*). *Again,* with any pneumonia associated with poultry, especially with splenomegaly, strongly suspect *C. psittaci* (Differential: *Histoplasma also* causes pneumonia and splenomegaly; it is associated with bird and bat droppings). Onset of psittacosis: Myalgias, rigors, headache, and high fever—to 105°F.
- *C. pneumoniae* (TWAR) causes community-acquired pneumonia in children > age 5 years and adolescents (It is not associated with bird exposure; rather, person-to-person spread). Bronchospasm is particularly prominent in respiratory infection caused by *C. pneumonia.*
- *C. trachomatis* causes the GU infections and trachoma (chronic external eye infection causing cataracts, but not glaucoma. It causes a chronic follicular keratoconjunctivitis with neovascularization, and is found especially in Asia and Africa). ~ 5% of pregnant women have *Chlamydia trachomatis* in their genital tracts; antibiotic ointment in infants' eyes at birth does not prevent *Chlamydia* conjunctivitis, but does prevent gonorrheal eye infection.

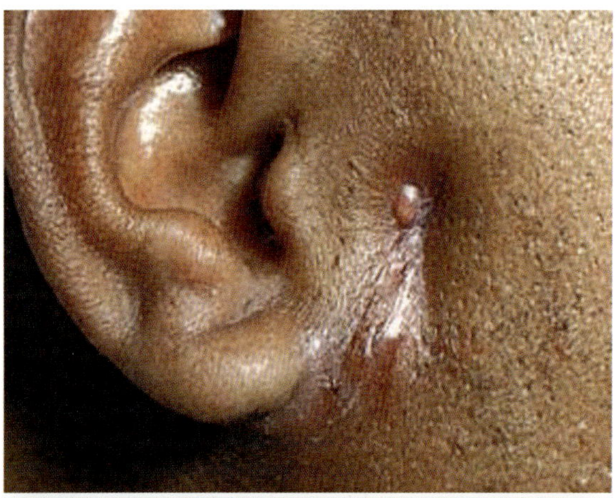

Figure 4-19: Actinomycosis

The same *C. trachomatis* can cause neonatal pneumonia! Chlamydial pneumonia is a common infection in the first 4 months of life; 10–20% will develop infection if born through an infected birth canal. Most infants do well with an afebrile pneumonia and a persistent staccato cough. Lymphogranuloma venereum is an STD caused by the same *C. trachomatis,* but a different immunotype.

ETC...

Sepsis is associated with an elevated WBC with left shift, increased PT and PTT, and metabolic acidosis; but overwhelming sepsis can cause leukopenia. Gram-negative septic shock is associated with warm extremities, because, despite the decreased blood pressure, there is no compensatory peripheral vasoconstriction (i.e., peripheral vascular resistance numbers are low). Cardiac index is elevated.

Antibiotic prophylaxis is recommended for procedures associated with high risk of infection (such as hysterectomies, abdominal, and bowel surgeries), procedures involving implantation of prosthetic material (such as joint replacement), and some procedures when infections, if they occur, would be especially serious (cardiothoracic). The drug of choice almost always is Cefazolin!

Staphylococcus, *Salmonella*, and *Serratia* are more likely to be seen in patients with chronic granulomatous disease (CGD). And again, *H. influenzae*, *S. pneumoniae,* and meningococci are more likely in patients with spleen or antibody dysfunction. For dysfunctional T-cell-associated infections, see AIDS-associated infections. *Aspergillus, Mucor,* and *Pseudomonas* infections are more likely in granulocytopenic patients (leukemia, chemotherapy, post-transplant) than in AIDS patients.

notes

Quick Quiz

1) A draining lesion of the face has sulfur granules noted on microscopy. What is the likely etiology?
2) What organism should you think of that causes pneumonia and splenomegaly and is associated with having parrot exposure?
3) What organism is common as an etiology for pneumonia in adolescents?
4) True or False: Antibiotic ointment in infants' eyes at birth prevents *Chlamydia* infection.
5) An infant presents at 6 weeks of age with a "staccato cough," no fever, and CXR consistent with pneumonia. What organism should you suspect?
6) What is the usual drug of choice when antibiotic prophylaxis is indicated before surgery?
7) What organisms are more commonly seen in chronic granulomatous disease (CGD)?
8) What presents with a "painless chancre"?
9) What stage of syphilis has "nickel and dime" lesions on the palms and soles?
10) Which test for syphilis will usually remain positive for life even with effective therapy?
11) Know how to interpret VDRL, RPR, MHA-TP, and FTA-ABS!

SPIROCHETES

SYPHILIS

Syphilis is caused by *Treponema pallidum.* Sequence of infection:

- **Primary** syphilis has diffuse metastases with a painless chancre (See Figure 4-21) within 3–40 days (depending on the number of inoculating organisms) and regional lymphadenopathy. In women, if the infection is cervical, it is often asymptomatic. Chancre lasts 2–6 weeks and then resolves.
- **Secondary** syphilis occurs ~ 2 months later with generalized lymphadenopathy, constitutional symptoms, and mucosal (35%) or cutaneous (90%) lesions that can mimic many other lesions ("the great imitator"). The skin lesions may be macular or papular, but are rarely vesicular. They can occur on the palms and soles, and frequently resemble "nickels and dimes." (See Figure 4-20). These signs/symptoms resolve in 3–12 weeks, and the disease goes into a latency period. Untreated, 1/3 of secondary syphilis cases eventually proceed to tertiary syphilis.
- **Tertiary** syphilis: CNS lues ("lues" is just another word for syphilis), aortitis (aneurysm rupture is the main cause of death from syphilis!), and tabes dorsalis (causes demyelination, resulting in foot slap and a wide-based gait). One CNS manifestation is the Argyll Robertson pupil, which is miotic (small) and irregular; it reacts normally to accommodation (contracts when focusing close, dilates when focusing on distant objects), but not to light.

Serology—there are two general types of tests:
1) Nontreponemal/reagin (VDRL and RPR)
2) Specific, Treponemal (MHA-TP and FTA-ABS) tests

20–30% of patients with primary syphilis are negative by either type, but the test will turn positive shortly thereafter. 99–100% of patients will be positive by either test in secondary syphilis.

Once positive, the specific treponemal tests (MHA-TP and FTA-ABS) stay positive for life. The nontreponemal tests become negative after treatment, unless treatment has been delayed for many years, in which case they may stay positive.

Scenarios [Know]:
1) –RPR +MHA-TP:
   a) Successfully treated for syphilis in the past, or
   b) Early infection, or
   c) False-positive—see below. Check for history of Lyme disease and repeat RPR in 6 weeks
2) +RPR –MHA-TP:
   a) Probably early infection, or
   b) Often a false-positive in low-risk population. Repeat in 6 weeks
3) +RPR, +MHA-TP: Infection

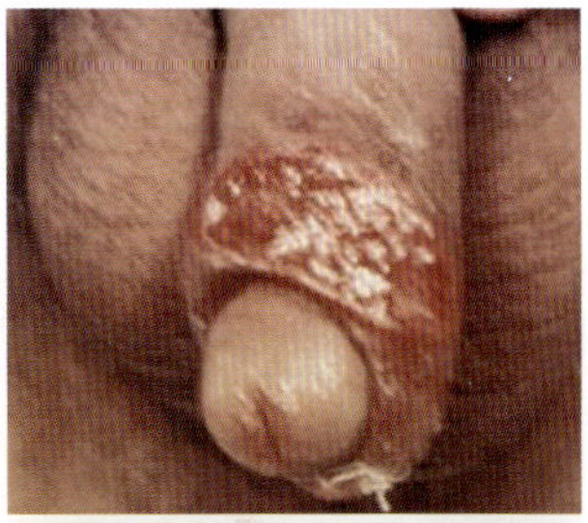
Figure 4-20: Syphilis

Antibodies to *Borrelia burgdorferi* (Lyme) cross-react and may cause a false-positive treponemal test (MHA-TP and FTA-ABS), but do not affect a nontreponemal test (VDRL and RPR).

A negative VDRL or RPR after treatment normally indicates

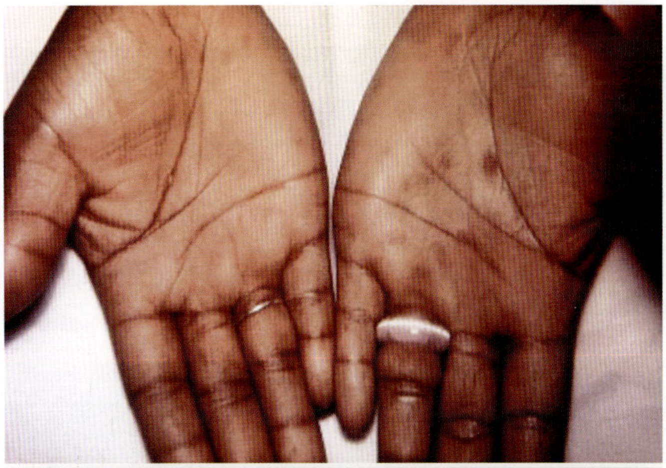
Figure 4-21: 2° Syphilis "Nickles and Dimes" Skin Lesions

notes

successful treatment. The nontreponemal tests may become negative in untreated persons with tertiary syphilis. So you can typically screen out secondary syphilis by a negative on either test; only the treponemal test can be used to screen out tertiary syphilis. I do not say "rule out" because, unfortunately, the false-negative rate in tertiary syphilis with the reagin (nontreponemal) tests is up to 30%!

Give all pregnant women a nontreponemal test in the 1st trimester. If at high risk, repeat test in the 3rd trimester, and at delivery.

Note: All standard antibody tests in a newborn are positive if the mother was positive, because of IgG crossover. The previously used newborn IgM test was not very sensitive because the maternal IgG tends to "overwhelm" IgM response.

Note: Use more sensitive and specific newborn IgM tests to check for *Toxoplasma*, rubella, and CMV.

Treatment of syphilis:

For primary syphilis and for the early latency period of secondary syphilis (< 1 year since acquiring the disease):

- Benzathine PCN G 2.4 MU IM or doxycycline 100 mg b.i.d. x 14 days.

Late latency secondary syphilis and tertiary syphilis with gummas or cardiovascular problems:

- Benzathine PCN G 2.4 MU IM q week x 3 or doxycycline 100 mg PO b.i.d. x 4 weeks.

Neurosyphilis:

- PCN G 18–24 MU IV qd for 10–14 days. This is sometimes followed by benzathine PCN 2.4 MU IM q wk x 3. An alternative is procaine PCN 2.4 MU IM qd with probenecid 500 mg q.i.d. x 14 days. If PCN-allergic, the best course is to desensitize the patient according to CDC protocol, and give the PCN. Use ceftriaxone as an alternative for PCN-allergic patients with 2 grams a day for 10–14 days. Oral doxycycline is not effective for neurosyphilis.

Treat pregnant women and newborns with syphilis only with PCN. If the pregnant woman is PCN-allergic, desensitize her, then treat with PCN. After treatment, do a quantitative nontreponemal/reagin test q month while pregnant.

The procedure for newborns with possible syphilis:

- If the mother was ineffectively treated, not treated with PCN, treated < 4 weeks before delivery, or there is a clinical suspicion, treat the newborn with PCN.
- If treatment of the mother was sufficient, follow the infant's physical examination, CSF exam and nontreponemal serologic titers—and treat if there is a rise in titer or other abnormality.

Non-venereal treponemal diseases include yaws, pinta, and bejel.

LEPTOSPIROSIS

Leptospirosis is a spirochetal disease transferred by contact with infected animals or contaminated water. It is considered to be the most widespread zoonosis in the world. It causes a wide range of symptoms, from myalgias, fever, and headache, with or without aseptic meningitis, to Weil syndrome: severe hepatitis with renal failure and hemorrhagic complications (renal or hepatic symptoms may predominate). Pulmonary symptoms are also common. The hepatitis is characterized by the bilirubin disproportionately elevated compared to the liver enzymes. The variety of presenting symptoms makes for a high incidence of initial misdiagnoses. Clue: Look for contact with dog or rat urine (a kid who swims in a pond with his dogs).

Diagnosis: Blood cultures may be positive in the initial septicemic phase (days 4–7), while urine cultures will be positive thereafter. Serology and PCR are probably more useful in real-world settings.

Treat with PCN or doxycycline.

LYME DISEASE

Borrelia burgdorferi causes Lyme disease. Transmission occurs by the *Ixodes scapularis* (previously *Ixodes dammini*) tick in the Northeast and the *Ixodes pacificus* tick in the California area. The protozoa *Babesia* is also transmitted by *Ixodes scapularis*. Lyme disease is generally thought to be confined to the Northeast, but it actually can be found in virtually all the lower 48 states. However, if you practice in Arkansas or Missouri, Ehrlichiosis is much more common than Lyme disease. The *I. scapularis* tick seems to be a better vector, so t he disease is seen most frequently in the Northeast, especially in the Martha's Vineyard and Nantucket areas. Rarely, it can cross the placenta and cause fetal infection and death.

For the most part, ticks transmit Lyme disease during the nymph stage, probably because nymphs are more likely to feed on a person and are rarely noticed because of their small size (< 2 mm). Thus, the nymphs typically have ample time to feed and transmit the infection (ticks are most likely to transmit infection after ~ 2 or more days of feeding). If a person reports a tick on him/her for a few hours the previous day, provide reassurance that no treatment is necessary.

Diagnosis is clinical: Erythema migrans is the pathognomonic skin lesion of the early localized disease (Stage I); it starts at the site of the bite and is a slowly spreading irregular erythematous lesion with either a bulls-eye or a clear center. See Figure 4-22. Other early symptoms include myalgias, arthralgias, fever, HA, and lymphadenopathy. Then, weeks–months later, early disseminated (Stage II) disease occurs with recurring erythema migrans (rare), neurologic problems (lymphocytic meningitis and/or neuritis), and heart problems

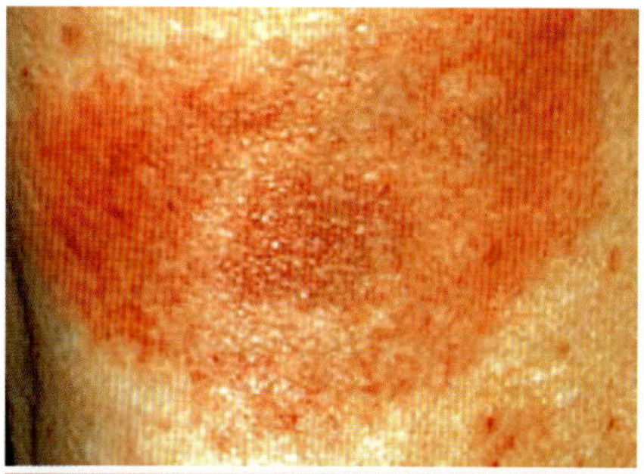

Figure 4-22: Erythema Migrans

notes

Quick Quiz

1) Know the treatment for syphilis at all stages.
2) How should you treat a pregnant woman with syphilis who is allergic to penicillin?
3) Swimming in a pond with an infected dog could predispose a child to what infection?
4) How do you diagnose leptospirosis in the first 4–7 days of infection? In the 2nd week of infection?
5) A child visits a "Lyme-prone" area for several hours. On return from his visit, a tick is noted. The tick was likely attached for between 2 and 3 hours. What is the appropriate therapy (if any) for this child?
6) Describe erythema migrans.
7) A child presents with isolated Bell's palsy and lives in rural Connecticut. What diagnosis should you consider?
8) In a patient with erythema migrans, should you check Lyme serology to confirm your diagnosis?
9) What are the treatments for Lyme disease at its various stages? Especially know the different therapies that depend on if the child presents with isolated erythema migrans, heart block, Bell's palsy, meningitis, or arthritis.
10) A 15-year-old adolescent in an endemic area for Lyme presents with chronic fatigue as a presenting and only symptom. Physical examination is normal. Is it appropriate to check Lyme titers?

(myocarditis, which may cause a rapidly alternating first-, second-, or third-degree AV block). The neuritis often presents as a peripheral neuropathy or a cranial nerve palsy, or both; consider it in a patient with a suggestive history and Bell palsy, foot drop, or both. Months to years later, late disseminated disease (Stage III) occurs most commonly with arthritis (oligo- or migratory—small or large joints—usually large), but there can also be chronic neurologic syndromes. A definite diagnosis may be difficult to establish. Serology is negative in 90% of early localized disease, so base the diagnosis on clinical findings.

Note for Board exam: They may give you a patient with erythema migrans, then ask if you want to check Lyme serology? The answer is no! Just **treat**! Again, erythema migrans is pathognomonic for the disease.

Lyme authorities recommend an ELISA, followed by a Western blot, for patients living in endemic areas who present with recurrent oligoarticular, inflammatory arthritis; then treat patients with positive results on either test.

Treat early disease and isolated Bell palsy with oral doxycycline 100 mg b.i.d., or amoxicillin (for children < 8 years of age) for 21 days. Initially treat Lyme arthritis with oral agents, as described above, then retreat with the same oral agent—or ceftriaxone—if there is no response. Nonresponders frequently are HLA-DR4 allele-positive. Treat cardiac and neurologic sequelae with ceftriaxone 75–100 mg/kg/day (max. 2 grams), or PCN G 300,000 U/kg/day divided q 4 hours (maximum daily dose 20 million U) IV x 21 days. No prophylaxis is indicated—i.e., do not give medications prior to camping out, or to "defend against" tick bites.

At one time, there was a recombinant outer surface protein (OspA) Lyme disease vaccine (LYMErix®), but it was pulled from the market.

NOTE: If on the Board exam, they present a patient with fatigue, joint stiffness (not arthritis), muscular aches and/or tenderness: Do *not* check Lyme titers, and do *not* treat for Lyme based on these nonspecific findings!

Other *Borrelia* infections are *B. recurrentis* and *B. vincentii*, which cause relapsing fever (in this, spirochetes are seen in the blood smears), and Vincent angina.

FUNGI

OVERVIEW

Fungi are roughly divided into two morphologic types: yeasts and molds. There is also a dimorphic type that changes from a yeast to a mold, and vice-versa, depending on temperature. The dimorphs are the type most likely to cause systemic disease in the immunocompetent host. The dimorphic fungi are also more limited in environment. The infecting form of fungi is usually spores (molds), which convert to yeasts in a moist environment at body temperature. The Deuteromycetes are a class of fungus that contains the yeasts *Candida* and *Cryptococcus*, the molds which cause skin and nail disease (dermatophytes), and the dimorphic fungi: *Histoplasma*, *Coccidioides*, and *Blastomyces*. *Mucor* is of the class Phycomycetes (nonseptate hyphae), and *Aspergillus* is of the genus Ascomycetes.

CANDIDA

Note

Candida albicans is a common infection in pediatrics, especially in newborns. It can cause problems ranging from simple superficial infection of the skin to life-threatening meningitis or sepsis.

Skin Infections

Cutaneous Candidiasis

Superficial skin infection is benign and usually occurs in locations of wet, macerated skin, such as the perineum in infants or diabetics, and intertriginous areas of obese children/adolescents. In infants, the peak age is 2–4 months; ~ 1/10 will be affected. *Candida* diaper rash has a classic presentation: a bright red, fiery rash with sharp borders and pinpoint, "satellite" papules and pustules. If you scrape one of the pustules and examine it under a microscope with KOH, you will see the classic pseudohyphae of *Candida*. Treat-

notes

ment: Keep the area dry and use topical antifungals (usually nystatin).

Nail infection is fairly common in thumb suckers and appears as dry, heaped-up gray granulomatous tissue around and on top of the nail.

Chronic mucocutaneous candidiasis is associated with a T-cell problem in which the T cell does not recognize *Candida*. It usually starts in those < 2 years old. Patients present with a bad chronic oral and facial rash, alopecia, and, occasionally, esophageal stricture. It is associated with polyglandular deficiency, in which there can be hypoparathyroidism, Addison disease, DM, hypothyroidism, and/or vitiligo. These patients respond well to fluconazole.

GI Tract Candidiasis

Oropharyngeal candidiasis, or "thrush," is one of the most common presentations of *Candida* infection in infants < age 5 months. After 5 months of age, it is seen in children who are receiving antibiotics, are immunocompromised, or are debilitated and malnourished. The lesions are classically described as "pearly white plaques" on the mucosal surface of the oropharynx. Removing the plaques results in pinpoint bleeding. Use topical therapy with nystatin or clotrimazole troches in the immunocompetent, and fluconazole in the immunocompromised. (Grandparents still like Gentian violet—"because you can see it is working"—especially when it gets all over the drooling child's clothes).

Esophagitis occurs in immunocompromised patients. They complain of pain with swallowing. Most start with fluconazole and, if no response, proceed to esophagoscopy with washings or biopsy, if indicated. *Candida* also can spread to the rest of the GI tract in the immunocompromised.

GU Infections

Cystitis

Candida infections of the urinary tract are common in immunocompromised children, and especially in those with an indwelling urinary catheter. DM and antibiotics are also risk factors. Urine smear and culture will diagnose the infection readily. Most give fluconazole, but for some, removal of the catheter may be the only treatment required.

Candiduria also may indicate obstructive uropathy or "fungus balls" of the kidneys/ureters.

Vaginitis

Candida vaginitis occurs in adolescent women, with increased frequency in those on birth control pills or who are pregnant. White vaginal discharge and pruritus, is common. Numerous topical agents are available; a single, 150 mg fluconazole dose has been successfully used to treat the infection.

Candida Sepsis

Treat *Candida* fungemia aggressively, and never blow off a positive blood culture with *Candida* as a "contaminant." Take special care to examine the skin and the eyes, because discrete lesions may occur at both sites. Retinal lesions present as white, cotton-like, chorioretinitis. Hepatosplenic candidiasis is also seen. CT is helpful, and may show hypodense abscesses. Prescribe amphotericin B for 4–6 weeks. (Many centers use fluconazole, but it is not FDA-approved for children in these conditions).

If a catheter is involved in the infection, you must remove it.

CNS involvement is usually secondary to dissemination from the blood stream, and rarely primary. Treat with amphotericin B and 5-fluorocytosine (5-FC).

Know that candidemia can result in 3 deadly syndromes:

1) Septic peripheral thrombophlebitis
2) Septic thrombosis of the great central veins (especially with central venous catheters)
3) Hepatosplenic candidiasis (mentioned above)—this should be considered in recovering leukemia patients, who present with fever and have negative cultures. CT scan shows focal areas of involvement in the liver.

Treat all of these by removing any infecting catheter, and giving amphotericin B. In addition, resect any suppurative peripheral vein. Suspect septic thrombosis of great central veins if there is edema of the upper body, and/or candidemia persists > 2 days after removal of the catheter.

CRYPTOCOCCUS

Cryptococcus usually causes minimally symptomatic, self-limited infections. Patients may have a low-grade fever, cough, and a pulmonary infiltrate—all of which resolve. It is not associated with any particular geographical location. Although it is found in old pigeon droppings, most patients have no recollection of being in contact with any. Cryptococcal pneumonia may form cavitary lesions and peripheral "cannon ball" skin lesions.

Dissemination is more likely in T-cell deficient patients (AIDS, corticosteroid therapy, Hodgkin disease, ALL, diabetes, and those who are post-organ transplant). These patients are especially likely to get cryptococcal meningoencephalitis—the most common presentation of severe cryptococcus infection.

Confirm presence of the organism with a CSF cryptococcal antigen test, or a CSF India ink test, which is positive when you see the large "halo" due to the thick capsule around the organism.

Treat cryptococcal meningitis with amphotericin B and 5-flucytosine (5-FC). You can treat less severely ill patients with fluconazole. HIV-infected patients and others chronically immunosuppressed require fluconazole for life after their initial therapy.

COCCIDIOIDES, HISTOPLASMA, BLASTOMYCES

Coccidioides and *Histoplasma* are dimorphs. Both usually cause few problems, except in immunocompromised patients.

notes

Quick Quiz

1) Describe the rash of *Candida* diaper dermatitis.
2) Describe the findings in thrush.
3) Which organ systems should be examined closely for dissemination if an infant presents with candidemia?
4) A child presents with *Candida albicans* bacteremia and central venous line infection. True or False: It is appropriate to try and "treat through the line" in hopes of "clearing the line" and saving it for later use.
5) What geographic locations are risk factors for *Coccidioides*? *Histoplasma*? *Blastomyces*?
6) What disease entity is *Malassezia furfur* associated with in adolescents? In infants?
7) In infants with *Malassezia furfur*, what type of hyperalimentations were they likely receiving?
8) Cutaneous sporotrichosis can be treated with which 2 agents?

The spores of *Coccidioides immitis* are found in the soil of the arid, southwest U.S. and northern Mexico (often called "Valley Fever"—think of San Joaquin Valley or Death Valley). Once inhaled, it converts to a yeast that, days to weeks later, causes a self-limited, flu-like illness with arthralgias, erythema multiforme, and/or erythema nodosum. It often has a sarcoid-like presentation. Disease often results in a pulmonary "coin lesion." In immunocompromised patients, the disease is usually more severe (see AIDS-related infections). Think of this disease in a patient from Arizona or California with a flu-like illness! For severe, progressive, disseminated infection NOT involving the CNS, treat with amphotericin B. For those with CNS infections, fluconazole is the drug of choice.

Histoplasma is confined to the Mississippi and Ohio River valleys, and is especially prevalent in bat and bird droppings. Do not confuse *Histoplasma* with the "Valley Fever" described above. Histoplasmosis can present with interstitial pneumonia, palate ulcers, and splenomegaly. 1/3 have anemia, neutropenia, or pancytopenia. The pneumonia and splenomegaly are similar to that seen in *C. psittaci* infection. *Histoplasma* occasionally causes a cavitary pneumonia similar to that seen in TB. Acute pulmonary disease generally does not require therapy. Treat chronic or severe acute disease with itraconazole and disseminated disease with amphotericin B, followed by itraconazole.

Blastomyces causes an illness similar to *Histoplasma* and *Coccidioides*. It is seen in Arkansas and Wisconsin hunters and loggers. (An outbreak occurred in some kids who were visiting a Wisconsin lodge and messed around with a beaver dam). On the Boards, if you see the words "beaver dam," think Blastomycosis! In addition, *Blastomyces* disseminate to the skin, causing crusted lesions. Bone lesions also are commonly seen in blastomycosis. Treat with itraconazole, or amphotericin B in severely affected patients.

DERMATOPHYTES

Dermatophytes are the skin and hair fungi. Treat ringworm (*Tinea corporis*) with topical clotrimazole or undecylenic acid. If these are not successful, itraconazole or terbinafine are the preferred oral agents. **Never** use amphotericin. These are discussed further in the Dermatology section.

MALASSEZIA FURFUR

Malassezia furfur is responsible for 2 disease types in children. First, it causes a superficial dermatosis called tinea versicolor. The lesions are hypo- or hyperpigmented patches that scale. Heat, moisture, and occlusive clothing make it worse. It is very common in adolescents. Look for "spaghetti and meatballs" on a skin scraping. Treat with topical 2.5% selenium sulfide or oral itraconazole/fluconazole.

The second disease type is a serious form, and occurs in NICU babies who are receiving IV lipids and TPN. These infants have fever, bilateral interstitial pulmonary infiltrates, increased WBC, and thrombocytopenia. On the Boards, a clue to this organism: If they tell you the organism required olive oil overlay to grow, or something with olive oil, it's *Malassezia furfur*! Treat by removing the catheter, stopping the lipid infusion, and starting fluconazole or amphotericin B.

SPOROTRICHOSIS

Sporotrichosis is caused by *Sporothrix schenckii*—a dimorphic fungus associated with plants. Cases have occurred in children on farms, especially if they deal with hay bales or straw in barns. Gardeners tend to get it, often after being pricked by a thorn.

Sporotrichosis can be a chronic problem. The disseminated type is more common in immunodeficient gardeners! Warn those post-transplant rose gardeners! Remember: *Mycobacterium marinum* can cause similar lesions over lymphatic channels.

Of the 4 types of clinical presentation, the cutaneous and the lymphangitic (nodules form on the skin over lymph channels) types are treated with ORAL potassium iodide or itraconazole, while the pulmonary and disseminated types are treated with amphotericin B or itraconazole.

ZYGOMYCOSIS

Mucor, Rhizopus, and Cunninghamella organisms can cause Zygomycosis. Pulmonary mucormycosis affects immunocompromised patients, causing pulmonary infarcts. In diabetics, sinusitis is more common. Rhinocerebral mucormycosis starts as a black necrotic spot in the nose or paranasal sinuses, and extends intracranially; it has a poor prognosis. Treat with amphotericin B and debridement. Know: Both *Aspergillus* and *Mucor* can cause a necrotizing, cavitating pneumonia.

notes

PARASITES

PROTOZOA

Overview of Protozoa

There are two main types of parasites—Protozoa and Helminthic organisms. See Table 4-3.

The protozoa are single-celled and can replicate within the body, so it takes only a small number of organisms to cause infection. Protozoa do not cause eosinophilia. The 3 types of protozoa are:

- Type I. Sporozoa: *Toxoplasma*, *Cryptosporidia*, *Isospora*, *Pneumocystis* (although recent data support this more as a fungus!), *Plasmodium*, and *Babesia*)
- Type II. Ameba
- Type III. Flagellates: Giardia, Trichomonas, Trypanosoma, and Leishmania.

ProtozoaType I. Sporozoa

Toxoplasma gondii

Toxoplasma gondii is the protozoa that causes toxoplasmosis. Cats are the definitive host, because all of the oocysts (infectious form) that eventually infect humans are shed in cat feces. It is common: 10–30% of human U.S. adults have had it and, in France, prevalence rates > 85%. Diagnose by finding an elevated IgM antibody.

There are 4 types of toxoplasmosis:

1) In the immunocompetent, it is most often asymptomatic, but may cause a "mono"-like illness with non-tender lymphadenopathy, night sweats, and atypical lymphs. Self-limited.

2) This type is serious in the immunocompetent only if acquired during pregnancy, when it causes congenital toxoplasmosis (causing mental retardation and necrotizing chorioretinitis). The fetus is more likely to have a congenital infection if the disease is acquired later in pregnancy (25%: 1st trimester; 54%: 2nd trimester; 65%: last trimester; but in contrast, the severity of clinical disease is inversely related to gestational age, so, those infected later in pregnancy are usually asymptomatic).

For severe congenital infection in a newborn, be on the lookout on the Board Exam for an infant with the following findings (know):

- Microcephaly
- Hydrocephalus
- Hepatosplenomegaly
- Maculopapular rash or thrombocytopenic purpura
- Retinochoroiditis
- Cerebral calcifications (periventricular—Note: Also commonly seen in CMV. But, if calcifications "circumvent" the ventricles, this is almost always CMV and not toxo!)

Treatment of the mother can begin during pregnancy if the diagnosis is made. If the infection occurs in weeks 7–34 of gestation, you could give spiramycin (though not licensed in the U.S., it is available in Canada and Europe) 1 gram q 8 hours for up to 18 weeks of gestation. If fetal infection is excluded, spiramycin is continued until term; if you confirm infection, switch therapy to pyrimethamine, sulfadiazine, and leucovorin. For maternal infections after 34 weeks gestation, the 3-drug regimen can be used.

For congenital infections, treat the fetus *in utero*, if possible, as discussed above. After delivery, treat the infant whether or not he/she has clinical signs/symptoms. Once you completely evaluate the healthy newborn, and you rule out infection, therapy can stop. The congenitally infected child must receive 12 months of therapy. Treat with a pyrimethamine loading dose of 2 mg/kg (maximum of 50 mg) daily for 2 days, then 1 mg/kg (max 25 mg) daily for 2–6 months, then 1 mg/kg 3 times a week to complete the 12-month course. Give sulfadiazine 100 mg/kg divided b.i.d. Give leucovorin (**folinic** acid, not *folic* acid) 5–10 mg 3 x a week if neutropenia occurs, increased to 5–20 mg daily. It is important to monitor CBC in these infants. At the end of 12 months, repeat eye exams at 3 and 6 months out to check for new chorioretinitis

Table 4-3

CLASSIFICATION OF PARASITES		
PROTOZOA (do replicate within the body) (no eosinophilia)	Sporozoa	*Toxoplasma*, *Cryptosporidium*, *Isospora belli*, *Plasmodium*, *Pneumocystis*, *Babesia*
	Ameba	*Entameba histolytica*
	Flagellates	*Giardia* - GI; *Trichomonas* - GU *Leishmania*, *Trypanosomes* - blood
HELMINTHS (do **not** replicate within the body) (+ eosinophilia)	Nemathelminthes (= nematodes) (= roundworms)	Pinworms, Hookworms, Whipworms (*Trichuris trichiura*), *Trichinella*, *Strongyloides*
	Platyhelminthes	Cestodes (tapeworms); Trematodes (flukes)

notes

Quick Quiz

1) At what stage of pregnancy is the mother more likely to transmit toxoplasmosis to her unborn infant?
2) At what stage of pregnancy is the infection more likely to cause serious sequelae?
3) What are the classic physical findings in congenital toxoplasmosis? What is the CT scan of the head likely to show?
4) What pharmaceutical agents are used to treat an infant with congenital toxoplasmosis?
5) What drug is used to treat *Isospora belli* infection?
6) What is the food associated with *Cyclospora* infection?
7) If you see "banana gametophytes" on a peripheral smear, what is type of malaria does the patient have?
8) Which type of malaria is more commonly associated with nephrotic syndrome?

lesions. How to prevent this? Make sure pregnant women do not eat rare or undercooked meat; and have them avoid cat litter duties in the house.

3) Immunocompromised patients tend to get CNS infection and multiple mass lesions caused by a reactivation of a latent infection. Patients with AIDS remain on therapy for life. Treat with pyrimethamine, sulfadiazine, and leucovorin.

4) Ocular toxoplasmosis causes retinal lesions that look like yellow-white cotton patches, and also causes irregular scarring and pigmentation (disseminated candidiasis produces white, cotton-wool patches). Treat with pyrimethamine, sulfadiazine, leucovorin, and corticosteroids until the infection has resolved.

Cryptosporidium

Cryptosporidium is a protozoan that causes infection, especially in the immunocompromised, but also in the immunocompetent. The oocytes are passed in animal and human feces (vs. just cats in toxo). Symptoms in immunocompetent patients usually consist of a watery diarrhea that is self-limited, lasting 1–2 weeks. In the immunosuppressed, it can persist indefinitely, and is refractory to medications. Recent information shows that a combination of paromomycin + azithromycin may be helpful. Diagnose by acid-fast stains (small and round). In the past, the organism caused major metropolitan outbreaks of diarrhea due to contaminated city water; be aware of this for the Boards!

Isospora belli

Isospora belli is another acid-fast protozoan that, in patients with AIDS, causes a watery diarrhea identical to *Cryptosporidium*. On the acid-fast stain, it is large and oval, whereas Cryptosporidium is small and round. Treat with TMP/SMX.

Cyclospora

Cyclospora is a newly described, acid-fast intestinal protozoan parasite, causing diarrhea in immunocompromised and immunocompetent patients. Clue: Raspberries from Guatemala! Systemic symptoms, such as malaise, myalgia, low-grade fever, and fatigue are commonly seen with *Cyclospora* infection. Treat with TMP/SMX.

Pneumocystis jiroveci (formerly *P. carinii)* is one of the most common causes of pneumonia in patients with AIDS. It is covered later in the HIV section.

Malaria

Malaria—*Plasmodium* is a protozoan that causes malaria. It affects the RBCs and is transmitted via the *Anopheles* mosquito. There are 4 types: *Plasmodium vivax*, *P. ovale, P. malariae*, and *P. falciparum*. Asplenic patients have more severe cases of malaria.

P. falciparum is the worst type of malaria. It is the cause of virtually all of the fatal infections. It also has widespread chloroquine-resistance. Most cases of *P. falciparum* are acquired in mid-Africa. The blood smear in *P. falciparum* shows "banana gametophytes." (See Figure 4-23). Often you see > 1 infected RBC on the slide, and even multiple parasitized RBCs.

This greatly contrasts with the other forms of malaria, in which the parasitized RBCs are often hard to find. Finding a banana gametophyte on the peripheral blood smear is diagnostic of *P. falciparum*. Even though *P. falciparum* causes the highest levels of parasitemia, the schizonts are not seen on peripheral smear. If you see schizonts, the patient has one of the other types.

The Duffy RBC antigen is the site of attachment for *P. vivax*. Any type of malaria can cause nephritis from immune complex deposition, but *P. malariae* is most commonly associated with nephrotic syndrome. Antibody production causes a decrease in parasitemia, but not in the number of intracellular parasites!

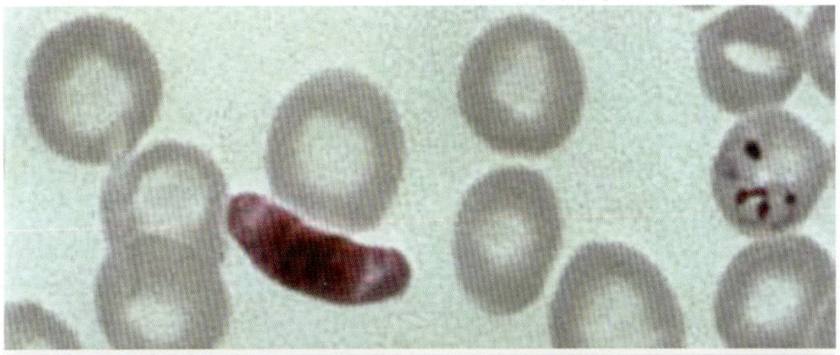

Figure 4-23: *P. falciparum*, "Banana Gametophytes"

notes

Table 4-4

MALARIA: TREATMENT AND PROPHYLAXIS		
TYPE OF MALARIA	TREATMENT	PROPHYLAXIS
Nonfalciparum malaria	Chloroquine and primaquine.	Chloroquine weekly. Give daily in endemic areas.
P. falciparum Chloroquine sensitive	Chloroquine Malarone	
P. falciparum Chloroquine resistant Not very ill.	Quinine sulfate p.o. plus either Fansidar, doxycycline, or clindamycin. or Mefloquine x 2 doses or Malarone x 3-5 days	Mefloquine: one dose weekly including 1 wk before and 4 wks after Malarone: one dose daily including 1-2 days before and 7days after
P. falciparum Chloroquine resistant Very ill.	IV quinidine gluconate +/- IV clindamycin. When better, change to p.o. quinine and clindamycin.	

Treatment (Table 4-4): Use chloroquine for infections of *Plasmodium vivax*, *P. ovale*, and *P. malariae*. Primaquine is adjunctive medication for infections with *P. vivax* and *P. ovale* to eradicate hypnozoites in the liver. Hypnozoites are the malarial forms responsible for relapse. Chloroquine-sensitive *P. falciparum* is treated with chloroquine, of course. If the *P. falciparum* is likely to be chloroquine-resistant, give quinine sulfate/gluconate, et. al., as shown in Table 4-4. Another option is mefloquine (Lariam®). Mefloquine is effective against the chloroquine-resistant, and even the Fansidar-resistant *P. falciparum*. It is also effective against the chloroquine-sensitive plasmodia.

Remember: The use of pyrimethamine/sulfadoxine (Fansidar®) is rarely associated with the risk of severe Stevens-Johnson syndrome (which is due to the sulfa)! Also remember: Primaquine induces hemolytic anemia in G-6-PD-deficient persons, so you must screen for G-6-PD deficiency before prescribing it.

For malaria prophylaxis, use chloroquine if there is no chloroquine-resistant Falciparum malaria present in the region in question. Start it 1– 2 weeks before arrival to the endemic area, and continue for 4–6 weeks after leaving the area. Use mefloquine, doxycycline, or Malarone® for prophylaxis in chloroquine-resistant regions. Primaquine can be given the last 2 weeks of a prophylaxis period with either chloroquine or mefloquine, and after travel to regions where there is *P. vivax* or *P. ovale*. [Know: The main causes of malaria in the U.S. are either not taking prophylaxis before traveling to endemic regions, or stopping prophylaxis too soon after returning from endemic areas!]

Malarone®, a fixed combination of atovaquone and proguanil, has recently been approved for the prophylaxis and treatment of uncomplicated *P. falciparum* malaria. For prophylaxis, the advantage is that it can be started just prior to leaving and stopped soon after return, and also has fewer side effects. The disadvantage is that it must be taken daily.

Babesia

Babesia microti is an intra-RBC protozoan parasite that causes babesiosis. This disease is a febrile, hemolytic anemia seen especially in debilitated elderly patients and asplenic patients. The organism is transmitted via the *Ixodes* tick from rodents (as is the spirochete *Borrelia*, which causes Lyme disease). It is mostly seen in the northeast U.S.—usually in summer or early autumn.

Symptoms, which may persist for months, include fever, profuse sweats, myalgias, and shaking chills. Hemoglobinuria is a predominate sign. Patients often are emotionally labile. Because of the symptoms and the parasitized RBCs, it may be misdiagnosed as malaria.

B. microti is distinguished from *Plasmodium* by the classic intra-RBC tetrad appearing as a "Maltese Cross," but which more often looks like 4 dots in a square shape (the malaria parasites have a ring form). (See Figure 4-24).

Mild babesiosis infections are usually self-limited. Treat moderate infections with clindamycin + quinine, or atovaquone + azithromycin. If severe, do an exchange transfusion, then give antibiotics. Again, asplenic patients have more severe disease.

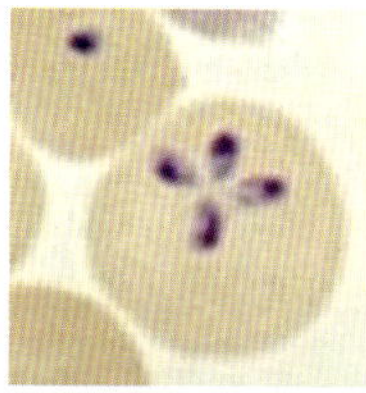

Figure 4-24

ProtozoaType II: Ameba

Human amebiasis is caused by the protozoa *Entamoeba histolytica*. Transmission is fecal-oral and can be food- or water-borne. In the U.S., the usual population groups in which it is found are the institutionalized, immigrants, and homosex-

notes

Quick Quiz

1) What drug must be taken after chloroquine for successful treatment of *P. ovale* and *P. vivax*?
2) How is *Babesia* infection distinguished from malaria?
3) Do you diagnose an amebic liver abscess with stool studies or serology?
4) What is the most common cause of diarrhea due to parasites in the U.S.?
5) How do you treat Giardia in a child who cannot swallow pills?
6) A child presents from South America with heart block and CHF. What parasitic infection is a possible etiology?

ual men. For intestinal disease, diagnose by examining the stool. However, the aspirate of an amebic liver abscess often shows no ameba or PMNs—Diagnosis: Serology!

For asymptomatic infection, a luminal agent is fine: Diloxanide furoate (available only from the CDC), paromomycin, or iodoquinol.

For liver abscesses or invasive colitis, metronidazole is the treatment of choice—even large amebic abscesses respond very quickly.

ProtozoaType III: Flagellates

Organisms

The flagellates: Giardia lamblia, Trichomonas vaginalis, Trypanosoma, Leishmania.

Giardia lamblia

Giardia is the most common disease-causing parasite in the U.S. It also is the most frequently identified diarrheal agent in waterborne-associated infections. Giardia infections are found in campers, travelers, children in day care, homosexuals, and in patients with IgA deficiency and/or hypogammaglobulinemia. It infects the duodenum. (Remember: *Shigella* is also found among daycare kids and homosexuals). 75% of infected persons are asymptomatic. Acute symptoms include a watery, smelly diarrhea and flatulence. Chronic giardiasis causes flatulence, sulfuric belching, and soft stools. Diagnose with microscopic examination of fresh **stool samples x 3** or **Giardia antigen test** on 1 stool. For chronic giardiasis, a string test may be required: Have the patient swallow a capsule on a string, leave it for several hours, then retrieve it and check for trophozoites. This is rarely done today.

Furazolidone (Furoxone®) and nitazoxanide (Alinia®) are anti-Giardia medications available in a suspension form. Metronidazole is frequently used, but it actually does not have this indication. The dose for metronidazole is 5 mg/kg t.i.d. x 7 days or a maximum of 250 mg t.i.d. x 7 days.

Trichomonas vaginalis

Trichomonas vaginalis causes an STD. Treat with metronidazole. More in the Adolescent section.

Trypanosomiasis

Trypanosoma causes trypanosomiasis. There are 2 main types. The African disease is sleeping sickness. It is caused by *Trypanosoma brucei*, and is transmitted via the tsetse fly. The American illness, Chagas' disease, is caused by *T. cruzi*; it is found in Central/South America and Mexico. Usually, it is self-limited, but the chronic form can cause problems with the heart (from heart block to CHF), GI system (especially achalasia, megaesophagus, and megacolon), and occasionally the CNS. Be suspicious on the Board exam of a child from Mexico or Central/South America who presents with unilateral firm edema of the eyelids (Romana sign, see Figure 4-25) followed by fever, generalized lymphadenopathy, and malaise. Myocarditis can follow. The heart failure and cardiomyopathy may occur years later after the initial infection.

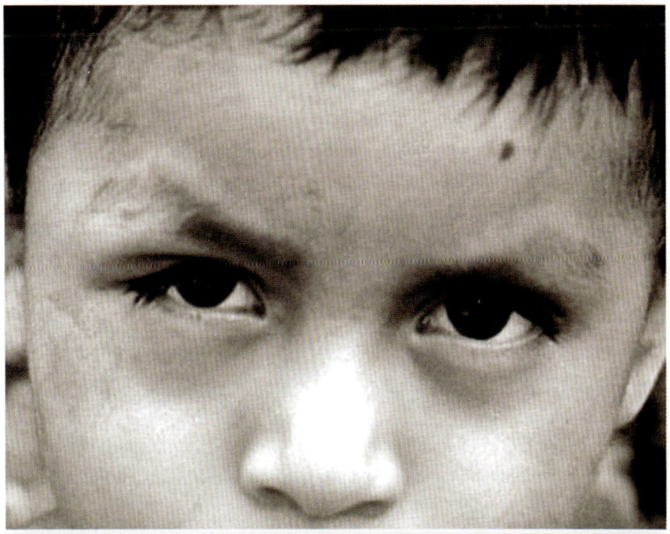

Figure 4-25: Romana Sign in Trypanosomiasis

Leishmaniasis

Leishmaniasis is caused by any of the following 4 species of the Leishmania protozoa: L. donovani, L. tropica, L. mexicana, and L. braziliensis. L. donovani is spread by a sand fly and causes visceral leishmaniasis, also called kala-azar. These patients get GI symptoms, hepatomegaly, and sometimes huge splenomegaly. The other species cause cutaneous and mucocutaneous forms of the disease.

Sodium stibogluconate (pentavalent antimony) is the treatment of choice—available from the CDC. Amphotericin B and itraconazole have been used with some success for cutaneous leishmaniasis.

notes

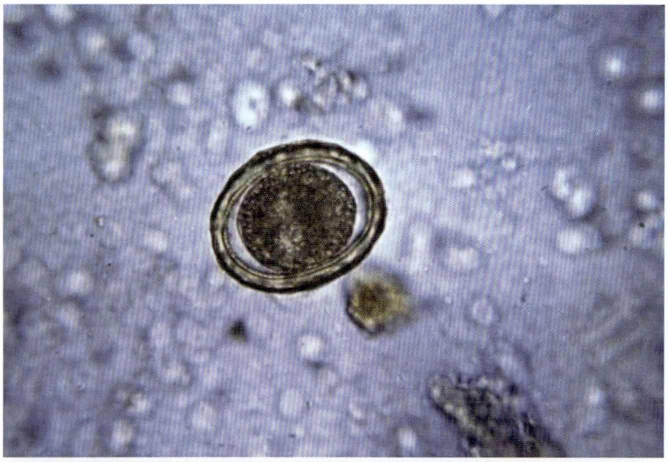

Figure 4-26: Nematode (Roundworm) Egg in Stool Sample

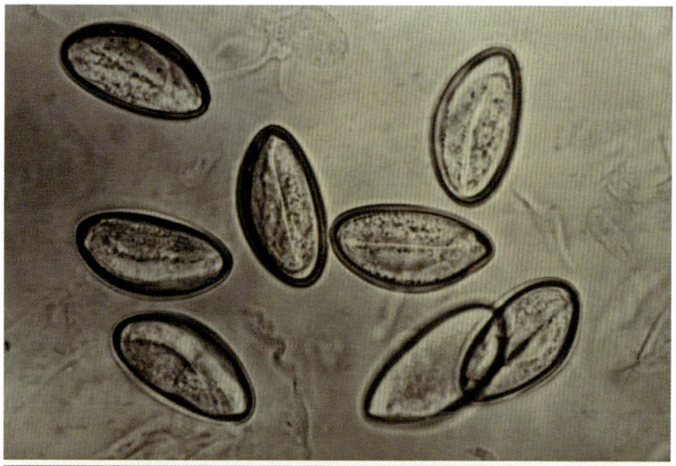

Figure 4-27: Pinworm Eggs

HELMINTHIC ORGANISMS

Overview

The helminthic organisms are the other major type of parasite (remember: 1. Protozoa and 2. Helminthic organisms). They are multicellular worms that, in general, do not replicate in the body—and DO cause eosinophilia. The two types of helminthic organisms are:

1) Nemathelminthes: the nematodes or roundworms, which include pinworms, hookworms, whipworms (*Trichuris trichiura*), *Trichinella, Strongyloides* and *Ascaris*.
2) Platyhelminths: include cestodes (tapeworms) and trematodes (flukes).

Nematodes (roundworm)

Ascaris lumbricoides

Ascaris lumbricoides is the largest intestinal roundworm that infects humans. Worms are 20–40 cm long. The female lays 200,000 eggs daily. Eggs then pass in the host's feces and become infective in the environment—only after the first-stage larva molts within the egg. Children often infect themselves and others while playing in the same areas where they poop. Mature worms set up shop in the jejunum, where they lay their eggs.

The larval form has a complex migration pattern in humans, and must cross from the duodenum into the mesenteric lymphatics, to the portal circulation, and reach the pulmonary vascular bed. There, they cut through the alveolar wall, go up the respiratory tree to the epiglottis, and are finally swallowed. During this period of going through the lungs, patients will frequently have cough, fever, and rales. Hemoptysis can occur. A key to look for is "shifting" infiltrates or atelectasis occurring with Löffler syndrome (which usually also has a high eosinophil count).

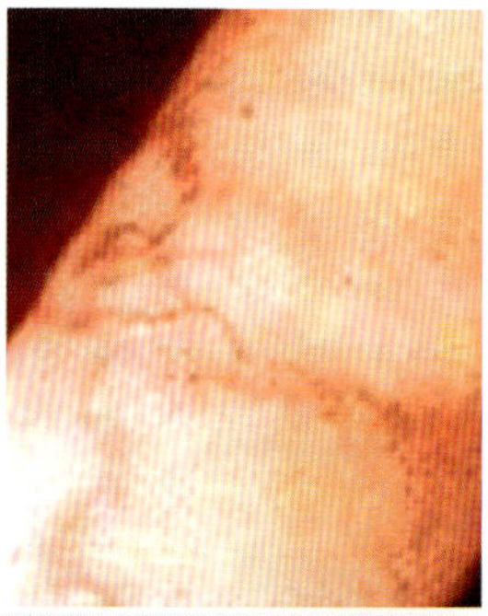

Figure 4-28

Diagnose by finding the eggs or worms in the stool. (See Figure 4-26 of the fertilized egg). Mebendazole is the drug of choice.

Pinworms (*Enterobius vermicularis*)

Pinworm infection is ubiquitous. It occurs when eggs (see Figure 4-27) are ingested by oral contact with contaminated hands, toys, or other fomites. Some feel that "slumber parties" are the pinworm's heaven. (All those kids jumping around on the bed, the eggs flying up in the air—aerosolized and easily ingested.). The eggs hatch in the duodenum, then travel to the cecum, where they have worm sex. The pregnant female worm travels to the large bowel and out the anus at night, leaving a trail of eggs on the surface of the skin. The female worms are 8–13 mm long. The prime time for the worms to exit the rectum is "10–11 p.m." (now, I don't know if that is Eastern or Central time, and I don't know if the worms observe Daylight Savings Time, and I doubt seriously if the ABP really will ask you what time, but that is your trivial trivia for the day!). All joking aside, the exam *will* ask you about this critter. Know that re-infection is common, as is autoinoculation. Treat with mebendazole 100 mg or albendazole 400 mg in a single dose, then repeat again in 2 weeks. Also, treat all family members. Be sure to launder the sheets and bedclothes, but don't shake those dirty sheets too much!

Hookworm (*Necator americanus*)

Hookworm infection in the U.S. is due mainly to *Necator americanus,* which causes anemia, weakness, and fatigue (also can cause cutaneous larva migrans, Figure 4-28). Know that children with hookworms may have failure to thrive! "Catch-up" growth usually occurs when the worms are killed.

notes

Quick Quiz

1) True or False: Most helminth (worm) infections cause a peripheral eosinophilia.
2) What is the largest roundworm that infects humans in the U.S.?
3) Know everything there is to know about pinworms.
4) What time of day do most pinworms emerge from the anus?
5) What is the only worm to replicate in humans?
6) What causes visceral larva migrans?
7) What is cysticercosis?

Whipworm (*Trichuriasis*)

Whipworm infection is due to infection of the large intestine with *Trichuris trichiura*. Infection is most predominant in the southern U.S. and occurs by ingesting eggs. If only a few worms are present, the infection is asymptomatic. If more worms are present, look for fever, abdominal pain, weight loss, and itching. Heavy infestations can cause diarrhea, blood-streaked stools, and rectal prolapse. Diagnose by finding the eggs in the stool. Treat with mebendazole.

Trichinosis (*Trichinella sp.*)

Trichinella spiralis larvae, which are usually found in pork (but also found in many carnivores), cause trichinosis. Although only ~ 50 cases per year are diagnosed in the U.S., the overall frequency of infection found on autopsy is ~ 4%! Symptoms are determined by where the worm is. After ingestion, the eggs hatch and the larvae invade the duodenum, which can cause abdominal pain, nausea, and vomiting. From here, they go into the blood stream and reach muscle tissue, which can cause muscle pain. If they reach the heart, myocarditis can occur. Ocular involvement is common, as is eosinophilia. Chemosis and periorbital edema suggest the diagnosis, which is confirmed by finding rising titers or muscle biopsy. Treat with mebendazole, thiabendazole, or albendazole.

Filariasis (*Wuchereria bancrofti*)

The mosquito transmits *Wuchereria bancrofti*. It is one of the causes of lymphatic filariasis (lymphatic blockage) and 2° elephantiasis! It may take thousands of bites by infected mosquitoes to inoculate enough of the organism to cause this. (Remember: With the exception of *Strongyloides*, helminthic organisms do not multiply in the human body.) Diagnose by presence of microfilariae in the blood.

Strongyloides stercoralis

Strongyloides stercoralis infection is common in certain areas of the U.S. and is very common in South America and Southeast Asia. Highly endemic areas exist in Southeast Asia and South America, where up to 60% of the population is infected. In the U.S., studies found infection rates of 3% among Kentucky school children and 6% at the Tennessee VA hospital.

It is (virtually) the only helminthic organism that replicates in the body. With this autoinfection, the infection can persist for decades. (*Strong*!)

Symptoms are usually GI, but there can be pulmonary symptoms during the infective part of the larvae's life cycle. Eosinophilia usually is present.

In immunosuppressed patients, potentially fatal, disseminated strongyloidiasis may occur, some call "hyperinfection"—presenting with abdominal pain and distension, neuro and pulmonary symptoms, and shock.

Diagnose with serial stool samples for larvae—not eggs. Treat with ivermectin or thiabendazole.

Toxocariasis (*Toxocara canis* and *T. cati*)

Toxocara canis (and sometimes *Toxocara cati*) causes visceral larva migrans. Older children may get retinal involvement. The normal host for *Toxocara canis* is dogs, and it is transmitted to humans by ingesting soil contaminated with dog excreta. In humans, the larvae do not develop into adult worms, but rather migrate through the host tissue—eliciting eosinophilia. Look for this in a child with "migratory pneumonia" and eosinophilia! In the U.S., *Toxocara* seropositivity is 20% in kindergarten children and 2% in the general population. Treat with albendazole or mebendazole.

Platyhelminthes (Cestodes and Trematodes)

Platyhelminthes include cestodes (tapeworms) and trematodes (flukes).

Cestodes are the flatworms (tapeworms). The pork tapeworm, *Taenia solium*, has two clinical entities:

1) If the cysticerci are ingested, taeniasis develops (a tapeworm grows in the intestines).
2) If an egg-contaminated food (from animal or human feces) is ingested, the patient will develop cysticercosis. The eggs hatch and the oncospheres go into the blood and, most significantly, cause cysticerci in the CNS and eyes. These cysts do nothing until the organism dies. In the brain (neurocysticercosis), the resulting inflammation usually causes seizures as the first symptom. Especially consider cysticercosis in a patient with new onset seizures who is an immigrant from Mexico, Central or South America, or who is from a household with an immigrant from these areas.

Niclosamide is the usual treatment for all intestinal tapeworms. Use albendazole (first choice) or praziquantel along with corticosteroids for neurocysticercosis. Note: if ocular or spinal cysts are present, do not treat—this causes irreparable damage!

notes

Trematodes are the flukes.

1) *Clonorchis sinensis* is the Chinese liver fluke. It is endemic in the Far East. Infection is caused by eating raw fish, and is often associated with biliary obstruction.
2) *Schistosoma haematobium* infects the bladder, causing urinary symptoms.
3) *Schistosoma mansoni* is a fluke found in Africa, the Middle East, and South America.
4) *Schistosoma japonicum* is found in Asia.

Schistosoma causes acute schistosomiasis (Katayama fever ~ 2 months after inoculation. This infection presents with fever, lymphadenopathy, diarrhea, hepatosplenomegaly, and marked eosinophilia. The most serious complication of schistosomiasis is cirrhosis with esophageal varices. Schistosomiasis does not cause the other stigmata seen with alcoholic cirrhosis (spiders, gynecomastia, or ascites).

Finding the eggs in the stool makes the diagnosis.

Give praziquantel for one day (!) for any *Schistosoma* and most other fluke infections.

VIRUSES

HSV

HSV-1

HSV-1 causes orofacial infections in ~ 40% of the population[1]. In the primary infection, the vesicular lesions and ulcers are usually localized to the oral mucosa, lips, and surrounding skin, whereas in recurrent infections, ulcers are usually on the outer lip. (See Figure 4-29). Peak incidence occurs at 1–5 years of age.

Herpes Viruses
The herpes viruses are double-stranded DNA viruses that include the herpes simplex viruses (HSV-I and HSV-2), CMV, Epstein-Barr, and varicella-zoster viruses.

Herpetic whitlow refers to an HSV infection of the fingers. It is painful and may be confused with a bacterial infection. Do not surgically open these infections. Herpes gladiatorum occurs in wrestlers or rugby players, and occurs in abraded skin that has contact with oral secretions infected with HSV. (See Figure 4-30).

Tzanck test is done by scraping down to the bottom cellular layer of a vesicle, placing the material on a slide, then staining with either Giemsa or Wright. In herpes simplex and varicella (including zoster), it will show multinucleated giant cells. (See Figure 4-31). Herpes direct fluorescent antibody testing (DFA) is also available and becoming more widely used.

It is possible to autoinoculate the virus; thus, the infection can spread from the lips (or other areas) to the eyes of a patient. Recurrent HSV-1 eye infection resulting in a keratitis is the most common infectious cause of blindness in industrialized nations. It presents with characteristic dendritic, branched, fluorescent-staining corneal ulcers.

HSV-2

HSV-2 causes "genital herpes." Actually, it causes ~ 75% of HSV genital infections—the rest are due to Type 1. Note that the prevalence of HSV-2 is 25% and, of those, only 25% have symptoms!! In 10% of patients, the initial occurrence of HSV-2 is associated with only a herpetic exudative pharyngitis. New data suggest that asymptomatic shedding of virus spreads many HSV infections.

Neonatal HSV

Most cases of neonatal HSV are from intrapartum contact, so a C-section is recommended if the mother has symptoms or signs of genital herpes, or its prodrome, at the time of delivery. The risk for transmission to the neonate is high (30–50%) among women who get their 1st episode of genital herpes near the time of delivery and

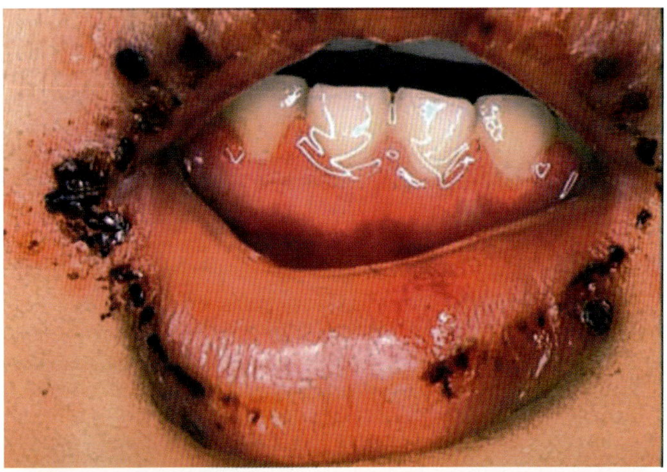

Figure 4-29: HSV-1 Infection

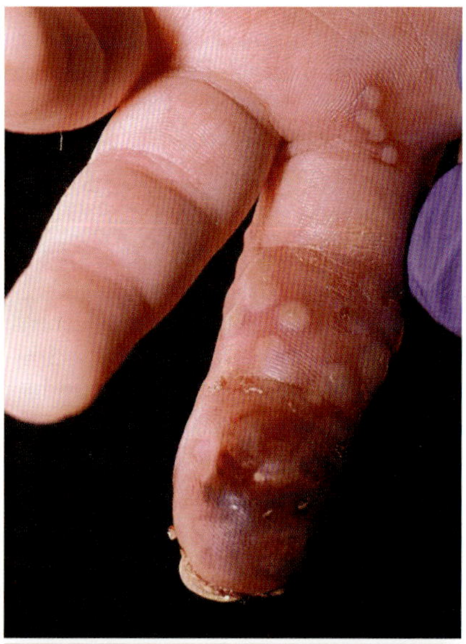

Figure 4-30: Herpetic Whitlow

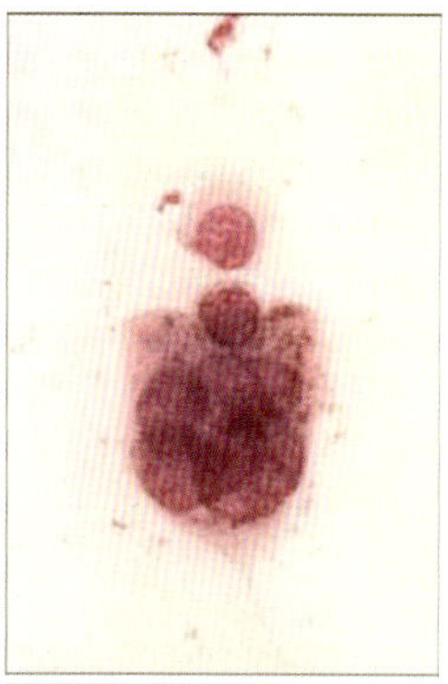

Figure 4-31

notes

Quick Quiz

1) Which fluke affects the bladder?
2) If a skin lesion is HSV, what will the Tzanck smear show?
3) What is the concern with HSV near the eye?
4) A pregnant woman has herpetic-like lesions in her vaginal area at the time of delivery. True or False: She must have a C-section.
5) A pregnant woman has recurrent herpes 4 weeks before delivery. At the time of delivery, she has no symptoms and no signs of lesions. True or False: She should have a C-section just in case she is shedding.
6) Which infant is more likely to be infected with HSV—one born to a mother with her first episode of HSV at delivery or an infant born to a mother with her 20th episode of HSV? Or is there no difference?
7) A college student presents with abnormal behavior, focal seizures, and signs of encephalitis. What radiologic test will best diagnose this if HSV is the etiology?
8) What is the incubation period for chickenpox?
9) When may a child with chickenpox return to daycare or school?
10) A child with cystic fibrosis is in the hospital for a "tune-up." He is exposed to a child with chickenpox 5 days before admission. The child has not received the varicella vaccine and has not had chickenpox. When should the child be placed in isolation, and when may he be removed from isolation if he is still hospitalized?

low (< 1%) among women with a history of recurrent herpes.

~ 40% of infections are localized to the skin, eye, and mucosa (SEM), 35% to the CNS only, and 25% disseminated. Infection in the neonate presents usually in weeks 1–2 of life. Skin lesions start as macules and quickly become vesicular on a red base. The lesions commonly occur at sites of trauma, such as fetal scalp monitor sites, eye margins, or over the presenting part. Never overlook HSV as a possibility in a neonate with a vesicular-looking lesion! With the eye, conjunctivitis, keratitis, or chorioretinitis may occur. SEM disease does well if the diagnosis is made quickly and acyclovir given early. It is common for skin lesions to recur during the next several years. Treat with IV acyclovir.

Encephalitis is the predominant cause of HSV-related mortality (the most commonly identified etiologies of encephalitis are arboviruses, but the majority of encephalitis etiologies are still not identified). Patients with herpes encephalitis usually present with constitutional symptoms, altered mental status, and may have focal neurologic signs. Because it has a predilection for the temporal lobe, patients may have temporal lobe seizure symptoms (abnormal behavior, smells burning rubber). > 60% are left with neurologic sequelae! The EEG and MRI are the tests most sensitive for diagnosis, but PCR is also very sensitive in some centers.

HSV is one of the many causes of erythema multiforme (See Dermatology section).

Treatment of HSV: Use acyclovir for all the types of herpes infections. Give IV in immunosuppressed patients (but be careful—it can cause acute renal insufficiency, though rarely in children!). Give acyclovir, or one of its analogs (famciclovir, valacyclovir), orally for genital herpes. Acyclovir (or famciclovir, or valacyclovir) can also be given to suppress chronic infection, or as a treatment for acute recurrence. Use foscarnet to treat HSV that is resistant to acyclovir; ganciclovir is not helpful for resistant HSV, because it is also inactivated by the same mechanism.

VARICELLA

Overview

Varicella-zoster virus (VZV; DNA) causes chickenpox (See Figure 4-32) and herpes zoster (shingles, see Figure 4-33). The incubation period is 10–21 days (up to 35 days if VZIG has been given). Children present with low-grade fever, headache, and malaise, followed in 24–48 hours with the vesicular exanthem, described as "dew drops on a rose petal." It appears most commonly on the trunk and extremities, but the face and scalp can be involved as well. The vesicles appear in crops for 3–5 days and are worse in areas of eczema or trauma. Eventually, the vesicles become cloudy with cellular debris and finally involute and crust over. Itching is the most common complaint. Healing usually occurs in 7–10 days without scar formation. Children may return to school or daycare when the lesions are crusted. Those exposed in the hospital should be in isolation from days 8 to 21 after exposure. For most children, varicella is a benign illness. Suspect bacterial infection if fever occurs after the initial 48 hours, or if there is progression of redness or tenderness around lesions that are crusting over. Other things to look for: Mental-status changes, hemorrhagic lesions, or significant abdominal pain or vomiting.

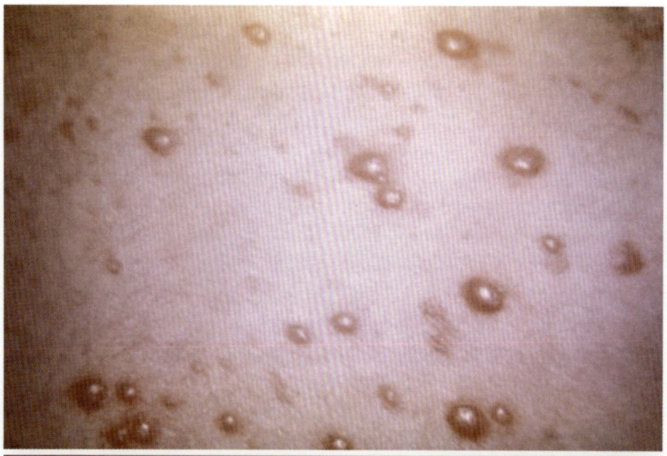

Figure 4-32: Chickenpox

notes

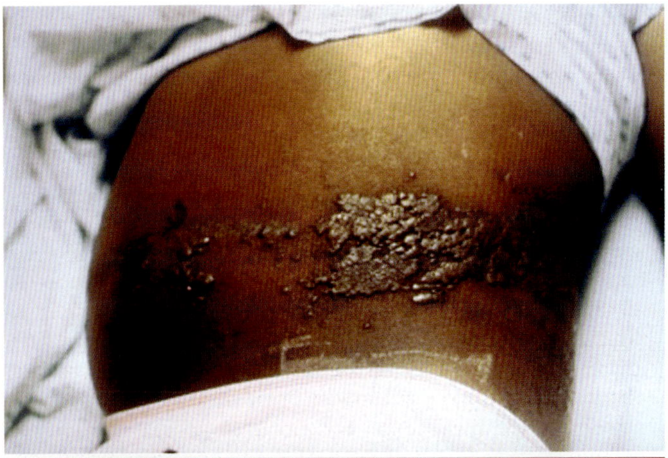

Figure 4-33: Shingles

Complications of Varicella

The most common complication is secondary bacterial infection. Most commonly, *Staphylococcus aureus* and *Streptococcus pyogenes* are involved. Infection can range from simple impetigo to necrotizing fasciitis. Also, deep tissue abscesses, bone infections, or severe lymphadenitis may occur.

Hepatitis, with mild liver enzyme elevations, is common in varicella. More extensive hepatitis is rare, but can occur. Reye syndrome has been associated with aspirin use and varicella infection.

Children have pneumonitis in ~ 10% of cases; it is usually mild. Adults and adolescents are more likely to have severe disease. Progression to pneumonia is more likely in these older age groups.

Thrombocytopenia can occur and result in bleeding problems.

The most common CNS complication is transient cerebellar ataxia and encephalitis. Cerebellar ataxia is self-limited and may occur before or after the onset of the exanthem. Encephalitis can be quite severe in some patients. Other, rarer CNS complications include aseptic meningitis, transverse myelitis, and Guillain-Barré syndrome.

Immunocompromised Patients

Children with congenital or acquired immune deficiencies, especially those who have defects in the ability to mount an antigen-specific T-cell immune response, are at risk for progressive, disseminated varicella infection. This includes those with lymphoproliferative malignancies, stem cell or solid organ transplant recipients, severe combined immunodeficiency, short-limbed dwarfism, Wiskott-Aldrich syndrome, ataxia-telangiectasia, and patients receiving chronic steroids.

Disseminated varicella begins with severe abdominal pain or back pain before the appearance of the rash. Fever is very high, may reach 104 to 106°F, and persists for several days. Liver involvement, pneumonitis, low platelet counts, coagulopathy, encephalitis, and renal dysfunction may all occur. Mortality is high. Infectiousness also is longer in these individuals.

Children with HIV or AIDS do not have the same risk of disseminated disease, but varicella can persist for weeks to months and may often recur. Varicella-zoster infection also is very common in these children.

Pregnancy

Symptoms of chickenpox are usually mild in children, but they may be severe in adolescents, adults, and especially in pregnant women. Pneumonia is more likely to occur in these older patients. Besides increased severity and pneumonia in the mother, if she is infected between 8 and 20 weeks gestation, her newborn is more likely to have birth defects. These defects can include classic cicatricial skin scarring and limb atrophy, microcephaly, cortical atrophy, seizures, chorioretinitis, and neurologic defects. Maternal zoster does not carry this risk.

Current recommendation for pregnant patients exposed to chickenpox: Give zoster immune globulin (ZIG or VZIG) within 4 days of exposure. If > 4 days, it does no good. Do not give varicella virus vaccine (Varivax®) to pregnant patients, because it is a live vaccine.

Infants born to mothers who develop varicella < 5 days before delivery, or 2 days after delivery, are at risk of severe neonatal varicella, because they are likely to have acquired significant virus in the absence of transplacental varicella antibody. Mothers who develop varicella > 4 days prior to delivery make varicella-specific IgG in sufficient time to permit placental transfer of antibody. This will generally prevent severe disease, but may not protect newborns against infection. Infants whose mothers have varicella at any stage of pregnancy, or infants who acquire varicella during the first few months of life, may manifest zoster early in life. Give term infants IV acyclovir in a dose of 15–20 mg/kg/dose q 8 hours. Decrease the interval in preterm infants to q 12 hours.

Most authorities recommend treating adults/adolescents with oral acyclovir 800 mg q.i.d. x 5 days if they present within the first 24 hours of the exanthem. Also, if the case is the second or later in the household, many will treat that child presumptively with acyclovir 20 mg/kg/dose 4 x a day x 5 days. Give immunocompromised patients IV acyclovir. (Toxicity: Acute renal insufficiency, but again very rare in children.) Avoid aspirin because of Reye syndrome risk. Also avoid ibuprofen, because of possible increased risk of *S. pyogenes* infection in children with chickenpox.

VZIG (Varicella Immune Globulin)

Consider VZIG for exposed, susceptible children at risk for severe disease. These include the following:

- Immunocompromised children
- Pregnant women
- Newborns whose mothers had varicella < 5 days before or 2 days after delivery
- Premature infants > 28 weeks gestation born to varicella antibody negative women

notes

Quick Quiz

1) What is the most common complication of chickenpox?
2) What is the most common CNS complication of chickenpox?
3) Which patients are more likely to get chickenpox pneumonia?
4) Which 2 antiinflammatory drugs should be avoided in chickenpox?
5) Who should be considered for VZIG therapy after exposure to chickenpox? In particular which term newborns should be considered for VZIG?
6) How does Herpes Zoster present?
7) How is CMV transmitted?
8) Do most children with congenital CMV infection have symptoms or signs?

- Premature infants < 28 weeks gestation (regardless of mother's varicella status)

What is significant exposure?
- Active case residing in the same household
- Active case sharing the same hospital room
- Face-to-face indoor play with an active case
- Intimate contact with a person with active zoster

Give VZIG as soon as possible, definitely within 96 hours of exposure. Be aware that VZIG may not prevent infection, and may prolong the incubation period up to 35 days. Do not give as a treatment to those with active infection.

Infection Control

Children with varicella are excluded from school until the lesions are crusted. Those exposed are potentially contagious from day 9 after exposure to the end of the incubation period (21 days). Therefore, any child admitted to the hospital with a history of exposure must be in a negative-pressure isolation room with airborne precautions during the incubation period.

In the hospital setting, a child with varicella is considered infectious and remains in isolation until all lesions are crusted over (or at least a minimum of 5 days if crusting occurs earlier).

Zoster (Shingles)

Herpes zoster (shingles) is caused by reactivation of the *Varicella-zoster* virus. A Tzanck smear will show multinucleated giant cells, which are pathognomonic for herpes viruses. A varicella virus DFA is diagnostic. Post-herpetic neuralgia is more likely with increasing age in adults > 60. Shingles recurs in < 5% of immunocompetent patients.

Most commonly, zoster affects 1 or 2 adjacent dermatomes with thoracic, cranial nerve, and lumbosacral areas most frequently involved. The lesions increase in number over 3–5 days and crust over by 2 weeks.

Prednisone, previously used with acyclovir, prolongs the course of Herpes zoster in immunosuppressed patients. Immunosuppressed patients often get severe cases of shingles. Although it was previously thought that prednisone decreases the incidence of post-herpetic neuralgia in the immunocompetent, well-designed studies have shown no benefit.

Use high-dose oral acyclovir alone to treat zoster; although it shortens the course of acute illness a little, it does not decrease the incidence of post-herpetic neuralgia. Only famciclovir and valacyclovir are shown to decrease the incidence of post-herpetic neuralgia. Valacyclovir is an L-valyl ester of acyclovir, has 3–5x greater bioavailability than acyclovir, and is almost completely converted to acyclovir after oral administration. For pain control, tricyclics, gabapentin, and lidocaine patches have some efficacy. Narcotics are effective and underused in this instance! Amitriptyline may be helpful for treatment of post-herpetic neuralgia.

If a patient presents with back pain and you think it is a Herpes zoster prodrome, what should you do? Answer: Nothing, except follow closely. Do not begin the acyclovir or its analogs until you see vesicles.

CMV

Overview

Cytomegalovirus (CMV) is a DNA virus that has been designated as human herpesvirus 5 (HHV-5). CMV infection is usually asymptomatic and is fairly common. Prevalence rates depend on geography and socioeconomic status. In Third World countries, 100% will have seroprevalence by their early 20s. By contrast, only 50% of the middle-upper socioeconomic population in the U.S. has anti-CMV antibodies by the age of 35.

CMV is transmitted through contact with infected urine, respiratory secretions, or blood. ~ 1% of all newborns are congenitally infected with CMV. Most of these infections are clinically silent and occur in mothers with existing immunity; however, clinically significant infections can occur. Breastfeeding is also a common method of transmission.

If the infant is not infected congenitally, or is in the perinatal period, he/she is likely to be infected in daycare. Daycare center prevalence rates approach 80%!

Congenital CMV Infection

Whether or not an infant will be infected depends largely on if the mother has IgG antibodies to CMV. If the infant is infected *in utero* when mom is reinfected with a new strain, or has reactivation of existing CMV, the chance of infection is much lower, ~ 1%, and of these infected infants, a majority will have no signs of infection.

notes

The most severe form of congenital CMV infection is cytomegalic inclusion disease. It presents with the following findings:

- IUGR
- Hepatosplenomegaly
- Thrombocytopenia
- "Blueberry muffin" baby (petechia/purpura as in congenital rubella syndrome)
- Microcephaly
- Cerebral atrophy
- Chorioretinitis
- Sensorineural hearing loss
- Periventricular intracerebral calcifications (especially look for: "Circumvent" the ventricles)

Some infants are born asymptomatic at birth, but can have subtle findings, including growth retardation. Some lesions may not occur for years! The greatest concern is that 15–20% of these children will have sensorineural hearing loss. No treatment has been shown to be conclusively effective for congenital CMV infection. At this time, routine use of ganciclovir is not recommended by the AAP or the Red Book Committee.

Perinatal CMV

Most perinatal CMV infections are asymptomatic and have no long-term risk of neurologic disease or hearing loss. Some infants may present with lymphadenopathy, hepatitis, or pneumonitis, but these also do not predispose to future hearing loss.

Mononucleosis-like Syndrome (Heterophile-Negative)

This usually occurs in adolescents with fever and malaise, mild hepatitis, and presence of atypical lymphocytes. Ampicillin/amoxicillin can cause a rash with this form.

Immunocompromised Hosts with CMV Infection

CMV is a very common infection in patients with decreased cellular immunity (post-transplant and AIDS). 75% of seronegative transplant recipients get CMV if the donor is seropositive. With a post-transplant, systemic CMV infection, the patient can have concurrent "-itises," which may include encephalitis, hepatitis, retinitis, colitis, pneumonitis, and adrenalitis (causing adrenal insufficiency). These are especially common and more severe if the recipient is seronegative prior to the transplant.

CMV is the usual cause of eye problems in adult and adolescent AIDS patients with low CD4 count. CMV can cause chorioretinitis, pneumonitis, esophagitis, and colitis. The CMV retinitis is distinctive; it has both retinal blanching and hemorrhage. Diagnosis is confirmed if CMV is cultured from the buffy coat smear. Diagnose CMV pneumonitis in transplant patients by finding inclusion bodies on the biopsy specimen. Finding CMV antigenemia or a positive-serum CMV PCR may be helpful also.

Treat CMV chorioretinitis (usually in AIDS patients) with ganciclovir (DHPG), foscarnet, or combination of both. Also, intraocular ganciclovir-release devices (with oral ganciclovir) have been effective. Cidofovir is also approved. However, all of these agents have only a suppressive effect, and must be given until the T-lymphocyte count increases to > 200.

Major toxicities of ganciclovir include granulocytopenia (30%!) and low platelets. ZDV (zidovudine, AZT) also causes granulocytopenia, and patients occasionally cannot tolerate both. The major toxicity of foscarnet is reversible renal failure; it also causes hypocalcemia, hypomagnesemia, and hyperphosphatemia (patients may present with seizures). Because they are only suppressive, these drugs do not cure the symptoms; once they are stopped, the disease resumes.

EBV (EPSTEIN-BARR VIRUS)

Epstein-Barr Virus (DNA) causes infectious mononucleosis. Incubation period is 1–2 months. Most (> 90%) patients have pharyngitis or tonsillitis, fever, lymphadenopathy, and abnormal liver function. Lymphocytosis is common with > 10% atypical lymphocytes: Enlarged with abundant cytoplasm, vacuoles, and indentations of the cell membrane. 1/2 have splenomegaly. Most develop a macular rash if given ampicillin. Heterophil antibody titers (monospot) decrease within 6 months, but the EB IgG antibodies are present for years. The atypical lymphs are T cells. Recurrence is unusual but possible—usually with high titers of antibody to EB early antigen (> 1:5000).

Children < 4 years of age rarely have the "classic" symptoms. Most present with rashes and hepatosplenomegaly. Otitis media, FTT, abdominal pain, and recurrent pharyngitis are common in young children. Prolonged fever may be the only manifestation. The monospot test is rarely positive in a child < 2 years and has ~ 50% sensitivity in children 2–4 years of age.

EBV-specific antibodies are a pain to learn, but please do so for the Board exam. You will have to discern what the heck it means. Here is a simplified version:

If the IgM-VCA is +, the patient has acute primary EBV or a very recent-past EBV infection. Forget everything else they are throwing at you.

EBNA + means the patient is convalescent or post-EBV.

IgG VCA doesn't help you at all. It is positive before the patient has symptoms and remains so for life. It will be positive if the patient is in convalescence, or had EBV years ago.

Anti-Early Antigen (anti-EA) isn't much help either. It can be positive in acute-primary, recent-past, chronic or reactivation, or in EBV malignancies. It should go away in convalescent or post-EBV infection. So someone convalescent should have only a + IgG-VCA (or maybe an EBNA).

Thus, the only really helpful test findings are an isolated + IgM-VCA: That means acute-primary or recent past infection; or an isolated + IgG-VCA generally means an infection in the non-remote past.

There are no antivirals effective for infectious mononucleosis. Corticosteroids are used sometimes for severe life-threatening complications—especially airway obstruction,

notes

Quick Quiz

1) Describe the clinical findings in an infant with congenital CMV infection.
2) What infection does CMV produce in adolescents?
3) What are the toxicities of ganciclovir?
4) What is the characteristic WBC finding in patients with EBV infection?
5) How do children < 4 years of age present with EBV?
6) How sensitive is the monospot test in a child 3 years of age for detecting acute EBV infection?
7) Which EBV antibody tests are positive in an acute infection?
8) Describe the infection associated with HHV-6 infection.
9) Describe a typical 10-year-old with Rubella.

neurologic complications, severe hepatitis, myocarditis, or hemolytic anemia. Give corticosteroids only to a minority of patients with EBV. Affected persons should avoid contact sports and other activities during the time of splenomegaly (usually 1–3 months).

EBV causes hairy leukoplakia; this mucocutaneous lesion may be seen as an early manifestation of HIV disease. High-dose acyclovir may offer some benefit in treatment of oral hairy leukoplakia. Chronic fatigue has no proven association with EB virus. EBV *is* associated with nasopharyngeal carcinoma and Burkitt lymphoma.

A patient with mononucleosis symptoms, who is heterophil-negative, usually has CMV.

HUMAN HERPESVIRUS 6

Human herpesvirus 6 (HHV-6) is a DNA virus. Nearly all children < age 3 years have been infected with HHV-6. Children can be asymptomatic, have fatal disseminated disease (rare), or anything in between. Most children have exanthem subitum or a febrile illness without a rash.

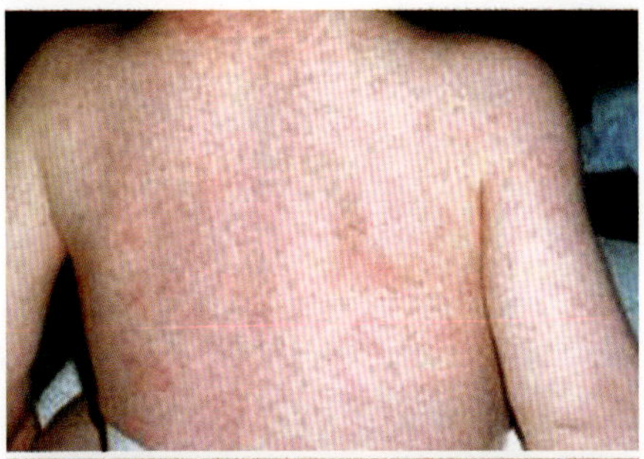

Figure 4-34: Exanthem Subitum

Exanthem subitum (Roseola infantum, "Sixth Disease") is very common. It presents as fever for 3–5 days, followed by the abrupt cessation of fever, and the appearance of a macular-to-maculopapular rash. (See Figure 4-34). Seizures are not uncommon during the febrile stage. Don't be fooled on the Board Examination by an 8-month-old with fever for 3 days, who is placed on amoxicillin and then has a "drug reaction." The answer is more than likely exanthem subitum!

CNS disease is usually mild, but HHV-6 likely accounts for a large percentage of febrile seizures occurring in children < 2 years of age.

HUMAN HERPESVIRUS 7 AND 8

HHV-7 and HHV-8 were "discovered" in the 1990s. HHV-7 is associated with roseola infantum (see above), and HHV-8 is associated with Kaposi sarcoma in AIDS and other immunocompromised patients.

RUBELLA (GERMAN MEASLES)

Rubella is "German measles" (ss RNA virus). In March 2005, the CDC declared that rubella had been eliminated from the U.S. There were 117 cases in 1989, 100 in 2001 and only 10 in 2004—all which were probable acquired in other countries. We will still review this because it may still appear on the Board exam.

Rubella is spread by person-to-person transmission of infected droplets. Patients are infectious starting a few days before the rash and a few days into the rash. Congenitally acquired infection is chronic, but postnatal infection is not. It peaks in the late winter and spring.

Clinically, rubella presents with adenopathy, rash, and low-grade fever.

The usual incubation period is 14–21 days. The tender adenopathy begins first and is usually postauricular (see Figure 4-35), occipital, and posterior cervical. Older children and adolescents complain of malaise, headache, sore throat, and

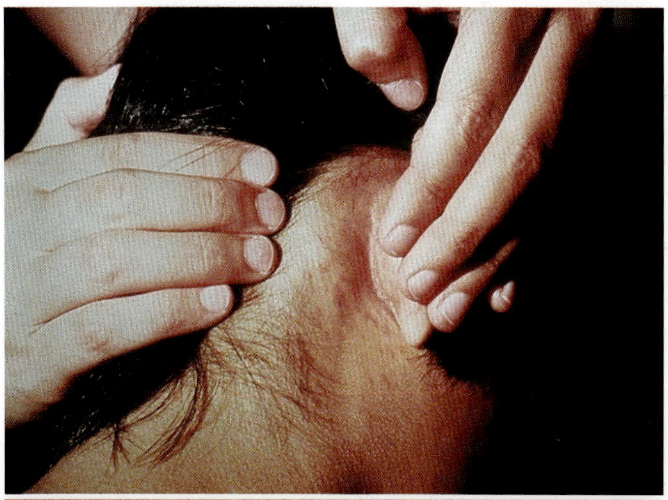

Figure 4-35: Rubella inf. with Postauricular Adenopathy

notes

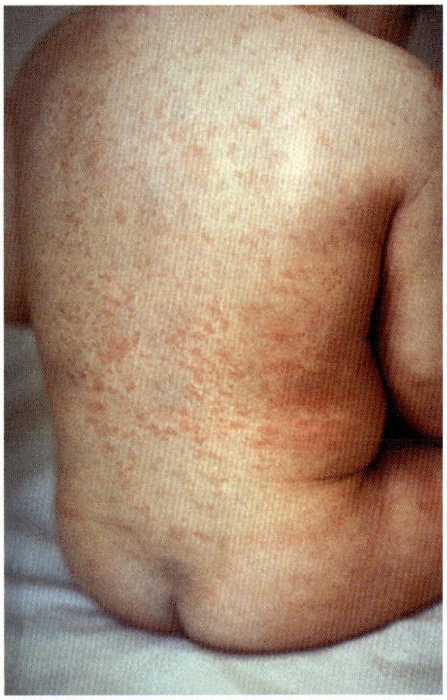

Figure 4-36: Rubella Rash

mild coryza during a 1–5 day prodrome before the rash develops.

The rash changes appearance throughout its course. It may be a "quick blush," but usually persists for 2–3 days. Most commonly, it begins as macules on the face that spread quickly to the neck, trunk, arms, and finally, the legs (see Figure 4-36). Usually, the rash is gone from the face by the time it has reached the legs.

Rubella also has an enanthem called Forchheimer spots. These are pinpoint or slightly larger red spots on the soft palate, and may occur during the late prodrome or at the beginning of the rash appearance. They are not specific for rubella, however, and can appear with other viral exanthems.

Fever is common but can be absent in some cases. Women tend to have polyarthralgia/arthritis, but this is rare in children. CNS involvement is less common than in measles.

Congenital rubella occurs when the mother is infected during pregnancy. The trimester the infection occurs has important prognostic predictors:

1st trimester: 90% fetal infection risk; cardiac, cataracts, and glaucoma common; hearing loss and neurologic manifestations

2nd trimester: 25–30% fetal infection risk; some risk of hearing or neurologic manifestations

Last weeks of gestation: Infection risk is 60–100%; but non-teratogenic

The difficulty is that these infants may present with multiple anomalies, be stillborn, or have no abnormalities at all.

The most severe syndrome manifestations include:

- Thrombocytopenic purpura, "blueberry muffin" lesions, which are reddish purple macular lesions, and the most common manifestation of congenital rubella. (See Figure 4-37).
- Radiolucencies in the metaphyseal long bones
- Hepatosplenomegaly
- Hepatitis
- Hemolytic anemia
- Bulging anterior fontanelle
- CSF pleocytosis
- Congenital heart disease: Most common is PDA with or without pulmonary artery stenosis; ASD and VSD
- Sensorineural deafness (due to damage to the organ of Corti); this may be the only manifestation if infection occurs after the first 8 weeks of pregnancy
- Cataracts with microphthalmia (see Figure 4-38)
- Congenital glaucoma
- Retinopathy with patchy deep pigmentation
- Mental retardation

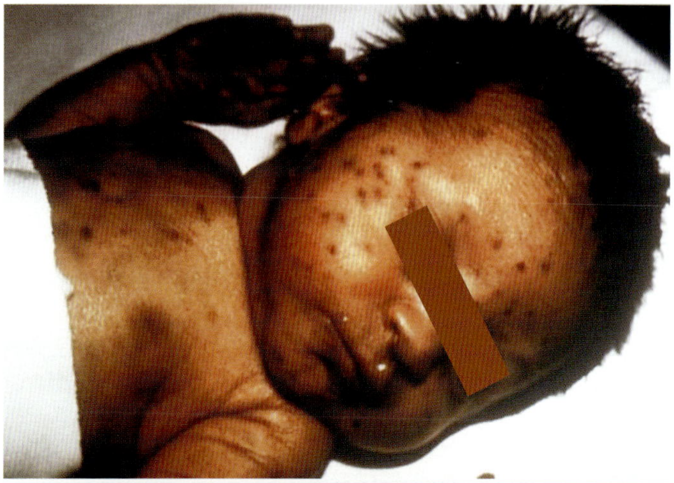

Figure 4-37: Severe Congenital Rubella Infection

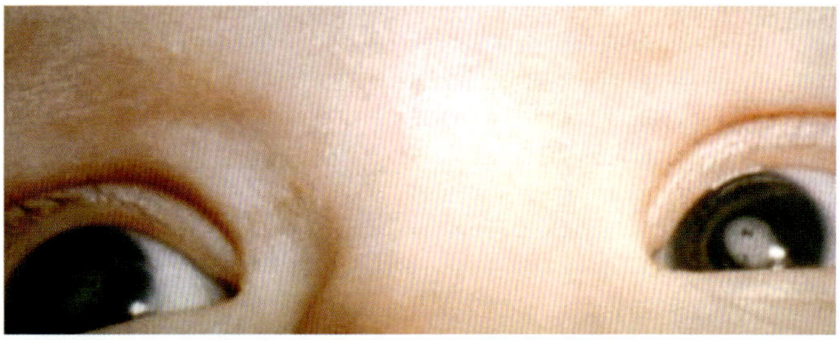

Figure 4-38: Cataracts from Congenital Rubella

A rare complication is progressive rubella panencephalitis, which is a severe, progressive neurologic deterioration that begins in the 2nd decade. It presents with mental deterioration, myoclonus, ataxia, and seizures, with progression to death in several years.

Children with a history of congenital rubella have a much higher risk of IDDM! By age 10, the risk is nearly 4x greater; by adulthood it is 10–20x greater.

Increased risk of thyroiditis has also been described.

notes

Quick Quiz

1) Describe the clinical findings in an infant with congenital rubella infection during the 1st trimester; the 3rd trimester.
2) Describe a newborn with severe congenital rubella infection.
3) Characterize the presentation for rubeola infection. Differentiate rubeola from rubella infection.
4) What vitamin deficiency worsens rubeola? In what way?
5) True or False: Rubeola can cause a "congenital rubeola syndrome."
6) What are the oral spots called in rubella? rubeola?
7) What can be given to prevent rubeola in a susceptible immunocompromised child?

Mortality is highest in the first 6 months of life. In those infants with congenital rubella and neonatal thrombocytopenic purpura, the mortality rate is ~ 40%. Most children die from sepsis or congestive heart failure.

RUBEOLA (MEASLES)

Rubeola is "measles". (See Figure 4-40). Symptoms start ~ 10 days after the initial exposure. Symptoms at the onset: the "3 Cs": cough, coryza, and conjunctivitis (with photophobia). The conjunctivitis causes edema of the lids, and the child has increased tearing. Stimson line may occur, which is a sharply demarcated transverse linear injection of the lower lid margins. Vitamin A deficiency (prevalent in Third-World countries) results in more severe eye disease, with corneal ulcers and loss of vision.

Children also have malaise and fever. Koplik spots (whitish spots on an erythematous base) appear on the buccal mucosa 2–3 days before the onset of the skin rash. The Koplik spots are usually gone by the time the skin rash appears (see Figure 4-39).

The skin rash starts at the hairline and spreads downward. It lasts ~ 5 days and then resolves, also from the hairline downward. Lymphadenopathy and splenomegaly are common.

Complications of the CNS are common; 10% of children will develop a CSF pleocytosis, and 50% will have EEG changes! Encephalomyelitis occurs in 0.1% (1/1000) of cases, and presents with seizures, altered mental status, and coma. Mortality approaches 10–25% with motor, mental cognition, or behavioral problems developing in 20–50% of the survivors.

Measles also can reactivate tuberculosis.

Gestational measles can induce premature delivery, stillbirth, or abortion, but does not cause a congenital syndrome of malformations, as is seen with Rubella.

Treatment with Vitamin A can be helpful in reducing eye abnormalities and pneumonia, especially so in individuals at risk for vitamin A deficiency.

Immune globulin (IG) can prevent measles from developing in a susceptible, at-risk child; but you must give it within 6 days of exposure.

Again: 3 Cs, Koplik spots, rash starting at hairline and spreading caudally.

RETROVIRUS

Retroviruses—RNA viruses. HTLV-1 causes T-cell leukemia. HTLV-2 causes a rare T-cell variant of hairy cell leukemia. HIV-1 (previously called HTLV-3) causes AIDS. HIV-2, found in West Africa and parts of the U.S., is a virus that causes an illness indistinguishable from AIDS (ELISA now picks up both HIV-I and -II). More on HIV later.

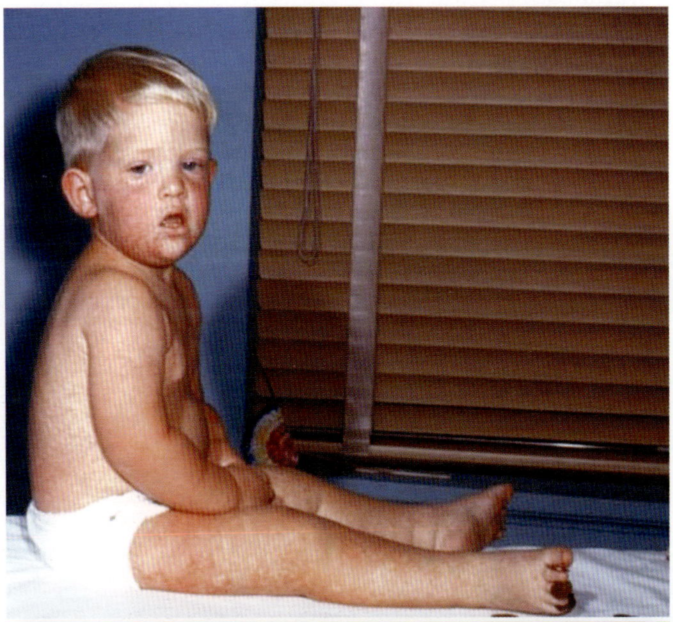

Figure 4-40: Rubeola (Measles)

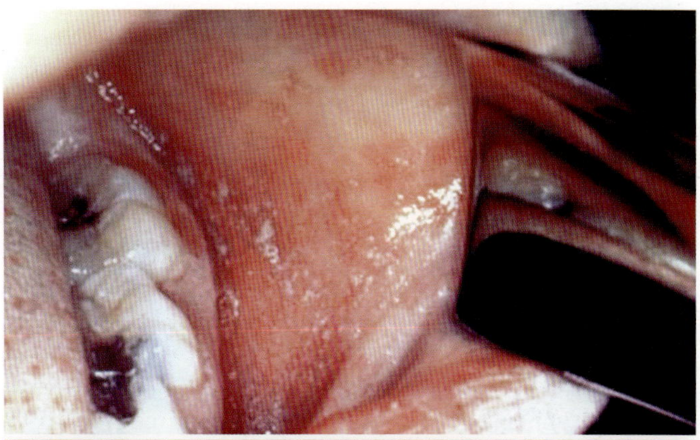

Figure 4-39: Measles, Koplik Spots

notes

RESPIRATORY VIRUSES

Rhinoviruses

Rhinoviruses are a common cause of URI—usually during the autumn. They are RNA viruses that replicate best at cooler temperatures (93–95°F), such as in the nasal mucosa. The numerous serotypes are responsible for the "common cold" in many.

Controlled trials have yet to prove that vitamins, minerals (including zinc—except in one adult study), or herbal remedies (Echinacea) are effective for reducing the duration of the typical cold.

Adenovirus

Adenovirus is a common cause of respiratory tract infection. It is a DNA virus with 41 serotypes recognized in humans. Most children are infected early with types 1, 2, and 5; serotypes 3, 7, and 21 are less common but important causes of respiratory infection.

Respiratory Manifestations: Infants present with coryza, conjunctivitis, otitis media, and pharyngitis, usually due to serotypes 1, 2, and 5. In infants with serotypes 3, 7, and 21, more severe infection is likely, with progressive, severe bronchiolitis, pneumonia, and long-term sequelae.

Pharyngoconjunctival Fever: This syndrome is frequently due to adenovirus 3 and presents with fever, pharyngitis, conjunctivitis, rhinitis, and cervical adenitis. It occurs most commonly in the summer and is transmitted while swimming—frequently causing epidemics in summer camp settings.

Epidemic keratoconjunctivitis: This occurs with conjunctivitis, corneal involvement, and preauricular lymph node enlargement. It too is seen more commonly in the summer and is associated with swimming.

Diarrhea: Adenoviruses 40 and 41 are common causes of infant diarrhea. ELISA or electron microscopy can detect the virus in stool. Some adenoviruses have been implicated in the diagnosis of intussusception.

Acute hemorrhagic cystis: Adenovirus types 11 and 21 are associated with acute hemorrhagic cystitis. The hematuria can last for several days or up to 2 weeks. Initially, it can be confused with post-streptococcal glomerulonephritis.

Meningoencephalitis: This can occur on occasion with adenovirus infection, particularly in the immunocompromised and patients with AIDS.

Treatment for all of the above is symptomatic. Antivirals are not helpful.

Because of the common association between adenovirus and "close quarters" in adults, military recruits are given the live, enteric-coated oral vaccine, but the vaccine is effective only for serotypes 4, 7, and 21.

Coronavirus

Coronavirus is an enveloped RNA virus. It is responsible for 3–5% of "common colds." It is more likely to be the etiology of the cold during the winter months.

SARS has now emerged as a concern, and is due to SARS-associated coronavirus (SARS-CoV). In 2003, there were > 8000 cases worldwide, and > 800 deaths. Be concerned about someone on the Board Exam who presents with recent travel to Asia (or an epidemic area like Toronto), and who has early "flu-like" symptoms—but quickly progress to severe respiratory distress. However, an elderly person is the more likely to be severely affected.

RSV (Respiratory Syncytial Virus)

Respiratory syncytial virus (RSV) infections occur yearly, during the autumn and winter. RSV infections are more severe in the infant, occasionally resulting in pneumonia. Only 1% of affected infants are hospitalized. Diagnose RSV by doing an ELISA test on nasal secretions. RSV is discussed in more detail in the Pulmonology and The Newborn sections.

Parainfluenza Virus

Parainfluenza virus is discussed in the Pulmonology section.

Influenza Virus

Influenza is still a major cause of death in the U.S. and can be quite severe in adult populations, particularly those > 55 years old or in children with underlying lung disease. Vaccination decreases mortality by 1/3!

There are 3 types of influenza viruses: Influenza A, B, and C. Influenza A & B cause the yearly epidemics of respiratory illnesses. Type A is widely distributed in animals, especially horses, hogs/pigs, and chickens/birds. Influenza C causes very mild, if any, symptoms.

Virus is spread by hand-to-nose, droplets of respiratory secretions, or small-droplet aerosol.

"Antigenic shift" refers to major changes in the viral hemagglutinin (HA) or neuraminidase (NA) on the outer surface. These "shifts" occur only in influenza A, and result in a new virus, to which humans or other animals have no natural immunity. These shifts resulted in the "pandemics" of the last century, and are among the concerns with the "bird flu" scare of this century. "Antigenic drift" refers to minor changes in the virus and occurs with both influenza A and B.

Influenza causes fever, chills, headache, and myalgias after 1–3 days of incubation. After 24 hours, rhinitis and lower respiratory symptoms develop. Tracheobronchitis is the most common manifestation of lower respiratory tract infection.

Most children recover without complication. However, 3 types of pneumonia are possible:

1) Viral bronchopneumonia: Usually occurs between days 3 and 5 of illness
2) Secondary bacterial pneumonia: Usually occurs 5–7 days into the illness; common bacteria include *S. pneumoniae* and *S. aureus*
3) Diffuse viral hemorrhagic alveolitis

Diagnose by isolating the virus or by an EIA-based antigen detection assay.

notes

QuickQuiz

1) Describe the eye diseases associated with adenovirus infection.
2) Which virus can cause acute hemorrhagic cystitis?
3) What causes SARS?
4) Describe the symptoms of influenza.
5) What 2 bacteria are likely to cause pneumonia in a patient with preceding influenza infection?
6) An outbreak of influenza A occurs in a child residential home. What should you do as the supervising physician?
7) What could you do if the same outbreak was due to influenza B?
8) An 8-year-old is to receive her first influenza vaccine this year. How should this be administered?
9) What causes hand, foot, and mouth disease?

Treatment of influenza:

- Amantadine and rimantadine are not only protective against infection with influenza A (A–A), but they also decrease the severity of infection if given within 24 hours of onset of symptoms. Adjust amantadine/rimantadine dosages for any renal impairment. Note that they are not approved for children < age 1 year.
- Oseltamivir (Tamiflu®—oral) and zanamivir (Relenza®—powder for inhalation) are the first of the neuraminidase inhibitors, a newer class of treatment for influenza A & B (FDA-approved 1999). If given within 48 hours of onset of symptoms, they decrease duration by 30%. If given within 12 hours, it decreases duration by 50%. It also prevents clinical disease in > 90% of household contacts. As of late 2005, with the "bird flu" lurking as a potential cause of the next pandemic, these two agents might be effective therapies, but unfortunately are likely to be in very short supply.

When an influenza A epidemic threatens an unimmunized nursing home or children's long-term care center, who should get amantadine or rimantadine? Answer: The entire population of the home...and give the influenza vaccine to all who have not yet been vaccinated for that season.

For children < age 9 years who have never been vaccinated, give 2 doses of vaccine, 1 month apart, to achieve adequate antibody levels. Vaccine efficacy is not established for children < age 6 months.

A live, mucosally administered influenza vaccine is now available. (Discussed in the Allergy and Immunology section.)

ENTEROVIRUS

Overview

The enterovirus group is made up of coxsackievirus A, coxsackievirus B, echovirus, and enterovirus. (Poliovirus, also an enterovirus, is considered below as a separate entity.) Enteroviruses occur year-round, but have increased infection rates between May and October in warmer climates. Transmission is by the fecal-oral route and person-to-person.

Infection is most common in children < age 4 years and in lower socioeconomic groups.

Clinically, enteroviruses can present in multiple ways.

Congenital and Neonatal Infections

Group B coxsackievirus can cause serious and fatal disseminated disease in newborns. It can be transplacentally transmitted as well. It can cause hepatitis, myocarditis, meningoencephalitis, and adrenal cortex failure. Illness onset is abrupt. Hepatic necrosis is common.

Febrile Illness

Nonspecific febrile illnesses are common with enteroviruses, especially in the first few months of life. GI symptoms are rare. If enteroviral infection is widespread in a community, a large number of infants < age 4 weeks will likely present with "fever without focus."

Rashes

Hand, foot, and mouth disease presents with fever and vesicles of the buccal mucosa, tongue and, less commonly, the palate, lips, and gums. A red maculopapular rash may appear on the hands and feet, and eventually may become vesicular. In infants, the diaper area is commonly involved. Coxsackievirus A16, A5, and A10, or enterovirus Type 71 are commonly involved.

Meningitis/Encephalitis

Fever, headache, and malaise are common in older children with meningitis/encephalitis. In all ages, fever to 104°F is common, and may be gradual or abrupt in onset. Fever lasts 3–5 days. Focal findings are rare. The CSF is nonspecific, may have a predominance of PMNs early on, and be confused with bacterial meningitis. Total protein is normal and glucose is usually normal, although it may be diminished.

No long-term sequelae have been demonstrated in infants with enteroviral meningitis / meningoencephalitis.

Of concern are patients with agammaglobulinemia, who cannot readily eradicate enterovirus infections from the CNS. These children have recurrent episodes and severe manifestations, such as seizures, hemiparesis, hearing loss, and mental deterioration.

Paralytic Disease

Polioviruses are commonly associated with paralytic disease, but group B coxsackievirus and enteroviruses 70 and 71 have also been associated with paralytic disease and encephalitis. Classically, if paralysis is to occur, it is asymmetric with lower extremity and involves larger muscle groups. Atrophy of involved muscles becomes apparent, usually within 2 months. Variable degrees of recovery occur in most by 6–18 months.

notes

Acute Hemorrhagic Conjunctivitis

Enterovirus type 70 and coxsackievirus A24 cause subconjunctival hemorrhage. Swelling, redness, and tearing with pain are common. It resolves within 1 week without specific therapy.

Herpangina

Herpangina is most commonly associated with coxsackievirus group A infection. It presents with tiny vesicles or punched-out ulcers on the anterior pillars of the tonsils, uvula, and pharynx. The lesions are 1–2 mm in diameter. They sometimes can enlarge and rupture with a shallow, yellow-gray ulcer. It presents with a high, abrupt fever, sore throat, and dysphagia.

Bornholm Disease (Pleurodynia, Epidemic Myalgia)

This acute illness presents with paroxysmal thoracic pain and is due to group B coxsackieviruses. The pain is pleuritic in nature and aggravated by deep breathing, coughing, or movement. It can last up to 14 days, but usually is over in 4 days.

Myocarditis/Pericarditis

Myocarditis or pericarditis may occur in older children with group B coxsackievirus or echovirus. It can be mild to fatal.

Diagnosis of all entities has been aided by PCR technology. Sensitivity and specificity approach 95% for many of the enteroviruses. Finding the virus in CSF or blood suggests an etiologic role.

No FDA-approved therapy is available at this time. Newer agents are being developed, but are not widely available for use.

POLIO

Polio—Polioviruses are part of the Enterovirus genus and belong to the family Picornaviridae, a small RNA virus. 90% are self-limited and a majority of those infected have asymptomatic or mild, nonspecific illness. CNS onset is characterized by an aseptic meningitis and/or an asymmetric, flaccid paralysis without reflexes. Paralysis begins proximally, and progresses to involve distal muscle groups—known as a descending paralysis. Brain stem, spinal, mixed spinal bulbar, or bulbar involvement can result in respiratory muscle paralysis. It has essentially been eliminated in the western hemisphere and developed countries worldwide.

The clinical case definition includes:

- Age < 6 years
- Fever at onset of the disease
- Descending paralysis with maximum extent of paralysis within 4 days
- Residual neurologic deficit at ≥ 60 days after onset of the paralysis

You easily recover poliovirus from stool, throat swabs, or occasionally CSF for up to 3–6 weeks.

No specific therapy is available. If bulbar paralysis is present, respiratory support is required.

Late symptoms of acute paralytic poliomyelitis or postpolio syndrome become apparent between 1.5–40 years. It presents with acute muscle pain, weakness, or new paralysis.

RABIES

Rabies is especially common in bats, dogs, wolves, ferrets, raccoons, skunks, and foxes. It is rare in squirrels, farm animals, and possums. On the Board exam (and real life), if the patient wakes up and a bat is in the room, even without evidence of a bite, the child should be prophylaxed for presumed rabies. In total numbers, the bites of rodents, rabbits, birds, and reptiles are seldom worrisome, and human rabies cases are rare. However, when it does happen, the fatality rate is ~ 100%. Rabies in humans presents as an acute encephalomyelitis, with symptoms of restlessness, excitation, and severe spasms of the larynx and pharynx—especially when the affected person sees food or water (hydrophobia).

Rabies is an RNA virus and a rhabdovirus. Bite wounds introduce the virus through infected saliva into abraded skin. Virus spreads via peripheral nerves to the brain, then via the sensory and autonomic nervous system to the eyes, salivary glands, skin, and viscera. The brain areas most commonly affected include the thalamus, hypothalamus, substantia nigra, pons, and medulla. Diagnose by finding pathognomonic Negri bodies (acidophilic inclusion bodies) in the cytoplasm of neurons.

80% of cases either have no known exposure to a rabid animal, or their exposure to a suspect animal did not involve a bite or mucous membrane exposure.

Incubation period is shorter for bites to the head than to the extremities. The initial phase is apprehension, anxiety, and insomnia, with fever also common. In the initial "excitation" phase, or "furious" rabies, the patient has apprehension and terror. This results in hydrophobia and often seizures. The excitation phase is followed by the paralytic phase, with coma and death following soon thereafter.

Microscopic examination of a biopsy of nerve fibers from the nape of the neck is the easiest way to diagnose, but it still takes several days for results to return. PCR is now available for saliva but not widely available.

After exposure to possible rabies via a bite or mucous membrane contamination—or contamination of a scratch or abrasion with saliva from an animal that is *suspected* of having rabies—initiate rabies immune globulin (RIG) and vaccine as soon as possible. For exposures from dogs, cats, and ferrets without evidence of rabies, these animals should be observed by a veterinarian for 10 days; if they behave normally by that time, immunization of the victim is unnecessary. Consider wild animals listed in the first paragraph (skunks, bats, foxes, etc.) rabid, and initiate vaccine and RIG unless the animal is captured, euthanized, and tests negative for rabies. Livestock, rodent, and lagomorph (rabbits, hares) bites rarely require treatment. Pre-exposure prophylaxis is indicated for cave ex-

notes

Quick Quiz

1) What virus can cause an acute hemorrhagic conjunctivitis?
2) List the clinical case definition for a child with polio.
3) How do you diagnose rabies?
4) Know the scenarios for rabies prophylaxis for bites due to: a) a wild animal; b) an immunized, non-rabid-appearing dog who had been provoked by a child and the dog is available for observation; c) a case where a "street" dog bit a child in an unprovoked attack and then ran away and cannot be located. (The child says, "he acted funny.")
5) Describe the clinical syndrome seen with mumps.
6) What complications of mumps can occur in adolescent males? In adolescent females?
7) What sensory loss may occur with mumps?
8) What infection does parvovirus B-19 cause?
9) Describe the rash of Fifth Disease.

plorers and veterinarians, but not for hunters, mail carriers, etc.

MUMPS

Mumps (RNA) occurs most commonly in winter and early spring. (See Figure 4-41). Although often asymptomatic, it can present with uni- or bilateral parotitis, aseptic meningitis, and/or encephalitis.

Mumps is most communicable 1–2 days before parotid swelling, and continues until 5 days after parotid swelling begins. Patients are not infectious after 9 days of parotid swelling.

Because of the use of vaccine in younger children, the incidence of mumps has decreased markedly, and the typical age of onset has increased to 10–14 years.

Vaccine "failure" occurs at a rate of 2–5%; use of the 2nd dose increases immunity considerably. Infection provides life-long immunity, and most believe that vaccine likely does also.

The swelling usually involves both parotids but sometimes is unilateral, and may also involve the submandibular glands, with or without the parotids. The entire parotid swells, including the uncinate lobe, which extends to the back of the ear lobe. Anorexia and abdominal pain are common, indicating either pancreas or ovarian involvement in the female.

15–35% of post-pubertal males with mumps get an epididymo-orchitis that is usually unilateral. Children as young as 3 years of age have been affected. Post-infection sterility is a rare occurrence. Mastitis occurs in 31% of adolescent females. Oophoritis occurs in ~ 7%.

CNS infection is very common. Headache, lethargy, and meningismus occur with CSF abnormalities. Most CSF counts are < 500 with most lymphocytes. The meningitis is usually self-limited without sequelae.

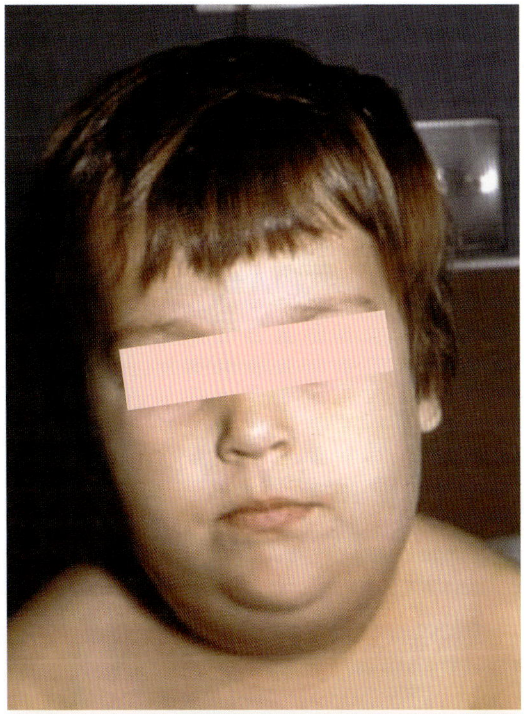

Figure 4-41: Mumps

Deafness is a complication of mumps and, in one study, occurred in 4% of those affected. Most were unilateral, and almost all recovered in a few weeks.

Mumps does not cause congenital malformation syndromes.

The mumps skin test is not effective for checking immunity.

To differentiate mumps from bacterial parotitis, check a Gram stain of the parotid secretions. There are many WBCs and organisms in bacterial parotitis, and none in mumps.

Note: Another cause of enlarged parotid glands is frequent vomiting. Always consider bulimia in an adolescent with parotid gland enlargement.

PARVOVIRUS

Parvovirus is a small DNA virus. One parvovirus, B19, causes various disorders, ranging from erythema infectiosum ("Fifth disease") to arthralgias/arthritis to aplastic anemia.

Erythema infectiosum (Fifth disease) is a mildly contagious, self-limited infection that causes a rash and arthritis. The facial component of the rash causes a "slapped cheek" appearance. (See Figure 4-42). This rash is much more common in children; the arthritis is more common in adults. The rash on the extremities is "lattice-like," and becomes more prominent in the sun or with a warm bath (See Figure 4-43). Most children are not that ill, but complain more of pruritus with the rash. The rash likely occurs in only ~ 1/2 of children with the infection.

notes

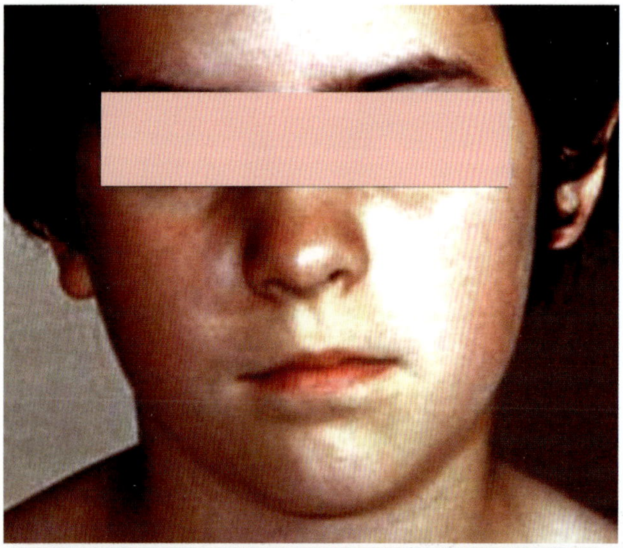

Figure 4-42: "Slapped Cheek" with E. infectiosum

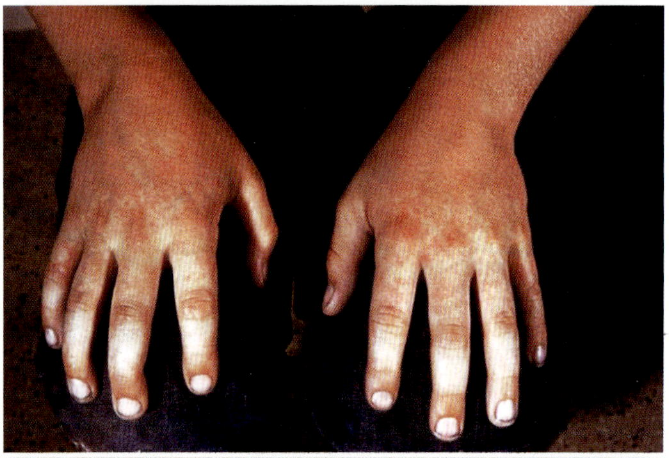

Figure 4-43: "Lace-like" Extremity Rash, E. infectiosum

The arthritis more commonly affects adults, especially women. Usually, it is a symmetric disease of the hands, knees, or wrists.

In patients with chronic, hemolytic anemias or AIDS, it can cause aplastic anemia. In these, the bone marrow shows characteristic "giant pronormoblasts."

Pregnancy with parvovirus B19 is a special case to consider. Most mothers who are infected during pregnancy have infants without abnormalities. However, ~ 5–10% will have fetal loss with intrauterine hydrops. To date, there is no reliable method to predict which fetuses will have poor outcomes.

Diagnosis is clinical. Test IgM antibodies to diagnose an acute infection.

Treatment is symptomatic. For those who are immunocompromised, IVIG is helpful.

Once the rash appears, the child is no longer infectious. However, children with aplastic anemia due to parvovirus B19 are highly infectious. If hospital admission is required, place the child in a negative-pressure room isolation with droplet precautions. Masks should be worn.

ARBOVIRUSES

Arboviruses are mainly transmitted by mosquitoes or ticks. Various arboviruses occur in the U.S., typically in the late spring and summer. Until recently, most cases occurred along the Gulf Coast in Louisiana and Florida. Now, with West Nile Virus, the arboviruses are seen from coast to coast. In 2003, West Nile was the most common arbovirus identified in the U.S. The state of Colorado had the highest number of cases.

Other viruses besides West Nile, including LaCrosse, St. Louis, Eastern Equine (EEE), Western Equine (WEE), Venezuelan Equine, Powassan, and Colorado tick fever viruses, occur on occasion in the U.S. Almost all have similar symptoms with fever, headache, chills, and various severity of encephalitis, or aseptic meningitis. However, many cases are asymptomatic; only ~ 1/100 infected may present with symptoms.

Diagnose by finding virus-specific IgM antibody in the CSF or serum.

HANTAVIRUS

A hantavirus-associated disease, called Hantavirus Pulmonary Syndrome (HPS), starts with severe myalgias, fever, headache, and cough, and quickly progresses to ARDS and death. > 50% die. The primary reservoir in the western and southwestern U.S. is the deer mouse. On the eastern coast and in the southeast, the cotton rat is the main reservoir. The infection occurs when the excreta or saliva are inhaled. Transfer of the virus can also occur through broken skin. No person-to-person transfer is known to have occurred.

Symptoms:

Early: Constitutional symptoms in all. ~ 1/2 have N/V, diarrhea, and abdominal pain.

Late: 4–10 days later; coughing and shortness of breath as ARDS develops.

No rash.

Suspect it on the Board Examination in an adolescent who lives in the desert southwest, presenting with severe hemorrhagic pneumonia, thrombocytopenia, and increased hematocrit.

DENGUE FEVER

Dengue fever, dengue hemorrhagic fever, and dengue shock syndrome are caused by 4 serotypes of the Flavivirus. It is a tropical disease that uses humans and the day-biting *Aedes* mosquitos (*Anopheles* carry malaria) in its life cycle. Dengue fever has had a resurgence in the past 10 years in South America and Mexico, with a few cases also in south Texas. No vaccine is available yet (but one is under development).

Symptoms are rapid onset of high fever, severe myalgias and arthralgias ("break-bone fever"), and severe headaches with N/V, followed by a macular red rash, which covers most of the body. A second rash that looks more like measles occurs

notes

Quick Quiz

1) When is a child with Fifth Disease not infectious anymore?
2) What is the risk for a pregnant woman infected with parvovirus B-19?
3) In what geographic area of the U.S. has hantavirus most commonly been reported?
4) What virus is associated with an increased risk of cervical cancer?
5) Which virus is associated with SSPE? Describe SSPE.
6) Describe a typical patient with new variant CJD.

later, along with a recurrence of fever ("saddleback fever"—up, down, up).

Suspect this in a traveler with these symptoms who has returned from tropical latitudes (including the Caribbean and Mexico).

Treatment is supportive.

SLOW VIRUSES

Overview

There are 2 classes of slow viruses:

1) Normal viruses, such as papilloma (warts) and papovavirus (PML)
2) Defective viruses, such as the defective measles virus, which causes subacute sclerosing panencephalitis

Papillomavirus

Papillomavirus causes warts. Genital warts are associated with an increased risk of cervical cancer. There are many variants. HPV #1, 2, and 5 are common causes of plantar warts. HPV #6, 11, 16, 18, and 31 are genital. HPV # 6 and 11 are the cause of the exophytic, grossly visible genital warts, but only HPV #16, 18, and 31 are associated with cervical cancer. (Remember: Higher numbers occur higher up on the body and are more cancer prone!) The HPV # 16, 18, and 31 that cause cervical cancer are usually subclinical! So do not jump to "cervical cancer!" when you see genital warts! All warts tend to recur. (Discussed in more detail in Adolescent section).

Papovavirus

Papovavirus—reactivation in the immunosuppressed host—results in Progressive Multifocal Leukoencephalopathy (PML), which is due to progressive demyelination of the white matter. Because it is multifocal, PML has varied presentations. Usually, the patient suffers altered mental status, followed by various focal motor/sensory defects. It is diagnosed by MRI.

SSPE

Subacute sclerosing panencephalitis (SSPE) is a rare form of encephalopathy thought to be due to a measles virus that changed, but was not eradicated, by the immune reaction to the primary infection. Occurrence is 1/300,000 cases of measles. Patients typically will have had measles at age < 2 years, and present with dementia, myoclonus, and new-onset seizures ~ age 10. Most die within several months of onset.

Prion Disease

Prions are proteinaceous infectious particles that lack nucleic acid and constitute a previously unknown means of transmitting disease. Previously, these diseases were thought to be caused by a "slow virus."

Prion diseases include Kuru, Creutzfeldt-Jakob disease (CJD), new variant CJD (vCJD), Gerstmann-Straussler-Scheinker (GSS) syndrome, fatal familial insomnia. In animals: Scrapie and mad cow disease (= bovine spongiform encephalopathy, = vCJD when transmitted to humans).

Human prion diseases can be sporadic (CJD), infectious (vCJD, Kuru, rare cases of CJD), or genetic (GSS syndrome, familial CJD, fatal familial insomnia).

Kuru is found in New Guinea, associated with cannibalism, and thought to be transmitted by ingestion of raw human brain tissue. It has an incubation period of up to 30 years. (No new cases since ritual cannibalism stopped).

Creutzfeldt-Jakob disease (CJD) is the most common prion disease. It is almost always sporadic, but ~ 5% are infectious (e.g., corneal transplants, cadaveric human growth hormone), and very few that are genetic. Its incubation period is ~ 18 months. Patients with CJD get myoclonus and severe dementia. Neurologic symptoms predominate. They generally die within 5 months! There is no effective therapy for either Kuru or CJD. The EEG is diagnostic.

A new variant of CJD (vCJD), transmitted from beef with bovine spongiform encephalopathy (mad cow disease), has been contracted by ~ 60 people in several European countries. No human cases of vCJD have been reported in the U.S. (But a cow imported from Canada to Washington State was infected). These patients have early-on psychiatric symptoms and late-appearing neurologic symptoms (~ 6 months out with ataxia). Once neurologic symptoms appear, progression to death is rapid. Test: Look for a young adult from England with progressive psychiatric symptoms and ataxia.

notes

HIV AND AIDS

OVERVIEW

Changes in the treatment and management of HIV infection are evolving rapidly. The following covers the basics—not the cutting edge.

The virus particle:

The HIV virus is composed of a dense, single-strand RNA core surrounded by a lipoprotein envelope. The RNA contains reverse transcriptase, which allows the RNA to be transcribed into DNA, which is then assimilated into the host's genome. The cell then becomes an HIV-producing machine.

The structure in the lipoprotein envelope that allows the HIV to attach to the CD4 cell is named gp120. As opposed to influenza, the envelope on HIV is very unstable. That's why it is much more difficult to make a vaccine against it.

HIV gp120 envelope glycoprotein binds to the CD4 receptors and co-receptors on the helper T cells, macrophages, and monocytes. The virus fuses with the cell, and the viral core material enters the cell. Immune dysfunction results from the ongoing destruction of CD4 lymphocytes, and will be more fully described under "Summary of Important Advances." The CD4 cells are the major regulator cells in the body. They can suppress the B lymphocytes, and regulate the CD8/suppressor cells.

With the decrease in CD4+ counts, B cells become deregulated and are no longer suppressed, causing a polyclonal increase in total serum immunoglobulins—even though overall antibody function is decreased! For this reason, infectious diseases in AIDS patients include not only the cell-mediated infections (PCP, viruses, *mycobacteria*, fungal), but also those seen with humoral deficiency (pneumococcus, meningococcus, *H. influenzae,* and *Giardia*).

The glial cells of the CNS may be directly affected by HIV, causing atrophy and dementia. The GI epithelium may be directly infected, causing a wasting enteropathy with diarrhea. Marrow progenitor cell infection may be the cause of anemia and thrombocytopenia.

Prevalence and transmission: HIV is found among 50% of IV drug users and 50% of gays seeking treatment for STDs. The number of HIV-infected children in the U.S. is currently estimated at 10,000–20,000. HIV is the 6th leading cause of death in children age 1–4 years. 90% of HIV-infected children and infants get their infection vertically. Most transmission occurs during labor and delivery. Of children born to untreated, HIV-infected women, 15–40% will be infected. Cesarean section appears to reduce the risk of perinatal transmission. Prevalence is < 1% in heterosexuals in the U.S., but in central Africa, heterosexual transmission is the primary route! It has also been transmitted in the course of treatment by an infected dentist. Percentages of patients with AIDS: Homosexuals (56%), IV drug users (24%), IV drug user & homosexual (5%), heterosexual contact (6%), hemophiliacs (1%), transfusion-associated (2%).

During their first year of life, infants with HIV do not have otitis media, rhinitis, fever, or diarrhea any more often than HIV-*un*infected children. However, they are more likely to have one of the following:

- Chronic candidiasis
- Parotitis
- Persistent lymphadenopathy
- Hepatosplenomegaly

~ 20% of untreated HIV-infected infants will present in the first 3–6 months of life with an AIDS-defining illness, such as *Pneumocystis jiroveci* (formerly *P. carinii*) pneumonia (PCP), serious bacterial infection, or serious fungal infection. CD4 count can even be normal at the time of PCP presentation in an infant.

Immune function is categorized in children based on age-specific CD4 counts:

Evidence of Severe Immune Suppression:

< 12 months of age: < 750 CD4 cells/μL (< 15%)

1–5 Years of age: < 500 CD4 cells/μL (< 15%)

> 6 Years of age: < 200 CD4 cells/μL (< 15%)

DIAGNOSIS

Diagnosis of HIV infection in children ≥ 18 months is by the presence of antibody to the virus by means of the ELISA test, which is 99% sensitive and 90% specific. Positive responders are confirmed by the Western blot. Antibody to HIV is usually detectable 2–3 months after inoculation, although there can be a window of up to 6 months! The earliest detectable sign of infection is a positive HIV DNA by PCR.

For children < age 18 months born to a mother who is HIV-infected, the presence of infection is more difficult to diagnose because of the presence of transplacentally acquired antibody to HIV. In these infants, diagnosis of HIV infection requires culturing the virus from the infant or demonstrating viral nucleic acids (HIV DNA by PCR). Also, HIV p24 antigen detection is specific, but is very insensitive, and has been replaced by PCR testing in most centers. Most centers will perform 3 PCR (or culture) tests over a period of 4 months, trying to determine if the child is truly infected. If all 3 are negative, and the last 1 has occurred ≥ 4 months of age, the child is considered uninfected.

There are several tests that measure HIV RNA by amplifying the RNA by oligonucleotide hybridization or enzymatic methods. These tests accurately determine viral load. They are discussed further below.

TREATMENT OF HIV INFECTION

Note

According to the latest content specifications (2005) dispersed by the ABP, knowledge of HIV medications is listed specifically: "Plan antiretroviral therapy for a patient with HIV infection." For many of you, this is WAY too much information. In fact, unless you are actively treating HIV patients, I

notes

Quick Quiz

1) What clinical findings occur more commonly in infants with undiagnosed HIV infection during the 1st year of life?
2) How do you diagnose HIV in a child ≥ 18 months of age? < 18 months of age?
3) What are the main side effects of zidovudine?
4) What are the main side effects of didanosine?

would just ignore this section and look at the yellow highlighted areas. I suspect that they will take this content specification out in the future, but for now it is still listed. Pay particular attention to the drug side effects that are highlighted; those are likely fair game for the Boards.

Treatment of HIV infection: Adherence is a key determinant in the degree and duration of viral suppression! AIDS: Note that it is extremely important to actively involve the patient and/or the parent in the treatment decision-making process. Guide decisions regarding initiation or changes in antiretroviral therapy by monitoring plasma HIV RNA (viral load) and CD4 T cell counts, in addition to the patient's clinical condition. First, we will review the 4 major classes of anti-HIV drugs, then the treatment protocols.

Drug acronyms:

NRTI = Nucleoside Reverse Transcriptase Inhibitor
Nucleotide RTI = Nucleotide Reverse Transcriptase Inhibitor
NNRTI = Non-Nucleoside Reverse Transcriptase Inhibitor
PI = Protease Inhibitors

Nucleoside Reverse Transcriptase Inhibitors

I. Nucleoside Reverse Transcriptase Inhibitors (ZDV, ddI, ddC, d4T, 3TC, and abacavir—NRTI). These drugs inhibit the replication of HIV by interfering with the reverse transcriptase enzyme. These are all analogs of normally occurring nucleic acid bases.

Zidovudine (ZDV) = Azidothymidine (previously called AZT) = Retrovir® This is the oldest of the antiretroviral drugs, but still remains very useful. It is well tolerated at currently used doses, but causes bone marrow suppression (anemia, granulocytopenia) and myopathy. A macrocytosis (elevated MCV) always occurs, but has no clinical consequence. ZDV does not usually cause problems for the kidneys or lungs, and does not cause pancreatitis.

As with all antiretroviral drugs, combination therapy is preferred, and is the standard of care. Use ZDV in combination with 3TC, ddI, and ddC, as well as protease inhibitors. Some studies have suggested antagonism between ZDV and d4T. The effectiveness of ZDV decreases over time due to development of resistance.

Give ZDV to pregnant HIV+ patients because ZDV decreases transmission of the HIV virus to the fetus by 25–35%!

Because ganciclovir and ZDV have overlapping bone marrow toxicities, in an AIDS patient with CMV retinitis, and on ZDV and ganciclovir, give Filgrastim® (G-CSF) to support the WBC. Sometimes, it is necessary to stop the ganciclovir and use foscarnet.

ddI (didanosine, Videx®) is useful in combination regimens—with ZDV, d4T, and protease inhibitors. Viral resistance develops more slowly than with other reverse transcriptase inhibitors. A newer, enteric-coated tablet has replaced the regular preparation, eliminating the GI side effects of diarrhea and cramping, and affording much better patient tolerance.

The most severe side effects of ddI are pancreatitis, which can be life threatening, and peripheral neuropathy. There is no bone marrow toxicity.

ddC (zalcitabine, Hivid®) can be used as part of a combination regimen (the combination with ZDV is best studied). It is very easy to take, and the only significant side effects are stomatitis, neuropathy, and—less commonly—pancreatitis. Since the availability of newer drugs, ddC is rarely used.

d4T (stavudine, Zerit®) has emerged as a very useful drug, because it is very well tolerated over long periods of time, with little toxicity. Well-studied combinations include ddI/d4T + d4T/3TC, with or without protease inhibitors. Recent data have implicated d4T in lipodystrophy and mitochondrial toxicity syndromes. Also, do not use d4T in combination with ddI in pregnant women—fatal lactic acidosis!

Side effects: pancreatitis and peripheral neuropathy.

3TC (lamivudine, Epivir®) is a very effective drug in combination therapy. Combinations with ZDV + d4T are often used. The drug is well tolerated.

Side effects are rare.

FTC (emtricitabine, Emitriva®) is the newest nucleoside reverse transcriptase inhibitor on the market. It is similar to 3TC, but stays in the blood stream for a longer period of time. It is not approved for pediatric use at this time.

Abacavir (Ziagen®) is very effective in combination therapy.

Side effects: The most serious reaction is a hypersensitivity, which usually occurs within 4 weeks. The reaction consists of a generalized rash and/or a flu-like illness, with fever, chills, N/V, myalgias, cough, and shortness of breath. Take any patient off abacavir who develops this reaction, and never prescribe it again for that patient; reactions will continue to worsen, and could even be fatal.

Combos: Currently there are several combo drugs including: Combivir®=ZDV + 3TC and Trizivir®=ZDV + 3TC + Abacavir. Trizivir can be used as single therapy since it contains 3 NRTIs.

notes

Nucleotide Reverse-Transcriptase Inhibitor

Tenofovir (Viread ™) is a nucleotide RTI very similar to the above nucleoside analogues, except that tenofovir is chemically pre-activated, and therefore, require less biochemical processing than the nucleoside RTIs. Tenofovir has once-daily dosing and a good side-effect profile—mainly asthenia/headache/N/V/D/flatulence. It must be taken with a NRTI and at least one PI or NNRTI.

Non-nucleoside Reverse Transcriptase Inhibitors

II. Non-nucleoside reverse transcriptase inhibitors (NNRTI).

Nevirapine (Viramune®) is the first of this class of drugs. It is not useful as a single agent, but is useful as part of a regimen with nucleoside reverse transcriptase inhibitors and/or protease inhibitors. Rash, which can be severe, is the primary toxicity.

Efavirenz (Sustiva®) is more potent than nevirapine. CNS toxicity is commonly seen. Efavirenz is teratogenic, so do not use—in any way—concurrent with pregnancy. Other side effects include rash and "weird dreams."

Delavirdine (Rescriptor®) is less potent and, therefore, rarely used.

Protease Inhibitors

III. The HIV protease inhibitors—PI— (saquinavir, indinavir, ritonavir, nelfinavir, amprenavir, lopinavir) inhibit the HIV protease enzyme that is involved with processing the completed virus. They are frequently used in combination with each other (e.g., saquinavir + ritonavir) or with the just discussed NRTIs +/– NNRTI to prevent the emergence of resistance. Fat redistribution and lipid abnormalities (increased triglycerides and cholesterol), as well as new-onset diabetes have been recognized with the use of PIs. However, in treating the lipid abnormalities, do not use simvastatin or lovastatin with any of the PIs! Avoid other interactions: Rifampin, astemizole, cisapride, and St. John's Wort.

Saquinavir (Fortovase®) is highly effective, has minimum side effects, and is useful in combination protease inhibitor regimens.

Ritonavir (Norvir®) is a very potent drug, but patient tolerability is poor due to side effects. The main side effects are N/V, flushing, distorted taste, and paresthesias. There are many drug interactions because of interference with the p450 enzyme system. Low-dose ritonavir inhibits metabolism of and therefore, significantly boosts levels of indinavir, saquinavir, amprenavir, and the NNRTI efavirenz. Ritonavir is now usually used in low dose to boost the levels of other PIs and efavirenz.

Indinavir (Crixivan®) has side effects that include an asymptomatic hyperbilirubinemia and a high incidence of nephrolithiasis. The drug should be taken on an empty stomach with adequate hydration—although boosting with ritonavir eliminates the food requirement.

Nelfinavir (Viracept) is a PI with good potency. Well tolerated. Most common side effect is diarrhea. If resistance to nelfinavir develops, treatment with indinavir or amprenavir may be effective.

Amprenavir (Agenerase®) is a new PI with a resistance profile that is unique among protease inhibitors. 1% get serious skin reactions, including Stevens-Johnson syndrome. GI side effects are common.

Fosamprenavir (Lexiva®) is just the prodrug of amprenavir. It is not approved for children.

Lopinavir/ritonavir (Kaletra®) is a co-formulation of lopinavir and low-dose ritonavir. Lopinavir is available only in this co-formulation. It is very potent and well tolerated.

Atazanavir (Reyataz®) is the newest protease inhibitor on the market. It is not approved for children.

Key words

Key word/phrases to remember for side effects:

- ZDV: bone-marrow suppression, myopathy
- The "D's" (ddI, ddC, and d4T): pancreatitis and peripheral neuropathy
- Abacavir (Ziagen®): potentially fatal hypersensitivity reaction
- Efavirenz (Sustiva®): teratogenic
- Indinavir (Crixivan®): kidney stones

Note: For the medications above, at least know the yellow highlighted areas! These are what they are most likely to ask on the Boards!

State of Treatment

I. Summary of important advances:

a) HIV RNA assays are available for accurately determining viral load. Prior to the availability of these assays, the HIV virus was thought to enter a prolonged latency period until the onset of symptoms. It turns out that there is continuous, high-level replication from the onset of infection to death.

b) Viral load is a good, long-term predictor of outcome. After primary infection, the rate of virus replication and turnover equilibrates to a certain set point for each individual—resulting in a pretty much constant plasma viremia of 100 to 10^6 HIV RNA copies/mL. This set point may endure for months or years, and it determines the rate of disease progression. Plasma viremia < 5,000 HIV RNA copies/mL is associated with near-normal CD4+ counts and minimal, if any, clinical progression of disease, whereas viral loads > 30,000 HIV RNA copies/mL indicate a greatly increased risk of disease progression. Barring treatment, a single HIV RNA count can establish a prognosis—similar to staging of certain malignancies.

Infected patients make up to 10^9 new HIV virions/day. The CD4+ lymphocytes, which are the principal cells targeted for reproducing HIV virions, have a half-life of only 1.6 days after infection. High levels of viremia cause tremendous, continuous CD4+ lymphocyte destruction—eventually causing decreased levels. Rather than using CD4+ cell level as a marker of disease activity (which is wrong—it is more an endpoint denoting prolonged disease activity), the present fo-

notes

Quick Quiz

1) Which anti-HIV medication is teratogenic?
2) What renal abnormality is seen in patients taking indinavir?
3) Which patients with HIV should be started on HAART?

cus of treatment is to decrease viral load, and thereby, prevent or minimize the CD4+ cell destruction.

c) The HIV protease inhibitors decrease viral load—sometimes tremendously—for prolonged periods when used in combination therapy.

d) HIV therapy should always be combination therapy. Treat with PI(s), with NRTI(s), and/or NNRTI(s). Combinations of nucleoside analogues given to asymptomatic patients with early HIV disease, and evidence of immunologic compromise (low CD4 counts), prolong survival and decrease AIDS-related problems. The combination therapy is superior to ZDV alone. Previously, it was unknown if treating early in the course of the illness would improve outcome.

II. Pending questions:

a) Does the level of HIV RNA achieved by antiretroviral therapy have the same predictive value as that of untreated patients in the study? Studies suggest this is true. Each of the studies found a decreased risk of disease progression with treatment-induced decrease in HIV RNA level, but did not address the actual levels.

b) How long-lasting is the effect of the protease inhibitor agents? HIV does mutate, but the lower the viral load, the less the likelihood of resistance developing, and the longer the regimen will be effective. Patients have been maintained without detectable virus for > 7 years.

c) What is the best combination of agents? Some guidelines exist (see below), but it's still vague...

d) When is the best time to start treatment? Some guidelines exist (see below), but it's still vague for asymptomatic patients…

III. The new Tx protocols are based on the above and:

- The probability that the decrease in viral load induced by combinations or HAART (highly active anti-retroviral therapy) have the same predictive value as the studies mentioned in Ib above.
- Determining CD4 and viral load is a key indicator for when to start therapy.
- Combination therapy is the standard of care; use monotherapy only in special circumstances.

Indications for Viral Load Testing:

- Syndrome consistent with acute HIV
- Initial evaluation of newly diagnosed HIV
- Every 3–4 months for patients on and not on therapy
- 2–8 weeks after initiation of therapy
- Clinical event or substantial decline in CD4 Count

Indications for using drug-resistance assays

Resistance testing appears to be a useful tool in selecting active drugs when changing antiretroviral regimens in cases of virologic failure or suboptimal reduction of viral load. Currently, 2 types of resistance testing are available—genotypic and phenotypic. These are expensive tests, but are becoming more popular in determining optimal regimens. The genotypic test will detect specific genes in the individual patient's HIV virus known to confer resistance toward a specific antiretroviral drug. The phenotypic test determines if the gene is operating and if resistance is being expressed. Currently, one is not recommended over the other, and some centers prefer to test for both. This is sort of like a crude antibiogram for the HIV virus—if resistance is determined, then you can switch from ineffective drugs. Drug resistance assay use is very expensive, and use is not well standardized in pediatrics (or adults for that matter!).

When to initiate antiretroviral therapy:

- Definite:
  Symptomatic (AIDS or severe symptoms): start therapy no matter what the CD4 or viral load
  Asymptomatic and CD4 is < 200 (or < 15% for age)

- Almost Definite:
  Asymptomatic and CD4 is 200–350 (or 15–24% for age)

- Most recommend:
  Asymptomatic with CD4 > 350 (24% for age) **and** viral load is > 55,000. (In untreated patients, the 3-year risk for progression to AIDS is > 30 %.)

Also know: A fingerstick from an infected needle requires immediate treatment with 3-drug antiretroviral therapy.

Be aware that the optimal time to initiate therapy is unknown among persons with asymptomatic disease and CD4 count > 200 (>15% for age). Make all decisions regarding the start of therapy on the basis of prognosis, as determined by CD4, viral load, and the willingness of the patient to adhere to therapy.

notes

Which combination of drugs to use:

"Strongly recommended" by the CDC:
Use one of the following:

- Efavirenz
- Indinavir
- Nelfinavir
- Nevirapine
- Lopinavir plus ritonavir
- Ritonavir
- Amprenavir

With 1 of the following:

- ddI plus 3TC
- Abacavir plus ZDV
- D4T plus 3TC
- ZDV plus DDI
- ZDV plus 3TC

Note: You are sweating this, right? How do you remember all of these? You don't!
Just know the few combinations not to use:

- ZDV + D4T
- ddC + ddI
- ddC + 3TC
- ddC + d4T

This is pretty easy to remember—ZDV + D4T is bad, and ddC combined with any NRTI *but* ZDV is bad.

If you are really having trouble—stick with this:
Throw out any answer that has:

- ZDV/D4T combined
- ddC anywhere in the choice
- Single-drug therapy

...and you are probably correct! Otherwise, you can combine these drugs into multiple permutations!

When to change HIV therapy:

This is again controversial. However, 2 things to know:

1. Don't change drugs based on 1 viral load; always repeat a high viral load to be sure it is not lab error.
2. Intolerance to the medication should prompt evaluation for change of therapy.

Possible reasons to change therapy are based on treatment failure (various definitions and not standardized):

- Therapy has not suppressed viral RNA to undetectable levels (< 50 copies) within 4–6 months of starting therapy
- An increase of ≥ 3-fold from the nadir of plasma HIV RNA
- Previously undetectable levels now surpassing 5–10,000 copies

The other problem: What drug to change to? Generally, just know you should probably change therapy based on resistance testing.

Postexposure prophylaxis (PEP)

First, determine the exposure risk: Was the source material blood or bloody fluid? If so, determine if it was a percutaneous exposure (yes—PEP recommended), mucous membrane, or skin with compromised integrity (PEP probably recommended). It is easier (and frequently asked on tests) to remember whom not to give PEP to: Do not give for intact-skin exposures and urine-source exposures. The latest guidelines from September 2005 are much more involved, but the basic principles remain. Use potent, combination therapy. Start treatment ASAP—within hours of exposure. The standard recommended regimen is ZDV, 3TC, +/- lopinavir/ritonavir for 4 weeks.

Pregnancy

At this time, ZDV is the only drug approved/recommended to prevent "vertical" transmission of HIV. Optimally, give the mother ZDV as one of her HAART drugs, as well as IV ZDV during labor and delivery. Treat newborns and, if possible, bottle feed instead of breast feed.

Most experts recommend that pregnant HIV+ patients receive highly active, anti-retroviral therapy (HAART), just as non-pregnant patients do.

Suppressing the viral load in the mother lowers the risk of transmission to the newborn. The bottom line for most pregnant women—treat them with HAART, include ZDV, if possible, and do not use efavirenz (teratogenic) or a D4T/ddI combination (increased risk of lactic acidosis in pregnant women).

HIV-ASSOCIATED INFECTIONS AND CONDITIONS

Introduction

Signs of HIV disease include persistent or recurrent seborrheic dermatitis, tinea infections, psoriasis, molluscum contagiosum, folliculitis, and mucocutaneous infections (hairy leukoplakia, herpes, oral or vaginal candidiasis). Know these. EBV causes hairy leukoplakia.

Kaposi lesions are a neoplasia of blood vessels, and are due to Human Herpesvirus 8. Lesions are heaped up and well localized, often with some surrounding bruising. Kaposi lesions may occur in adolescents, but are very rare.

Don't forget the Acute Retroviral Syndrome: This is a flu- or mononucleosis-like syndrome that occurs 2–4 weeks after initial infection, and lasts 1–2 weeks. Suspect the sexually active or IV drug-using adolescent! Patients present with fever, lymphadenopathy, pharyngitis, rash (usually erythematous maculopapular with lesions on face, trunk or extremities, including palms and soles), mucocutaneous ulcerations involving the mouth, esophagus or genitals, and myalgias/arthralgias. Consider it in a young person who has multiple sexual partners/IV drug users and presents with signs/symptoms of mono or scarlet fever.

notes

Quick Quiz

1) True or False: ZDV/D4T combined or ZDV therapy alone is acceptable for a child with symptomatic HIV.
2) A nurse is emptying a Foley catheter bag and some urine from an HIV patient spills on her un-gloved hand. Should she take postexposure prophylaxis?
3) What are 2 important considerations when considering a change of HIV therapy?
4) Describe the acute retroviral syndrome in an adolescent.
5) What is the most common opportunistic infection in pediatric AIDS patients?
6) When should you start PCP prophylaxis?
7) What is the treatment for PCP?

PCP and HIV

Pneumocystis jiroveci infection produces subclinical infection in most "normal" children by the age of 4 years. Typically, only the immunocompromised are seriously affected by this organism.

Infantile form: The infection occurs in premature and debilitated infants age 2–6 months. Onset is insidious with cough and mild tachypnea. Fever is absent. Over a period of 1–4 weeks, the infection progresses to a diffuse, bilateral, interstitial plasma cell pneumonitis with cyanosis and retractions. Without effective therapy, 1/2 of these infants die.

Immunocompromised older children and adolescents: *Pneumocystis jiroveci* pneumonia (PCP) is the most common opportunistic infection in patients with AIDS. It is the presenting illness in 50% of untreated patients. It is probably the most common lung infection overall in these patients, but, because prophylaxis is so effective, PCP incidence in these patients is decreasing to less than that of *S. pneumoniae* in some places.

Presentation of PCP: insidious onset of fever, shortness of breath, dry cough. ABG: pH > 7.40. A-a gradient is wide. Hypoxia is common. PCO_2 is low (from respiratory alkalosis). LDH is elevated (> 400) and liver enzymes are normal. The CXR usually shows a diffuse "batwing" infiltrate, although it may also be lobar or unilateral. Occasionally, the CXR is normal. Again, PCP usually has an insidious onset; if an AIDS patient presents with an acute onset of pulmonary symptoms, first get sputum for Gram stain and C+S, and start empirical treatment for community-acquired pneumonia. Patients who are most susceptible for PCP have fallen below their age-appropriate CD4 count threshold, so give all of these patients PCP prophylaxis!

The threshold for starting PCP prophylaxis (know):

- All infants 1–12 months of age who are HIV-infected or are HIV-indeterminate.
- HIV-infected children ages 1–5 years with a CD4 count < 500/mm3 (<15%).
- HIV-infected children ≥ 6 years with CD4 count < 200/mm3 (15%).

The best method of diagnosis is by methenamine silver stain of samples taken by bronchoscopy or BAL, although induced sputum is effective in up to 50% in some hospitals. CMV is usually grown along with PCP from BAL/bronchoscopy samples; only rarely is this significant.

Treat mild PCP with oral TMP/SMX, or atovaquone if the patient is unable to tolerate TMP/SMX.

Treat more severe PCP—$PO_2 < 70$ or A-a gradient > 35— with po or IV TMP/SMX or IV pentamidine and high-dose corticosteroids (start on the first day). Inhaled pentamidine is not recommended for **treatment** of PCP. If there is no response after 1 week, or if severe side effects develop, switch. Alternative treatments are dapsone + trimethoprim, clindamycin + primaquine, or atovaquone alone for mild-to-moderate cases. PCP patients must receive 21 days of effective therapy. Remember: Include steroids for any patient with a $PaO_2 < 70$!

Side effects: Both TMP/SMX and pentamidine can cause neutropenia/leukopenia. TMP/SMX side effects include skin rash, nausea/vomiting, and occasionally fever. Pentamidine causes fever, nausea, vomiting, and diarrhea. Pentamidine also causes azotemia and renal failure. Recurrent courses of pentamidine destroy the islet cells of the pancreas, causing hypoglycemia that may not be reversible. (If a patient treated with pentamidine is seizing, check fingerstick glucometer!) Hyperglycemia may also occur with pentamidine. Patients on aerosolized pentamidine are at risk for apical pneumothorax. For some AIDS patients, the reactions to either TMP/SMX or to pentamidine are intolerable, and the medication must be changed.

Prophylaxis of PCP: give TMP/SMX with a dose of 5 mg/kg, based on the TMP portion divided b.i.d. daily. If this is not tolerated, give dapsone or atovaquone. Atovaquone has a lower incidence of side effects than TMP/SMX. ~ 4% of patients discontinue therapy because of rash.

1) TMP/SMX is more effective,
2) TMP/SMX gets extrapulmonary *Pneumocystis jiroveci*, whereas aerosolized pentamidine does not.
3) TMP/SMX also prophylaxes against toxoplasmosis.

Mycobacterium and HIV

Tuberculosis is also common in AIDS patients, sometimes without infiltrates, and hardly ever with cavitation. Patients usually respond very well to treatment. Do a TB skin test on all persons who are seropositive for HIV. Treat a positive PPD (> 5 mm) without sign of disease with INH for 9 months. Treatment of active TB in a patient with AIDS is the same as for regular patients.

M. avium Complex (MAC, *M. avium-intracellulare*) is a common infection in patients with AIDS. It is usually disseminated, causing a wasting syndrome with fever, weight loss, and night sweats. There is no cure. Clarithromycin or azithromycin in combination with ethambutol, and sometimes, other

notes

agents, including rifabutin, quinolones, clofazimine, or amikacin can be beneficial in terms of decreasing fever or improving bone marrow function.

Pulmonary: OTHER

Cryptococcus also involves the lung and can be disseminated, but it also commonly goes to the CNS. Cryptococcal meningitis is strongly associated with AIDS, Hodgkin disease, ALL, diabetes, and post-organ transplant. Treat with amphotericin B +/- flucytosine, then oral fluconazole. Fluconazole is a good choice for all but critical disease. Flucytosine (5-FC; 5-fluorocytosine) is sometimes not used along with amphotericin B in patients with AIDS, because of the problem with bone marrow suppression.

Histoplasma can either affect the lung or disseminate in AIDS patients (only non-AIDS patients have the calcified lung lesions). It can affect many organ systems, including the bone marrow. Think of this when an HIV-positive patient presents with interstitial pneumonia, palate ulcers, splenomegaly, and bone-marrow suppression. This infection is very common in natives of El Salvador. Treat with itraconazole or amphotericin B.

Coccidioides: Again, involves the lungs, but it also can disseminate. It is associated with arthralgias, arthritis, hilar adenopathy, erythema multiforme, and erythema nodosum (similar to sarcoidosis). Treatment suppresses, but usually does not cure, this disease, so chronic, suppressive treatment is needed (weekly fluconazole {1st choice} or amphotericin B).

[Know: Both *Aspergillus* (especially associated with marijuana use) and *Mucor* can cause a necrotizing, cavitating pneumonia in AIDS patients.]

Pseudomonas infections are seen more in granulocytopenic patients (leukemia, chemotherapy, and post-transplant) than in AIDS patients.

GI and HIV

Organisms to consider in AIDS patients with GI infections: *Candida*, especially with esophagitis. Not all *Candida* esophagitis is associated with thrush. If the patient does not respond to treatment for *Candida*, consider CMV esophagitis. Chronic diarrhea in AIDS patients is usually caused by *Cryptosporidium*, *Salmonella, Shigella*, *Cyclospora*, and *Isospora belli*. *Cryptosporidium* shows up as small, round, red organisms ("round bodies") against a green background on acid-fast staining of the specimen. There is no effective treatment of Cryptosporidiosis. *Cyclospora* and *Isospora belli* are also acid-fast (*I. belli* is large and oval); both are treated with TMP/SMX.

Neuro and HIV

Subacute, diffuse encephalitis (caused directly by HIV) is a common neurologic problem seen in AIDS. CNS disease is much more common in children, and occurs quite early.

In as many as 1/4 infants with HIV, CNS disease manifests as static encephalopathy, presenting as developmental delay in the first year of life. In ~ 1/3, progressive encephalopathy occurs, with loss of milestone and moderate-to-severe cognition defects. It appears that HAART (highly active anti-retroviral therapy) prevents or retards progressive encephalopathy.

Toxoplasma gondii is the most common cause of "AIDS-associated enhancing focal-space-occupying-lesions" (but the differential diagnosis also includes CNS lymphomas). CT scan shows CNS abscesses due to *Toxo* as ring-enhancing lesions. They are usually multiple, but may be single. If these are seen in any AIDS patient, start empiric treatment for CNS toxoplasmosis: 1) long-term pyrimethamine + a sulfonamide, 2) clindamycin, or 3) trimetrexate. This is rare in children.

Again: for suspected cryptococcal meningitis, get a cryptococcal antigen test (or India ink) of the CSF or the blood! (more sensitive in HIV patients). Especially consider *Cryptococcus* in the meningitis patient who has AIDS, Hodgkin disease, ALL, diabetes, and those who are post-organ transplant. Treat cryptococcal meningitis initially with amphotericin B, then oral fluconazole.

Syphilis, even if previously treated, may reactivate in AIDS patients and cause neurosyphilis!

Any eye problems are probably due to CMV retinitis.

Stopping Prophylaxis Guidelines (Adolescents and older only)

Stopping Primary Prophylaxis (No history of these infections)

PCP: If CD4 > 200 for ≥ 3 months in response to HAART, you can discontinue PCP prophylaxis.

MAC: If CD4 > 100 for ≥ 3 months in response to HAART, you can discontinue MAC prophylaxis

Stopping Secondary Prophylaxis (+ history of these infections)

PCP: If CD4 > 200 for ≥ 3 months in response to HAART, you can discontinue PCP prophylaxis

MAC: Controversial on whether if and when you can stop MAC prophylaxis with a history of MAC

Other Issues in Children

IVIG therapy is recommended in those children with documented defects in the production of functional antibody, or a history of recurrent bacterial infections while receiving antiretroviral therapy and PCP prophylaxis.

COMMON ID SYNDROMES

FEVER WITHOUT LOCALIZING SIGNS IN INFANTS AND CHILDREN

Febrile Infants < 60 days of Age

Fever in this age group can indicate bacteremia in 2.5% and meningitis in 1%. Group B streptococcus and *E. coli* are the most common causes of bacteremia, meningitis, and osteomyelitis in this age group. *Listeria* may be an infrequent

notes

![Quick Quiz]

Quick Quiz

1) In a neonate < 60 days old, name the bacteria most commonly associated with bacteremia. UTI? Diarrhea?
2) In children with fever without a focus between the ages of 3 months and 36 months, when should urine cultures be considered for girls? For boys?
3) What laboratory test is the most important diagnostic test in endocarditis: a blood culture or echocardiogram?
4) True or False: Most children with endocarditis have an underlying heart defect.

cause as well. UTIs are usually due to *E. coli*, and bacterial gastroenteritis is most commonly *Salmonella*.

Viruses also commonly cause infection in this age group, and include HSV and enteroviruses.

For all infants with fever in this age group, do a complete history and physical, CBC, U/A, and blood/urine cultures. CSF evaluation is controversial in 30–60-day-old infants; some recommend it while others do not. CXR is not indicated unless symptoms warrant it.

If the infant appears "well," was previously healthy, and the laboratory values show a normal WBC with absolute band count < 1500, < 11 WBC/hpf on spun urine, and < 6 WBC/hpf on stool smear (if diarrhea is present), you can observe the infant (inpatient or outpatient) with or without antibiotics. If you give the antibiotics, you must do a lumbar puncture.

If the infant appears ill, antibiotics and hospitalization with lumbar puncture are mandatory. Further workup depends on the symptoms/signs.

Infants 61–90 Days of Age with Fever

Management is the same as the younger infant, but most are likely to be managed as an outpatient.

Children 3–36 Months of Age with Fever

Obtain blood cultures if you suspect occult bacteremia, or if the patient is to receive empiric antibiotics. Many recommend getting blood cultures for temperatures > 39.0° C (102.2° F) without localizing signs of infection and with a WBC > 15,000. If *H. influenzae* or *N. meningitidis* is found with "occult" bacteremia, admit the child, and perform full blood, urine, and CSF cultures. If *S. pneumoniae* is found and the child returns and is well, repeat the blood culture and continue observation. If the child is ill or worsening, repeat the blood cultures and do CSF, and give ceftriaxone.

Do lumbar puncture if you suspect meningitis. UTIs are present in 7% of boys ≤ 6 months of age and 8% of girls < age 1 year who present with fever and no localizing signs. Do urine cultures on all boys < 6 months and girls < 1 year. CXR are beneficial if the child has symptoms/signs. Obtain stool for those with bloody or mucoid diarrhea.

Admit any toxic-appearing child, begin antibiotics, and do blood, urine, and CSF cultures. A well-appearing child with fever < 39°C is unlikely to have occult bacteremia, and does not require further laboratory testing.

COMMON ID SYNDROMES: ENDOCARDITIS

Introduction

Bacterial Endocarditis—See Cardiology section for prophylaxis indications and medications. Blood cultures are vital in diagnosing endocarditis of any type, and should be drawn before empiric antibiotics are started. Blood cultures are usually positive (95%!) due to continual bacteremia. If they are negative (and patient has not been partially treated with antibiotics), think of fungi, Q fever (*Coxiella burnetii*), *Legionella*, *Chlamydia psittaci*, and the HACEK organisms (discussed below) as possible causes. Surgery is required for endocarditis with fistula, abscess, pericarditis, or persistent fever, and for cases in which the resulting valve dysfunction causes ventricular failure. In the heart, the electrical conduction pathway passes just beside the aortic valve. A conduction disturbance in a patient with aortic valve endocarditis is another indication for surgery. Vegetations alone usually are not an indication for surgery.

Again: CHF with endocarditis is an indication for cardiac surgery. Mortality in endocarditis surgery correlates with the preop severity of ventricular failure. The most common cause of cardiac death due to endocarditis is congestive heart failure.

ABE vs. SBE

There are two methods of classification of endocarditis in adults, but these are less commonly used in children. The classic method is based on acuity of presentation: acute vs. subacute. The more recent method is based on pertinent etiologic factors: Native valve, prosthetic valve, addict (i.e., IV drugs), and culture-negative. These may have acute or subacute presentations. Addict and culture-negative can also be thought of as subsets of native valve and prosthetic valve endocarditis.

In one series, 92% of children with endocarditis had an underlying heart defect (congenital or rheumatic). Congenital defects made up > 80% of the total, with Tetralogy of Fallot and VSD the most common. Other lesions included aortic stenosis, PDA, and transposition of the great vessels.

Viridans streptococci are responsible for 40% of cases of infective endocarditis in children, with 20–30% due to *Staphylococcus aureus*. *S. aureus* is more likely to infect normal heart valves. Next most common, at nearly 5%, is coagulase-negative staphylococci, followed by Gram-negative bacilli and *Enterococci*. *S. Pneumoniae* cause only ~ 3% of endocarditis in children.

In adolescent and adult IV drug addicts, the major organism is, again, *S. aureus* (50%), with MRSA a major component, followed by enterococci (15%). The following 3 have a fre-

notes

quency of 7–8% in this group: Streptococci, Gram-negative (usually *Pseudomonas* or *Serratia)*, and candida.

In prosthetic valve endocarditis occurring up to 1 year after surgery, by far the most common organism is *S. epidermidis*, (55–60%).

Acute bacterial endocarditis (ABE) is caused by virulent bacteria, often attacking normal valves. It has an acute course, in which there is often rapid cardiac valve destruction and resultant ventricular decompensation. There is ~ 50% mortality with *Staphylococcus aureus* endocarditis despite early intervention! Children are most likely to present with fever, splenomegaly, and heart murmur. (But remember: Most of these already had a murmur from their previous cardiac defect)

Other findings that are common in adults are rare in children:

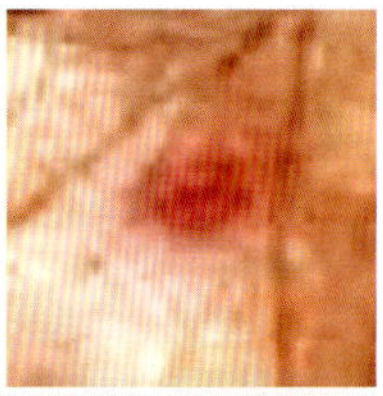

Figure 4-44

- The peripheral manifestation of ABE is Janeway spots, which are small nontender macules on the palms and soles. (See Figure 4-44). With *Staphylococcus*, peripheral ecchymoses sometimes appear. Embolization (again, especially with *S. aureus*) of the heart vegetations leads to metastatic infection (especially to the CNS and kidneys).
- Subacute bacterial endocarditis (SBE) usually occurs in patients with underlying cardiac disease. Manifestations include low-grade fever, heart murmurs, conjunctival petechiae, splenomegaly (in 2/3), splinter hemorrhages, Roth spots, and Osler nodes. But again, in children, only fever, splenomegaly, and heart murmurs are common.
- Roth spots are pale retinal lesions, surrounded by hemorrhage. Osler nodes (= OUCHlers nodes) are ~ 0.5 cm, tender nodules on the palms, fingertips, and soles. Roth spots and Osler nodes are late developments of SBE, and are seen less frequently today, because SBE is diagnosed and treated earlier. Remember: The Janeway lesions (nontender macules) are found in ABE, usually not SBE.

Streptococcus bovis, one of the group D streptococci, is the only type that is easily killed by PCN alone. *Enterococci* require an aminoglycoside plus a beta-lactam antibiotic (2 'cidal antibiotics).

There are some cases of fastidious, Gram-negative organisms causing SBE. They are called the "HACEK" organisms (*Haemophilus*, *Actinobacillus*, *Cardiobacterium*, *Eikenella*, and *Kingella*), and usually are sensitive to beta-lactams. These are often the cause of "culture-negative" endocarditis, since they may require > 7 days to grow to detectable levels in culture media. Treat with PCN + gentamicin or ceftriaxone, or per culture results.

Also remember: endocarditis in adults, caused by either *S. bovis* or *Clostridium septicus*, is often associated with colon cancer, so do a thorough GI workup in these patients.

Prosthetic Valve

Prosthetic valve endocarditis (PVE) can be acute or subacute in presentation.

Early PVE (< 2 months) is usually due to seeding during the surgery. An acute presentation means emergent surgery is usually necessary. Even with surgery, it still has a 40% mortality.

Late type of PVE (> 2 months) has a subacute presentation. The infection often invades the annulus and requires surgery. *S. epidermidis* is the culprit in 55–60% of the cases of PVE in the 1st year after surgery. If the infecting organism is viridans Streptococci, the prosthetic valve infection may be cured with antibiotics alone.

Treatment of Bacterial Endocarditis

Treatment of native valve endocarditis:

1) PCN-sensitive streptococcus (*S. bovis*): 2 weeks of PCN G or ampicillin + gentamicin or 4 weeks of PCN/ampicillin, cefazolin, or ceftriaxone. Note: For this, vancomycin is less effective than beta-lactam antibiotics, and should be used only for severe PCN allergy. Reliably compliant patients may be discharged from the hospital on a once-daily IM dose of ceftriaxone.
2) PCN-insensitive streptococcus (usually *Enterococcus faecalis*): the treatment is 4 weeks of gentamicin + PCN G, ampicillin—or vancomycin, if PCN-allergic.
3) Treat *S. aureus* endocarditis with oxacillin, vancomycin, or cefazolin; again: if the *S. aureus* is methicillin-resistant, use vancomycin + gentamicin +/- rifampin.

Treatment of prosthetic valve endocarditis:

1) Methicillin-resistant Staph (especially *S. epidermidis*) requires vancomycin, rifampin, and gentamicin—all 3—for 14 days, followed by vancomycin + rifampin for 4 weeks. The gentamicin prevents the emergence of resistance to rifampin. Remember: Gentamicin is nephro- and ototoxic.
2) *S. aureus*: Naf/ox or cefazolin + gentamicin for 5 days, followed by the beta-lactam for a total of 6 weeks.

COMMON ID SYNDROMES: CNS

Bacterial Meningitis

Overview

Acute Bacterial Meningitis—If suspected, do the following CSF tests: Gram stain, C+S, cell count with differential, protein, and glucose. Previously, CIE (counterimmunoelectrophoresis) or latex agglutination was used, but they are not cost-effective for initial workup and are, therefore, no longer indicated in initial workups. The culture results are the gold standard, unless the patient previously was on antibiotics. CIE or latex agglutination tests for the following: *H. influenzae*, pneumococcus, meningococcus, Group B *Streptococcus*,

notes

Quick Quiz

1) What organism most commonly causes endocarditis in children?
2) In patients with "normal valves," which organism is most likely to cause endocarditis?
3) What are Janeway spots? Osler Nodes? Roth spots?
4) What are the treatments for native valve endocarditis?
5) Which organisms are the most common cause of meningitis in a 1-month-old? 6-year-old? 17-year-old?
6) Regarding meningitis, name empiric antibiotic therapy for each of these age groups.
7) What is the antibiotic therapy for pneumococcal meningitis?

Klebsiella, and *E. coli*. The sensitivity of these varies from 20%– 90%.

The etiology of meningitis is age-dependent. Overall (see Table 4-5), *S. pneumoniae* is the most common cause of meningitis. Next is *Neisseria meningitidis*, and then *Listeria monocytogenes*. > 60 years old is when listerial meningitis becomes more prevalent again.

The main culprit in the meningococcal group is B (B for Bad, B for Bad). There are effective vaccines against A, C, Y, and W-135, but not type B.

In neonates (< 1 month old), think Gram-negative, group B streptococcus (*S. agalactiae*), and *Listeria*.

In children prior to 1990, *H. influenzae* had been, by far, the most common cause. The Hib vaccine has had a wonderfully dramatic effect on this disease in the U.S. Its prevalence has decreased from ~ 40% to ~ 2%!!

Treatment of Bacterial Meningitis

In partially treated Gram-positive meningitis, the bacteria stain poorly, and they may even look Gram-negative! A bloody tap (contaminated) has increased protein and decreased glucose.

Effective treatment requires an antibiotic that both crosses into the CSF and has bactericidal activity.

Antibiotics that do not cross into the CSF well at any time are:

- Erythromycin
- Tetracycline
- Aminoglycosides
- Cefoxitin
- 1st generation cephalosporins

On the Board exam, if you see any answers to meningitis questions with these last antibiotics in them, pick something else!

Start empiric treatment of meningitis while Gram stain and/or culture results are pending. If the LP cannot be done immediately, start antibiotics even before the LP! Know:

- Meningitis in children > 3 months is empirically treated with ceftriaxone or cefotaxime (3rd gen cephalosporin). But add vancomycin if *S. pneumoniae* is suspected (e.g., previous antibiotics)!
- For empiric treatment of the neonates (< 3 months), add ampicillin (for *Listeria*) to the above treatment. So, start these children on triple antibiotic therapy if you suspect pneumococcus!
- More specifically, in neonates (< 1 mo), use cefotaxime as the 3rd gen cephalosporin, because ceftriaxone may exacerbate hyperbilirubinemia.

Table 4-5

BACTERIAL ETIOLOGIES OF MENINGITIS IN THE U.S.

0-2 mos	%	3 mos to 15 yrs	%	Adult	%	Notes on > 60 yrs
Gram-neg (*E. coli* & *Klebsiella*)	20-30	***S. Pneumoniae***	30-50	***S. Pneumoniae***	30-50	*S. Pneumoniae* *N. meningitidis* See more: *Listeria* *E. coli* *H. influenzae* *Pseudomonas*
Strep (Group B) (*S. agalactiae*)	40-50	***N. meningitidis***	10-35	***N. meningitidis***	10-35	
Listeria	2-10	***H. influenzae***	0-7	***Listeria***	2-11	
Staphylococci *S. pneumoniae* *H. influenzae* *N. meningitidis*	2-5 0-5 0-3 0-1	Streptococci Gram Negative Staphylococci *Listeria*	2-4 1-2 1-2 1-2	Gram negative Streptococci Staphylococci *H. influenzae*	1-10 5 5 1-3	

Remember, for the newborn and the adults > 60 yrs, empiric treatment is usually ceftriaxone or other 3rd gen cephalosporin AND AMPICILLIN (cephalosporins have NO effect against *Listeria*!).

notes

If you have a suspicion of one of the following, the empiric therapy may change:

- For presumed pneumococcal meningitis (especially if Gram stain is suspicious), be sure to add vancomycin to the 3rd gen cephalosporin; rifampin if vancomycin-allergic.
- Treat presumed meningococcal meningitis with high-dose PCN (3rd generation cephalosporin if PCN-allergic,) and ensure contacts receive prophylaxis.
- The 3rd generation cephalosporins cover Gram-negative meningitis.

Prophylaxis with rifampin is also indicated for invasive *Haemophilus influenzae* disease.

In adolescent patients with AIDS, ALL, or Hodgkin disease, think *Cryptococcus*, and do a cryptococcal antigen and/or India ink. Consider amebic meningitis first when the meningitis patient has been swimming in brackish (cow ponds) water.

Aseptic Meningitis

Aseptic, chronic meningitis is manifested by headache, meningismus, and CSF lymphocytosis. Many, many causes. On the CSF, do the same tests as for acute meningitis, and add testing for *Coccidioides* in endemic areas, VDRL, acid-fast smear and culture, and either the India ink or cryptococcal antigen test. Test results that make aseptic meningitis unlikely are CSF glucose < 40, CSF protein > 150, and CSF WBC > 1200. Viral causes are the most common (hence, the most common cause of meningitis) of aseptic meningitis—including enteroviruses and mosquito-borne arboviruses in the summer/early fall, mumps in the spring, and HSV. Suspect *Coccidioides* and *Histoplasma* in endemic areas (arid southwest and Mississippi/Ohio River valleys, respectively). Chronic neutrophilic meningitis is unusual—think of *Nocardia*, *Actinomyces*, or fungus as possible causes. Treat cryptococcus, common in AIDS, Hodgkin disease, and ALL (i.e., cell-mediated), with IV amphotericin B + oral flucytosine (5-FC; 5-fluorocytosine), followed by oral fluconazole.

Classic presentation and findings for a viral meningitis:

- Fever
- Headache
- Nuchal rigidity
- Nonfocal exam
- Normal CT
- LP showing increased lymphocytes

TB Meningitis

Tuberculous meningitis is sometimes manifested by cranial nerve palsies, especially the 6th cranial nerve. Look especially for basilar enhancement on CT scan of the head. Other causes of aseptic meningitis include spirochetal (secondary syphilis and Lyme disease).

Lyme Meningitis

Lyme meningitis can cause peripheral and cranial nerve palsies (especially of the 7th cranial nerve), so think of Lyme disease when a patient presents with Bell palsy and/or foot drop, and a suggestive history. Treat meningitis with ceftriaxone 2 gm qd x 21d. Bell palsy can be treated with oral agents alone. Alternative is high-dose PCN G.

Encephalitis

Acute encephalitis—The causes of most of the acute encephalitis cases are unknown! The most commonly identified cause of encephalitis in the U.S. is arboviruses (West Nile, LaCrosse, etc.) HSV is responsible for the highest number of deaths due to encephalitis.

Spinal Epidural Abscess

Spinal epidural abscesses may be caused by either hematogenous spread or local extension (from osteomyelitis...). *S. aureus* is the most common cause. Patients present with fever, spinal pain, and nerve compression problems. Do an MRI. CT is not as good as MRI because it is susceptible to bony artifacts. Drainage is usually required.

Neurosyphilis

CSF-VDRL test is the test of choice for neurosyphilis; it is 100% specific, but only 50% sensitive. A positive test confirms neurosyphilis, but a negative test cannot be used to rule it out. CSF FTA-ABS is very sensitive—unfortunately, it is so sensitive that a positive result often reflects contamination of CSF with peripheral blood—so it is not used. Often, treatment must be based on suspicion.

Brain Abscess

Diagnosis: CT scan with contrast is the procedure of choice (> 95% sensitivity). If the abscess is accessible, you would usually aspirate it and give antibiotics. You may need to surgically excise the lesion. Lumbar puncture is absolutely contraindicated if signs of increased intracranial pressure are present—such as focal neurologic signs. Overall, the risk of herniation is as high as 20%.

Cysticercosis (caused by ingesting the pork tapeworm, *Taenia solium*) is the most common cause of brain lesions in developing countries, and imported cases are often seen in the U.S. Symptoms, especially seizures, are seen when the cysticerci (larval forms of *T. solium*) die, causing an inflammatory reaction. Toxoplasma is the most likely etiologic agent if the patient is immunodeficient—especially if there are multiple lesions. It is usually due to a reactivation of dormant cysts.

Location of the abscess is often related to the source. Frontal lobe—think paranasal sinus: pneumococcus, *H. influenza*, and anaerobes. Temporal or cerebellum—think middle ear: pneumococcus, *H. influenza*, *S. aureus*, Gram-negative. Both frontal and parietal abscesses can be due to hematogenous spread from such things as lung infections and endocarditis.

Treatment of brain abscesses is always initially empiric:

- High-dose ampicillin or ceftriaxone combined with metronidazole to cover aerobes and anaerobes.
- PCN-allergic: Give metronidazole along with a 3rd generation cephalosporin.

notes

Quick Quiz

1) What CT finding is classic for tuberculous meningitis?
2) What virus causes the most deaths in acute encephalitis?
3) What organisms are common in brain abscesses in the United States?
4) True or False: You should treat the diarrhea caused by *E. coli* O157:H7 to decrease the risk of HUS.
5) What organisms are suggested by finding fecal WBCs in a stool smear?
6) What is the usual organism for traveler's diarrhea?
7) What is the characteristic type of diarrhea seen with rotavirus infection?
8) A famous children's resort cruise line has an outbreak of diarrhea among its passengers. What is the likely viral etiology?

- If you suspect *Enterobacteriaceae* (i.e., ear focus), give a 3rd generation cephalosporin and metronidazole.
- If there was a neurosurgical procedure, penetrating head trauma, or acute endocarditis, think *S. aureus* and add vancomycin (high incidence of MRSA).

Nocardia pulmonary disease can spread and cause focal lesions in the brain. It is also a rare cause of neutrophilic aseptic meningitis (see above).

COMMON ID SYNDROMES: GI

E. coli is the most common cause of bacterial diarrhea (usually without blood or WBCs) affecting both the resident children and travelers in developing countries. There is an enterohemorrhagic, Shiga-toxin-associated, *E. coli* (serotype O157:H7) that causes localized outbreaks of hemorrhagic colitis, TTP, and HUS (hemolytic uremic syndrome)—usually after eating undercooked beef or unpasteurized milk. Do not treat diarrhea caused by *E. coli* O157:H7 with antibiotics, because you increase the risk of HUS.

Travelers' diarrhea is usually caused by enterotoxigenic *E. coli*. Prophylaxis with bismuth subsalicylate (Pepto-Bismol®): two tablets q.i.d. (yecch!) or daily quinolone or TMP/SMX.

Vibrios—think seafood and shellfish. *V. cholerae* 01 (causes cholera) is occasionally associated with Gulf Coast crabs. The *non*-01 *V. cholera*, *V. parahaemolyticus*, and other *Vibrios* are even more frequent causes of shellfish-associated diarrhea. These are usually self-limited. *Vibrio vulnificus* causes skin infections and sepsis, especially in the immunocompromised or those with chronic liver disease.

Antibiotic-associated colitis is caused by *Clostridium difficile* (antibiotic-associated diarrhea is usually just a side effect of the medicine with change in normal flora). Symptoms can occur up to 3 weeks after the antibiotics are stopped. To diagnose, do a stool assay for the *Clostridium difficile* cytotoxin. A toxin assay is required, because 5% of healthy persons (50% of infants < 1 year old) have *C. difficile* in their stool and not all of the *C. difficile* organisms produce the cytotoxin.

Cryptosporidia is known to cause prolonged diarrhea in AIDS patients and a self-limited diarrhea in travelers. It is found with acid-fast stains of the stool (small, round, red organisms on a green background). Animals (including humans) are the reservoirs.

Viral causes of diarrhea:

Rotavirus is frequently found in children. It is the most important cause of severe diarrhea in infants, and is easily found in their stools. It is non-bloody in character. It most commonly occurs between November and April and is transmitted by fecal-oral spread, with an incubation period of 1–3 days. A previous rotavirus vaccine was associated with an increased risk of intussusception, and was pulled from the market.

Adenoviruses types 40 and 41 make up the 2nd most common cause of gastroenteritis in children. Adenovirus is similar to rotavirus in that it mainly affects children < age 2 years, but adenovirus infection is year-round. Incubation is 3–10 days, which is longer than most other GI viruses.

Norwalk-type viruses (now called Noroviruses) are associated with clams and oysters, causing "winter vomiting disease," but it can also be water-borne. Identify Norwalk viruses with an ELISA test. Infections are usually epidemic, and recent cruise ship outbreaks underscore this. It is also spread fecal-orally with a 1–2 day incubation period.

Workup: Fecal WBCs suggest an invasive-type bacterial etiology, and are seen in *Shigella*, *Salmonella*, *Campylobacter jejuni*, *Yersinia enterocolitica*, and amebic GI infections—but remember: fecal WBCs are also seen in IBD. You can find all of these on C + S. Additionally, you can find *Vibrios* on stool and O & P. So, do a fecal WBC and stool C + S and O & P if you need to workup a diarrhea.

Note: Start cultures for *Shigella* (usually *Shigella sonnei*) as soon as possible after the bowel movement, because *Shigella* dies soon after exposure to air.

Treatment Protocol Overview: If there are fecal WBCs, do a stool C + S and O & P. Some will give fluoroquinolones (if ≥ 18 years of age) or TMP/SMX empirically, although antibiotics may prolong *Salmonella* infection and are contraindicated in *E. coli* 0157 infections. Do not give antimotility agents for any diarrhea when there are fecal WBCs. *Campylobacter* is resistant to TMP/SMX, so give erythromycin or quinolones instead. Prolonged, intermittent diarrhea with malaise and flatus suggests giardiasis or *Cyclospora*.

Treatment for antibiotic-associated colitis: Stop the antibiotics and give 7–10 days of metronidazole or oral vancomycin. Other treatments are bacitracin, rifampin, or bile binding resins (cholestyramine...), which bind the toxin. Usual treatment is metronidazole, because it is just as effective as oral vancomycin yet much less expensive. Relapse rate on either drug

notes

is ~ 30%. This is usually due to the spores becoming active; just repeat the same treatment! Use bacitracin, rifampin, and cholestyramine as adjuncts in complicated cases.

Treatment for travelers' diarrhea only:

Mild: Loperamide and single-dose quinolone. In children < age 18 years, trimethoprim-sulfamethoxazole may be used for several days.

Severe: Same, except quinolone b.i.d. x 3 days or trimethoprim/sulfamethoxazole for longer period.

COMMON ID SYNDROMES: GU INFECTIONS & STDs

Note

There are many causes of STDs. Know the treatment of all STDs! Many of them have similar manifestations, consisting of genital ulcerations with regional adenopathy (gonorrhea does not have these). These are covered in the Adolescent section.

Urinary Tract Infection

Acute urethral syndrome (dysuria, frequency, and pyuria) is most commonly caused by *E. coli* and, in adolescents, also by *Chlamydia trachomatis*. *S. saprophyticus* causes cystitis in adolescents also. This is a coagulase-negative staphylococcus.

The symptoms of acute urethral syndrome may be due to urethritis, vaginitis, or cystitis. In women, sexual intercourse can cause *E. coli* to be pushed up the urethra, predisposing them for an acute cystitis. Besides sexual activity, other UTI-predisposing factors in women include spermicide diaphragm use and an inherited abnormality called Lewis nonsecretor phenotype.

UTIs are rare in boys and adolescent males and are not associated with male sexual activity, except in homosexuals. In boys, UTIs are usually a result of an abnormality in the urinary tract, such as obstruction and vesicoureteral reflux. Both sexes with DM, neurogenic bladders, or indwelling catheters have an increased frequency of UTIs.

Diagnostic criteria have changed. Urine cultures are required in children, but no longer required on all young women with symptoms of an acute UTI. If there are no complicating factors, pyuria alone is an indication to treat in adolescents and young women.

Treatment of UTIs in older children and adolescents:

- Routine UTI: TMP/SMX x 3 days. (TMP/SMX is more effective than amoxicillin).
- Uncomplicated pyelonephritis: the treatment is oral TMP/SMX x 14 days.
- Complicated pyelonephritis (including pregnant patients!): IV ampicillin + gentamicin, TMP/SMX, fluoroquinolones (not in pregnant or < 18), or 3rd generation cephalosporins. Use gentamicin or 3rd generation cephalosporin alone if the Gram stain shows no Gram-positive cocci. Recommend follow-up urine analysis after the antibiotic treatment ends. Fluoroquinolones are alternate therapy for complicated, or recurrent, cystitis or pyelonephritis.
- NOTE: Spring 2004, the CDC approved ciprofloxacin for 2nd line therapy of UTI and pyelonephritis in children ages 1–17. (Still, probably not likely to be on ABP in 2006; maybe for 2007).

Organisms to know: *Proteus* infections are associated with stones (i.e., do a KUB to check for stones) and hyperammonemia. Group B streptococcus (*S. agalactiae*) infections are seen in pregnancy and infants < 3 months.

Pregnant: Treat asymptomatic bacteriuria in pregnant women (1/3 go on to pyelonephritis!!), neutropenic patients, diabetics, and transplant patients. Also, always admit pregnant patients with pyelonephritis and treat as a complicated pyelonephritis (above). Pregnancy-safe antibiotics to use for pyelonephritis are ampicillin, aminoglycosides, cephalosporins, and TMP/SMX; but you should not give TMP/SMX in late pregnancy or early nursing mothers, because it might cause kernicterus in the child. Also, do not use tetracycline/ doxycycline or quinolones.

There is an increased frequency of urinary tract infections in patients with DM, SS disease, hyperparathyroidism, or gout. In the last 2, the UTI is secondary to stone formation and obstruction. UTIs are the most common nosocomial infections. With normal catheter care, most indwelling urinary catheters stay sterile up to 7 days. They used to be changed after 7 days, but it did not make any difference.

COMMON ID SYNDROMES: SOFT TISSUE INFECTIONS

Vibrio are found especially in shellfish. *V. vulnificus* causes large hemorrhagic bullae, followed by necrosis and lymphadenopathy +/- septicemia. Patients who are immunocompromised, or have chronic liver disease, are especially susceptible.

Mycobacterium marinum is also called "fish tank bacillus." It causes nonhealing skin ulceration in people who work around fish tanks. Infection may present as a single granuloma, but the organism often invades the lymphatics and can cause a series of lesions over a lymph vessel similar to the lesions seen in sporotrichosis. Lesions tend to localize in the distal extremities because the organism does not grow well at body temperature. Diagnosis: Look for acid-fast bacilli in the lesion biopsy. Treat with ethambutol + rifampin or clarithromycin + rifampin.

Erysipelothrix rhusiopathiae is another cause of skin infection in fishermen and meat handlers. Treat with PCN G, ampicillin, or fluoroquinolones.

notes

Quick Quiz

1) What is a risk factor for UTIs in boys?
2) Which bacterial cause of UTI is associated with kidney stones?
3) What is the "fish tank bacillus"?
4) What is the most common cause of osteomyelitis in children? In neonates? In patients with Sickle Cell disease?
5) What does a negative bone scan tell you about the likelihood of osteomyelitis?
6) How long does it take before you can see plain x-ray changes in osteomyelitis?
7) What is the most common cause of septic arthritis?
8) What is a common cause of septic arthritis in a sexually active teenager who is menstruating?
9) What is responsible for most nosocomial infections?
10) What are the organisms that commonly cause IV catheter related infections?

COMMON ID SYNDROMES: BONE INFECTIONS

Osteomyelitis

Acute hematogenous osteomyelitis occurs in children < age 6 years, and is more common in boys. Frequently, there is a history of minor trauma or intercurrent URI. Hematogenous osteomyelitis most commonly affects the long bones, with the lower femoral and upper tibial metaphyses being the most commonly affected, followed by the proximal femoral metaphysis and distal metaphyses of the radius and humerus.

Acute infection is usually caused by *S. aureus*. *H. influenzae* used to be very common, but now has disappeared.

In neonates, *S. aureus*, group B Streptococcus and Gram-negatives are most common.

In IV drug abuser, think *Pseudomonas*, especially if the infection involves the vertebrae or pelvis.

If a puncture wound through a tennis shoe again think *Pseudomonas*.

In sickle cell patients, think *Salmonella*.

Blood cultures are usually (2/3!) positive in acute osteomyelitis. A negative pyrophosphate bone scan usually excludes osteomyelitis, but positive scans are also seen with other infections, fractures, and malignancy. Usually it takes 10–14 days to see plain x-ray changes in osteomyelitis.

With sinus tract osteomyelitis, C + S of the sinus tract drainage is sufficient if you find *S. aureus*, but it is not sufficient otherwise. Then you must use bone biopsy/scraping.

With suspected spinal osteomyelitis, do a needle biopsy as the first diagnostic procedure.

Except for small bone disease, the necrotic bone must be removed before a chronic osteomyelitis can be cured with antibiotics.

Treat acute hematogenous osteomyelitis with IV antibiotics directed at the pathogen for 5–14 days, followed by oral antibiotics to complete 4–8 weeks. Length of therapy is based on clinical response, the pathogen found, and any complications.

Septic Arthritis

Septic arthritis is most common in children < age 3 years. It typically involves a single large joint, and more commonly affects boys.

Children present with pain and refusal to move or bear weight on the joint. Fever is common. *S. aureus* is the leading cause.

In neonates, group B Streptococcus and Gram-negatives are implicated as well.

In children < age 5 years, *S. aureus*, *S. pyogenes*, and *S. pneumoniae* are the most common; > 5 years, *S. pneumoniae* diminishes as a common cause.

Don't forget: *N. gonorrhoeae* in the sexually active adolescent, especially if she is menstruating! *Salmonella*, again, is common in sickle cell patients.

Do joint aspiration quickly to discern the diagnosis. WBC > 50,000 is common with mostly PMNs. Also obtain blood cultures. MRI or ultrasound of the joint may be helpful in discerning the presence of fluid.

Treatment involves drainage of the infected joint and starting antibiotics directly against the most likely organism. Open drainage is sometimes recommended. Continue antibiotics for 3–6 weeks.

COMMON ID SYNDROMES: NOSOCOMIAL INFECTIONS

Order of frequency: UTI > post-op wound infection > pneumonia.

Nosocomial pneumonia is usually bacterial, and has the highest mortality rate of all the nosocomial infections. It is usually caused by Gram-negative organisms; next most frequently, *Staphylococcus aureus*. Resistance may develop quickly if you use only a single, broad-spectrum antibiotic. If there is an outbreak of bacterial pneumonia (or almost any illness) in the ICU, the most likely vector of transmission is the hands of the ICU workers.

Catheter-related infections—there are 3 types, and all 3 can cause bacteremia/fungemia: 1) asymptomatic, 2) localized, and 3) septic thrombophlebitis (rarest). Secondary endocarditis is more likely to occur in patients with catheters that extend into the heart. IV lines become infected after ~ 3 days! Metal needles are less likely than plastic angiocatheters to become infected. IV catheter infections are usually due to *S. epidermidis* and *S. aureus*. Some other causes are *Candida*, *Corynebacterium jeikeium* (especially in bone marrow transplant units) and Gram-negative rods.

Treatment: Remove catheter and give antibiotic therapy for 2 weeks. Septic thrombophlebitis often requires removal of the affected vein. If there is Gram-positive septicemia, start with

notes

vancomycin in case it is methicillin-resistant. Exception—if there is a Gram-positive bacteremia in a patient with a Hickman or Broviac, you can try to treat with antibiotics for 2–4 weeks without removing the catheter. Again, start with vancomycin until culture results are back.

ANTIBIOTIC THERAPY

OVERVIEW

Review of Protein Synthesis

Most antibiotics work either by interrupting protein synthesis or cell wall synthesis (See Figure 4-45). First, let's look at a review of protein synthesis.

Protein Synthesis: Transcription:

The DNA particle must be unwound from its supercoiled arrangement before it can be "read" by RNA polymerase. This involves cutting the strand, holding onto the cut ends to prevent them being damaged, allowing the double helix to uncoil and the DNA to be copied, then precisely gluing the cut ends back together again. The key enzyme that carries out this process in bacteria is DNA gyrase.

RNA polymerase moves along a section of DNA (a gene), uncoiled by the DNA gyrase and, following the coded messages on the deoxyribonucleotides, forms a string of complementary-paired ribonucleotides, i.e., a piece of RNA—more specifically pre-mRNA. With the removal of an intron, the pre-mRNA becomes mRNA (messenger RNA). This is called transcription because the DNA code is transcribed into a complementary RNA code.

Protein Synthesis: Translation:

Ribosomes are the translation units that convert the coded message in the mRNA to a specific sequence of amino acids. A 30S ribosomal subunit attaches to the mRNA at the "ribosome binding site," then moves along it until it reaches the start codon (AUG). Here a tRNA (with anticodon UAC) carrying an altered methionine (f-Met) binds with this subunit and mRNA to form the "initiation complex." A 50S ribosomal subunit then comes along and binds to this complex to form the 70S ribosome.

Amino acid-specific transfer RNAs (tRNA) attach to the 20 amino acids used in making protein. The bottom loop of these "inverted cloverleaf-shaped" tRNAs have 3 unpaired bases called anticodons.

As the 70S ribosome moves along the mRNA, tRNAs attach one at a time, bringing these amino acids with them. These amino acids are bound together, forming a gradually lengthening protein chain.

When the ribosome reaches the end of the coded message, translation stops. The ribosomal subunits then separate and detach from the mRNA, and the completed protein is released.

Antibiotics That Block Protein Synthesis

There! Now we can see what is affected by the antibiotics that interfere with protein synthesis:

Rifampin binds to RNA polymerase and blocks initiation of the transcription of DNA to mRNA.

Quinolone antibiotics specifically target the DNA gyrase of bacteria. This allows the DNA gyrase to cut the double helix, but then prevents the cut ends from being rejoined.

Metronidazole, a very important anti-anaerobic and antiprotozoal agent, probably has a similar primary mode of action to the quinolones, although it also affects cell membrane function.

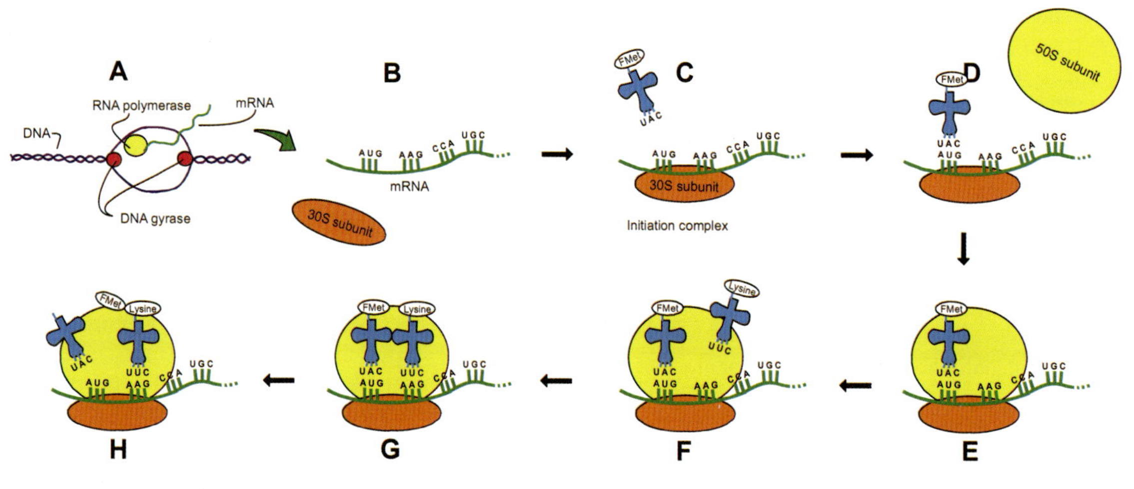

A represents transcription. DNA gyrase is targeted by **quinolones** and **metronidazole**. **Rifampin** binds to RNA polymerase.
B to **C** shows attachment of the 30S subunit to the mRNA. **Tetracyclines** bind reversibly and **aminoglycosides** bind irreversibly to the 30S subunit.
C to **D** show attachment of the 50S subunit to form the 70S ribosome. **Oxazolidinones** and **macrolides** bind to the 50S subunit.

Figure 4-45: Antibiotic effects on Protein Synthesis

notes

Quick Quiz

1) Which antibiotic targets the DNA gyrase of bacteria?
2) Which antibiotics binds to the 50S subunit?.
3) Which antibiotics interfere with folic acid production/recycling in the bacteria?
4) What are the bacteriostatic antibiotics?
5) What organism is common in cat bites?
6) What are the criteria for implementing antibiotics for a bite?
7) What is the drug of choice for bite wounds?
8) Name common infections for which penicillin is still the drug of choice?

Aminoglycosides bind irreversibly (bacteriocidal) to the 30S subunit and prevent the 50S subunit from attaching.

Tetracyclines bind reversibly to the 30S subunit, distorting it so that the anticodons of the tRNAs cannot align properly with the codons on the mRNA.

Oxazolidinones is a new class of antibiotic, of which linezolid (Zyvox™) is the first available. The drug binds to the 50S ribosomal subunit, thereby preventing attachment to the initiation complex.

Macrolides bind reversibly to the 50S subunit. They prevent peptide bond formation between the amino acids and hence, keep the 70S ribosome from translocating down the mRNA.

Antibiotics Affecting Cell Wall Synthesis

Peptidoglycan is an exclusively bacterial polymer and is a component of bacterial cell walls. There are a variety of antibiotics that act at one or more stages of peptidoglycan synthesis.

Beta-lactams (see next section) are a class of antibiotics that focus on attacking the cell wall. They contain a structure similar to that in the amino acids, which crosslink and stabilize the bacterium cell wall. Because there is no analogous structure in human cells, these antibiotics can be given at much higher doses without fear of toxicity.

Also:

To replicate DNA, folic acid is required. Bacteria are required to make their own folic acid from paraaminobenzoic acid (PABA). Trimethoprim and the sulfonamides block this process.

Know: Antibacterial agents must be 'cidal for effective treatment of endocarditis, meningitis, and for treatment of infected neutropenic patients. Bactericidal antibiotics are the beta-lactams (PCNs, imipenem, and cephalosporins), fluoroquinolones, vancomycin, aminoglycosides, rifampin, and metronidazole. Bacteriostatic agents are erythromycin, tetracycline, and clindamycin. Chloramphenicol is unusual in that it is normally bacteriostatic, but it is 'cidal against *H. influenzae*, pneumococci and meningococci!

BETA-LACTAM ANTIBIOTICS

Overview

The first of the beta-lactam antibiotics was penicillin (PCN) and now includes the semisynthetic PCNs (methicillin, oxacillin, and cloxacillin), carbapenems, and cephalosporins. Because the bacteria rupture when the integrity of the cell wall is decreased, these drugs are also bactericidal.

Penicillins

Penicillin, as noted above, has the beta-lactam ring. It is very active against meningococci, most streptococci (groups A and B, viridans group, and *S. pneumoniae*) *Pasteurella* (dog and esp. cat bites), *Listeria*, and many *Neisseria* species. It is also active against many anaerobes (such as *Clostridium*), but not *B. fragilis*. Know: Even though PCN is indicated for meningococcal infections, rifampin or quinolones are better for eradication of the carrier state. Rifampin concentrates in the upper respiratory mucosa.

More on cat/dog bites—when to give antibiotics:

- Moderate or severe bite wounds
- Crush injury
- Puncture wounds (nearly all cat bites)
- Facial bites
- Hand and foot bites
- Genital area bites
- Immunocompromised kid

Besides *Pasteurella*, *Staphylococcus aureus* is a likely organism, so most recommend amoxicillin-clavulanate potassium as the drug of choice for bite wounds; if PCN-allergic, use cephalosporin or TMP/SMX + clindamycin. For human bites, the main organisms are Streptococci, *S. aureus*, *Eikenella corrodens*, and anaerobes. Always treat human bites with antibiotics.

PCN is still the drug of choice for many infections (know):

- Periodontal infections
- Erysipeloid (*Erysipelothrix rhusiopathiae*)
- Group A and group B streptococci
- Rat-bite fever
- Syphilis
- Yaws
- Leptospirosis
- Actinomycosis
- Meningococcal meningitis and meningococcemia

Ampicillin has a spectrum similar to that of PCN, but its spectrum extends to include certain Gram-negative rods—especially some *E. coli*, *H. influenzae*, *Salmonella*, *Shigella*, and *Proteus mirabilis*. However, it does not get *Klebsiella*, and many of the *H. influenzae*, *E. coli*, and *P. mirabilis* are now resistant to it.

Ampicillin is the drug of choice for:

notes

- Listeria monocytogenes meningitis
- Salmonellosis—if sensitive
- UTIs due to susceptible organisms
- Enterococcal infections

Penicillinase-resistant semisynthetic PCNs like nafcillin and cloxacillin are needed against *S. aureus*, because 85% have beta-lactamase (Note: Penicillinase is just a specific type of beta-lactamase). Unfortunately, there has been a rapidly expanding resistance to these in staphylococci (i.e., "methicillin-resistant"). Nafcillin is similar to methicillin, but it is not as likely to cause interstitial nephritis (so methicillin is rarely used). These (nafcillin and cloxacillin) are drugs of choice only for staphylococcal infections.

Antipseudomonal PCNs (AP-PCN: Ticarcillin-clavulanate, piperacillin-tazobactam) are better against the Gram-negative organisms (including *Pseudomonas*) and anaerobes (including *B. fragilis*).

Antipseudomonal PCNs: They are the only PCN drugs effective against infections caused by:

- *P. aeruginosa*
- Acinetobacter

Cephalosporins

Note:

Cephalosporins also contain the beta-lactam ring but are penicillinase-resistant. In general, cephalosporins have no activity against enterococci, *Listeria*, and methicillin-resistant staphylococci.

...1st Generation

1st generation cephalosporins (cefazolin, cephalothin, cephapirin) are active against most *Staphylococcus aureus* (including the lactamase-producing strains, excluding the methicillin-resistant strains) and most *Streptococci*. Really, there is no anaerobic activity or reliable CNS penetrations, so do not use for meningitis or ventriculoperitoneal (VP) shunts. 1st generation also get many of the community-acquired *E. coli*, *Klebsiella*, and *Proteus* (the Gram-negative coverage is superior to ampicillin). Cephalothin increases the nephrotoxicity of concurrently administered aminoglycosides. Commonly given for:

- Skin and soft tissue infections
- Some surgical prophylaxis

...2nd Generation

All **2nd generation** cephalosporins are more active against the gram-negative organisms (e.g., good against *H. influenzae*) and less active against Gram-positive bacteria.

Parenteral: All of the 2nd generation cephalosporins—cefoxitin, cefotetan, cefamandole, etc. (except cefuroxime {Zinacef®}) have variable activity against gut anaerobes. None of the 2nd generation cephalosporins consistently cross into the CSF, so they are not used to treat meningitis.

2nd generation cephalosporins have good activity against *H. influenzae*, *Neisseria*, and Gram-positive organisms. They are among drugs of choice for:

- PID
- Abdominal surgery

Know that 3rd generation cephalosporins have largely replaced 2nd generation, except for abdominal/pelvic infections, because of the better anaerobic coverage of the 2nd generation cephalosporins.

...3rd Generation

3rd generation cephalosporins are especially resistant to beta-lactamase, and are especially effective against *N. gonorrhoeae* and *H. influenzae*. They also get most of the *Enterobacteriaceae* (*E. coli*, *Klebsiella*, *Proteus*, *Enterobacter*, and *Serratia*).

They are not active against *S. aureus* as are the 1st generation. Of the cephalosporins, only some 3rd generations are active against *Pseudomonas*—especially ceftazidime (Fortaz®), but it is not reliably effective against *S. pneumoniae*.

Ceftriaxone (Rocephin®) has the longest half-life and is effective against most *S. pneumoniae*, but is not effective against *Pseudomonas*.

There are four 3rd generation cephalosporins that can cross an inflamed blood-brain barrier, and thus, are indicated as the primary therapy for meningitis caused by Enterobacteriaceae. These are 1) ceftriaxone, 2) cefotaxime (Claforan®), 3) ceftizoxime (Cefizox®), and 4) ceftazidime.

Remember: Ceftriaxone is used as a single agent for empiric treatment of meningitis while lab results are pending (except in neonatal, elderly, and pregnant patients— add ampicillin (for Listeria, enterococci); and presumed *S. pneumoniae* meningitis—add vancomycin).

...4th Generation

"4th" generation cephalosporin. Cefepime (Maxipime®) is a broad-spectrum antibiotic with enhanced stability to cephalosporinases. It has the Gram-negative activity of 3rd generation cephalosporins and Gram-positive activity of 1st generation cephalosporins. Plus, it has limited anaerobic coverage.

Carbapenems

Imipenem is a very-broad-spectrum carbapenem antibiotic. It is very active against *B. fragilis*. It kills most *Enterobacteriaceae*, *Pseudomonas*, and Gram-positive organisms, and is inhibitory for *Listeria* and *Enterococcus faecalis*. The few organisms resistant to it include *Enterococcus faecium*, *Pseudomonas cepacia*, *Corynebacterium jeikeium* (JK), *Stenotrophomonas maltophilia*, and methicillin-resistant staphylococci. Now, ~ 20% of *P. aeruginosa* are also resistant. [Know: Imipenem can lower the seizure threshold, so it should be used only as a last resort in seizure patients, or in patients with renal insufficiency.]

Imipenem is always formulated with equal amounts of cilastatin (combo = Primaxin®). Cilastatin causes metabolism of

notes

Quick Quiz

1) True or False: IV cefazolin is a good choice for VP-Shunt infections.
2) What antibiotics are good for PID?
3) Which is better for *S. pneumoniae*—ceftriaxone or ceftazidime?
4) Which is better for *Pseudomonas*—ceftriaxone or ceftazidime?
5) What group of patients should not receive imipenem?
6) Why is cilastatin combined with imipenem?
7) What is the "red man" syndrome?
8) Which antibiotics have "the post-antibiotic effect"?

imipenem to be blocked in the renal tubule, thereby increasing its half-life to…one hour! Cilastatin has no effect on beta-lactamases.

Meropenem is a similar carbapenem with a longer half-life, so there's no need for an enzyme inhibitor. It is also less likely than imipenem to cause seizures.

Aztreonam

Aztreonam is a monobactam, which is good only against aerobic and facultative, Gram-negative bacteria. Its spectrum is similar to aminoglycosides (Gram-negative aerobes). It is effective against most *Enterobacteriaceae* and *Pseudomonas*, but it is not active against Gram-positive cocci or anaerobes.

Beta-lactamase Inhibitors

Beta-lactamase Inhibitors:

- Sulbactam
- Clavulanic acid
- Tazobactam:

These bind irreversibly to the beta-lactamase made by some bacteria. These inhibitors increase the activity of drugs against beta-lactamase producing bacteria such as *B. fragilis*, *Klebsiella*, and *S. aureus* (variably).

Formulations using the beta-lactamase inhibitors:

- Clavulanic acid mixed with amoxicillin (Augmentin®, Clavulin®)
- Clavulanic acid mixed with ticarcillin (Timentin®)
- Sulbactam mixed with ampicillin (Unasyn®)
- Tazobactam mixed with piperacillin (Zosyn®, Tazocin®)

OTHER ANTIBIOTICS

Vancomycin

Vancomycin is, in general, bactericidal. It is effective against most Gram-positive organisms, including methicillin-resistant staphylococci, *Clostridia*, and *Corynebacterium*. There are some vancomycin-resistant strains of enterococci and recent reports of vancomycin-resistant *S. aureus*. (Yikes!) *Staphylococcus haemolyticus* and a few *Staph epidermidis* are resistant (causing serious trouble in some endocarditis patients).

Vancomycin sometimes causes the "red-man syndrome," which consists of tachycardia, flushing, occasional angioedema, and generalized pruritus. You can prevent this either by slowing down the infusion time or by pretreatment with antihistamines (but not H2-blockers). Nephro and ototoxicity used to be a concern, but current formulations of vancomycin do not have significant toxicity, unless combined with an aminoglycoside.

Aminoglycosides

Aminoglycosides are effective against many Gram-negative organisms. They require the aerobic mechanism of the cell to be effective, so are no good against anaerobes. Aminoglycosides have a persistent, anti-Gram-negative effect after removal of the drug—known as the post-antibiotic effect! So, it is possible to dose aminoglycosides q24 hours with equivalent or better results than the same daily dosage given more often. Because they irreversibly inhibit ribosomal protein synthesis, they are bactericidal.

Aminoglycosides are effective against *Yersinia pestis* plague (streptomycin), *Francisella tularensis* (streptomycin or gentamicin), *M. tuberculosis* (streptomycin), and *M. avium-intracellulare* (amikacin). Gentamicin is used in combination with a beta-lactam antibiotic for the treatment of subacute bacterial endocarditis. Gentamicin is often given along with rifampin to prevent the rapid development of resistance to rifampin (as in prosthetic valve endocarditis). It is also given to febrile neutropenic patients, along with either a 3rd generation cephalosporin or an antipseudomonal penicillin.

Major side effects of aminoglycoside treatment are ear toxicity and kidney toxicity—these are more likely if either amphotericin B or cephalothin is also used!

Fluoroquinolones

Fluoroquinolones (ciprofloxacin, norfloxacin, ofloxacin, levofloxacin, sparfloxacin, moxifloxacin, gatifloxacin) are a set of very-wide-spectrum antibiotics that inhibit bacterial DNA synthesis. They are very good against Gram-negative, aerobic organisms—including rods. They are not FDA-approved for children < age 18 years, except in special cases (CF, anthrax exposure, and in 2004, ciprofloxacin is approved as 2nd line therapy for UTI and pyelonephritis).

Indications for fluoroquinolones:

- Ciprofloxacin, ofloxacin, and the newer agents can be used for systemic infections.
- Fluoroquinolones are also good against all the usual causes of bacterial gastroenteritis (Salmonella, Shigella, Campylobacter, and Yersinia enterocolitica).

Fluoroquinolones are not effective in:

- They are not good against anaerobes (*B. fragilis*, et al).
- Ciprofloxacin and ofloxacin have only intermediate activity against Gram-positive organisms, including *S. pneumoniae*.

notes

Hence, they are not a good choice for empiric treatment of pneumonia. (On the other hand, levofloxacin, moxifloxacin, and gatifloxacin are alternative choices for community-acquired pneumonia. The newer fluoroquinolones are also effective treatment for atypical pneumonias.)

- They are not used for MRSA, because of the widespread, rapid development of resistance to them.
- Again, they are not given to small children (FDA says no one < 18 years of age, except for anthrax and UTI, while the CDC has approved quinolone use in adolescents for STDs)
- Never use in pregnant patients.

[Know: Some fluoroquinolones increase the levels of theophylline and cyclosporine by decreasing metabolism, and increase the effect of warfarin by an uncertain mechanism. They do not increase the elimination of any drug.] Although ciprofloxacin and enoxacin, like erythromycin, delay theophylline clearance, norfloxacin and ofloxacin apparently do not.

Macrolides

Erythromycin is a drug to consider for community-acquired pneumonia, because it is effective against *S. pneumoniae* (although there is increasing resistance), *Mycoplasma pneumoniae*, and *Legionella pneumophila*. It is also effective against *Chlamydophila pneumoniae*, *Campylobacter* (diarrhea), diphtheria, and pertussis. It is not so good against *H. flu* and is not effective against Q fever (*Coxiella burnetii*), which is treated with tetracycline or chloramphenicol. Like the quinolones, erythromycin increases the effect of theophylline, cyclosporine, and warfarin.

Azithromycin has the **same** indications as erythromycin—and it has better *H. flu* coverage. It has a very long half-life (so once-per-day dosage), and is available in an IV form.

Rifampin is bactericidal. It is never given alone to **treat** an acute infection, because organisms rapidly develop resistance to it. Rifampin is used for prophylaxis, as in meningococcus.

Oxazolidinones

Oxazolidinones is an entirely new class of antibiotic, of which linezolid (Zyvox™) is the first available. They have a unique mechanism of action for the blocking of protein synthesis. The drug binds to the 50S ribosomal subunit, thereby preventing attachment of the 30S+mRNA subunit—so the 70S ribosome initiation complex is not made, and no protein is produced.

Linezolid is active against Gram-positive organisms, including MRSA (methicillin-resistant *S. aureus*). It is also effective against VRE (vancomycin-resistant enterococci) and anaerobes! Linezolid is available in oral (with 100% bioavailability!) and IV preparations. The oral form makes it a desirable alternative to vancomycin for MRSA. However, concerns of developing resistance and the cost make this drug an unlikely first-line agent.

Streptogramins

Quinupristin/dalfopristin (Synercid®) is the first of this new class of antibiotics. It was the first antibiotic approved for the treatment of serious infections with Vancomycin-resistant Enterococcus *faecium*. The main side effects with this antibiotic are severe myalgias and arthralgias.

ANTIVIRAL AGENTS

Acyclovir is a nucleoside analog used for the treatment of herpes simplex and varicella-zoster viruses. Valacyclovir and famciclovir have similar indications.

Ganciclovir (previously DHPG) is used for the treatment of CMV infections in AIDS patients, especially for the chorioretinitis and colitis. Leukopenia is a side effect. Because it has only a suppressive effect against CMV, it usually needs to be given until the CD4 lymphocytes are > 200.

Foscarnet is used in patients with acyclovir-resistant Herpes infection, or as an alternative to ganciclovir for CMV.

Ribavirin is indicated for the treatment of RSV (not used much anymore), and is used as part of combination therapy for Hepatitis C.

Amantadine and rimantadine are effective against influenza A.

Oseltamivir (Tamiflu®—oral) and zanamivir (Relenza®—powder for inhalation) are neuraminidase inhibitors, a new class of treatment for influenza A & B.

ANTIFUNGAL AGENTS

Overview

There are 3 major classes of antifungal medicines: polyenes, imidazoles, and triazoles.

Polyenes

Systemic polyene: Amphotericin B is the standard treatment for most systemic mycoses. Systemic amphotericin B can be given only IV, and it has many side effects: fever, renal failure, phlebitis, acidosis, low K+, and Mg. Again! Amphotericin B is associated with electrolyte abnormalities—especially hypokalemia, hypomagnesemia, and renal tubular acidosis. Some recommend giving a test dose first. Every-other-day treatment is just as effective as daily dosage. Hypotension with the first dose may occur (decrease in peripheral vascular tone).

Lipid-associated amphotericin B preparations are less nephrotoxic but much more expensive. Depending on the center, some have switched to lipid-associated formulations, while others prefer to use them only when toxicity has become a problem with regular amphotericin.

Topical polyene macrolides: Nystatin and amphotericin topical formulations are good only against cutaneous candidiasis (not ringworm…). Both are also available in liquid form for oral and esophageal candidiasis.

notes

Quick Quiz

1) What electrolyte abnormalities are associated with amphotericin B use?
2) Which systemic imidazoles are usually given for severe fungal infections?
3) What is the drug of choice for schistosomiasis?
4) Which antibiotics should you never use in a pregnant woman?

Imidazoles

Systemic imidazole

Ketoconazole for systemic use is given orally—increased gastric pH (low acid) decreases absorption. Absorption is not affected by food. Ketoconazole does not penetrate CSF well. It is occasionally used for palliative treatment of Cushing syndrome caused by ectopic production of ACTH (i.e., cancer), because it blocks the 11-hydroxylase enzyme in the adrenal gland, thereby decreasing the amount of cortisol produced.

Ketoconazole increases levels of indinavir and digoxin, and potentiates benzodiazepines. Side effects of ketoconazole include nausea and hepatitis. It also causes a decrease in androgen production, so patients may have decreased libido and males may get gynecomastia.

Ketoconazole is cheaper than fluconazole or itraconazole, but has largely been replaced by them for serious fungal infections. It has many interactions with common drugs—sometimes dangerous.

Topical imidazoles:

Clotrimazole and miconazole are available in both cutaneous and vaginal preparations. Other cutaneous imidazoles are ketoconazole, econazole, sulconazole, and oxiconazole. Other vaginal formulations are butoconazole and tioconazole. Spectrum and efficacy is the same. All are effective in the treatment of cutaneous candidiasis, tinea versicolor, and ringworm.

Triazoles

Systemic triazoles:

Itraconazole (Sporanox®) is a triazole analogue of ketoconazole and is generally more effective and safer. The liquid formulation has much better bioavailability. Food enhances absorption. Indications are the same as ketoconazole (histoplasmosis, blastomycosis, coccidioidomycosis, esophageal candidiasis, and chronic mucocutaneous candidiasis), but also include aspergillosis, cryptococcosis, sporotrichosis, and onychomycosis.

Fluconazole (Diflucan®). Main side effect is N/V. A single 150 mg oral dose is effective in vulvovaginal candidiasis! Fluconazole is also effective treatment for oral and esophageal candidiasis and candidemia. It has excellent penetration into the CSF, and it is often used for maintenance therapy in AIDS patients with cryptococcal meningitis—after an initial 2-week course of IV amphotericin B. Fluconazole is the treatment of choice for chronic coccidioidomycosis.

Voriconazole (Vfend®). The FDA approved the clinical use of voriconazole in May 2002 for primary treatment of acute, invasive aspergillosis, and salvage therapy for rare, but serious, fungal infections caused by the pathogens *Scedosporium apiospermum* and *Fusarium spp.*

Topical triazoles:

There is only one vaginal formulation: **ter**conazole.

Other Antifungals

Other systemic antifungals:

Flucytosine (5-fluorocytosine; 5-FC) is highly soluble and penetrates well into the CSF. Upon entering a fungal cell, it is metabolized to the antimetabolite 5-fluorouracil. If used alone, drug resistance develops quickly. For this reason, and because it may have a synergistic antifungal effect with amphotericin B, it is combined with amphotericin B to treat cryptococcosis and serious forms of candidiasis. It can cause serious GI, hepatic, renal, and bone marrow toxicities—the latter usually presents as neutropenia and thrombocytopenia. Drug levels should be monitored. Slight decreases in renal function can increase 5-FC to toxic levels.

Caspofungin acetate (Cancidas®) is the first of a new class of drugs called echinocandins—a glucan synthesis inhibitor. It is approved for invasive aspergillosis in severely immunocompromised patients.

Other topical antifungals:

Undecylenic acid and tolnaftate are effective only against ringworm. The following cutaneous preparations have the same efficacy and clinical spectrum as the imidazoles: Naftifine, terbinafine, haloprogin, and ciclopirox olamine.

ANTIPARASITIC DRUGS

Praziquantel (Biltricide®) is the only drug effective against all species of Schistosoma, and so is the drug of choice for schistosomiasis. It is also good against flukes and tapeworms (i.e., used to treat neurocysticercosis—caused by the pork tapeworm, *T. solium*).

Albendazole is now used for cysticercosis and schistosomiasis.

Niclosamide is also used for the treatment of tapeworm, but it affects only those in the intestine.

Pentamidine, which is used for treatment (IV form) and prophylaxis (inhaled form) of *Pneumocystis jiroveci* (which is most likely a fungus), has many side effects, including azotemia (1/4), leukopenia, pancreatitis, and hypo- or hyperglycemia. It causes no significant skin reactions.

Anti-malaria drugs (see malaria section above).

notes

VACCINES

For Vaccines, see Health Supervision section.

ANTIBIOTICS AND THE PREGNANT OR BREASTFEEDING WOMAN

Many antibiotics cross the placenta or into breast milk. Only tetracycline has definite contraindications in the breastfeeding mother. And tetracycline and quinolones are definitely not used in pregnant women. Also, many avoid the use of aminoglycosides and chloramphenicol in pregnant or nursing mothers because of the concern of side effects with these drugs in the infant. Sulfa drugs are generally avoided near term.

notes